D1590431

# *A Black Physician's Struggle for Civil Rights*

*EDWARD C. MAZIQUE, M.D.*

# *A Black Physician's Struggle for Civil Rights*

## *EDWARD C. MAZIQUE, M.D.*

*Florence Ridlon*

University of New Mexico Press
Albuquerque

Printed in the United States of America.

11 10 09 08 07 06 05 1 2 3 4 5 6 7

Library of Congress Cataloging-in-Publication Data

Ridlon, Florence, 1946–
A black physician's struggle for civil rights : Edward C. Mazique, M.D. / Florence Ridlon.
p. cm.
Includes bibliographical references.
ISBN 0-8263-3339-7 (cloth : alk. paper)
1. Mazique, Edward Craig, 1911–1987. 2. African American physicians—Biography. 3. Minorities—Medical care—United States—History—20th century. 4. Right to health care—United States—History—20th century. 5. Health services accessibility—United States—History—20th century. I. Title.
R695.M35R53 2005
610'.89'96073 B—dc22

2004023086

Book design and composition by Damien Shay
Body type is Utopia 9.5/13.
Display are Papyrus and Utopia Black.

*To* **Maude Mazique**

The heart of the Mazique family

She gave selflessly and with great joy

Her unending zest for life gave us all hope

We love her and miss her

*To* **Robert W. Wheeler**

The heart of my family

Who supports us all with his compassion and faith

And makes all our endeavors possible

# CONTENTS


LIST OF ILLUSTRATIONS ix

PREFACE xi

ACKNOWLEDGMENTS xv

INTRODUCTION xix

CHAPTER ONE 1
Mississippi Roots

CHAPTER TWO 11
A Country Boy

CHAPTER THREE 59
Shedding the Shackles of Natchez

CHAPTER FOUR 95
The Nation's Capital—A City of Inconsistencies

CHAPTER FIVE 121
Being a Doctor Is Not Enough

CHAPTER SIX 145
The Battle Continues

CHAPTER SEVEN 171
A Year at the Helm

CHAPTER EIGHT 195
Health Care for All

CHAPTER NINE 221
Battles on the Home Front

CHAPTER TEN 237
The Turmoil of the Sixties

CHAPTER ELEVEN 257
City of Hope, City of Despair

CHAPTER TWELVE 285
Continuing Challenges and New Honors

EPILOGUE 321

NOTES 331

BIBLIOGRAPHY 373

INDEX 383

# LIST OF ILLUSTRATIONS

| | | |
|---|---|---|
| Fig. 1. | List from James Railey's will in 1861 | xxiv |
| Fig. 2. | Alex Mazique I and Laura Craig Mazique | 14 |
| Fig. 3. | The Boyd family | 16 |
| Fig. 4. | The Mazique family in Mississippi | 20 |
| Fig. 5. | The Maziques and Wilkersons in Wildsville, Louisiana | 21 |
| Fig. 6. | Alex Mazique Jr. | 23 |
| Fig. 7. | Edward C. Mazique with his dog | 42 |
| Fig. 8. | Natchez College graduation, 1929 | 55 |
| Fig. 9. | Edward C. Mazique as a Morehouse undergraduate | 75 |
| Fig. 10. | Morehouse College senior class officers for 1932–1933 | 77 |
| Fig. 11. | Edward C. Mazique and G. M. Sampson at State Teachers College, Forsyth, Georgia | 92 |
| Fig. 12. | Jewell Crawford Mazique and Edward C. Mazique | 104 |
| Fig. 13. | Edward C. Mazique with his mother, Addie Wilkerson Mazique, and his wife, Jewell | 115 |
| Fig. 14. | The young Dr. Mazique in his office | 118 |
| Fig. 15. | Edward C. Mazique with his mother and his siblings and their wives | 129 |
| Fig. 16. | Dr. Mazique, as president of the National Medical Association, addresses the Arkansas Medical Association in June 1960 | 179 |
| Fig. 17. | Dr. Mazique consulting with President John F. Kennedy | 206 |
| Fig. 18. | Dr. Mazique in discussion with Abraham Ribicoff, Director of Health, Education and Welfare | 212 |
| Fig. 19. | Western Union telegram from the White House | 215 |
| Fig. 20. | Dr. Mazique poses with his mother and sister Maude | 225 |
| Fig. 21. | Dr. Mazique with his mother | 227 |
| Fig. 22. | The Mazique family in 1979 | 228 |
| Fig. 23. | Dr. Mazique and Margurite Belafonte on their wedding day with family and friends | 234 |
| Fig. 24. | Cover of July 1986 *American Magazine* | 296 |
| Fig. 25. | Dr. Mazique and Margurite Mazique with staff and administrators from Providence Hospital | 298 |
| Fig. 26. | Dr. Mazique and his sister Maude at Morehouse in 1974 | 303 |
| Fig. 27. | Dolores Pelham, Maude Mazique, Margurite Mazique, and Edward C. Mazique | 307 |
| Fig. 28. | Dr. Mazique in the 1980s | 318 |
| Fig. 29. | Dr. Mazique and sister Maude in Natchez with cousins James Boyd and Brenda Boyd Anderson | 327 |
| Fig. 30. | Maude Mazique and Dr. Mazique with the author, 1984 | 329 |

# PREFACE 

I first met Dr. Edward Craig Mazique in 1981 when my husband, Robert W. Wheeler, was an HEW Fellow in Washington, D.C., and I was finishing my dissertation for my doctorate in sociology. Margurite Mazique, Dr. Mazique's wife, was in charge of the Fellows program. When Margurite learned that Bob and I were interested in writing a book on the contributions of black athletes to the world of sports, she suggested we meet her husband. This book is a natural outgrowth of our meeting and getting to know Eddie, as we soon came to call him.

In 1982, when Bob and I started the Jim Thorpe Foundation to seek the reinstatement of Jim Thorpe's pentathlon and decathlon wins in the 1912 Olympics to the record books, Eddie served on our board. In 1984 we achieved our goal when the International Olympic Committee president, Juan Antonio Samaranch, presented duplicate gold medals to Mr. Thorpe's family prior to the Olympic Games in Los Angeles.

At this juncture, it was time for us to move on to a new project. After having gotten to know Eddie over the previous several years, there was no question we were eager to focus our attention on Eddie's remarkable life. As he told his stories, we recognized an opportunity to do sociology in the C. Wright Mills tradition by investigating the interplay of biography and history. Telling Eddie's story would enable us to focus on the major events of African-American history from slavery to civil rights. Here was a person whose life was constantly hampered by individual and institutionalized racism. Yet despite the societal pressures that would have defeated another person he excelled beyond any reasonable expectations.

Eddie was a great storyteller. Mostly he saw the humor in any situation, but even when the events he related were sad or humiliating, he displayed no animosity. At times you could see anger about the way the system was organized, but never bitterness. When Eddie discussed his youth in the South, he slipped back into the southern vernacular. At first Eddie was horrified when he realized I planned to leave the quotations about his early years in Natchez, Mississippi, unrevised. After we talked about the pros and cons of such editing, he agreed to leave the quotations intact. Eddie was a precise and eloquent speaker, as will be apparent to the reader from later quotations from his interviews, speeches, and articles. However, in talking of those early days, he took on a different persona, a persona that was an important part of his more sophisticated personality.

Much of the book is in Eddie's own words. I think his words convey better than I ever could what Edward Craig Mazique was really like. No citations were used for Eddie's conversations with me since they were a compilation from years of interviews. From May 1984 through the time of his death in December 1987 we spent numerous hours doing long interviews. We had countless telephone conversations and a great deal of written correspondence. Eddie invited me into his life. I joined him at his office, on house calls, and at his numerous professional meetings. He brought me to family gatherings, shopping, and fishing. I saw him in the presence of congressmen and garage attendants, and he gave them equal respect and attention.

Eddie not only gave me access to his private and personal life but he also provided me with his papers. I viewed all his clippings, speeches, personal files, letters, and photographs. When in the notes I make mention of Eddie's private papers, it is to this collection that I am referring.

In addition to all of Eddie's papers, my research consisted of interviews with numerous individuals including friends, relatives, colleagues, patients, teachers, students, and coworkers. They ranged from congressmen to nurses to judges to newspaper editors to bank presidents to agency heads to laborers and labor leaders. Research on original documents was done at the courthouse and the library in Natchez, Mississippi. Further research was conducted through the Historic Natchez Foundation and at numerous libraries, including the National Medical Library in Bethesda, Maryland; the Schomburg Center for Research in Black Culture in New York City; the Library of Congress in Washington, D.C.; the University of North Texas; Fairleigh Dickinson University; Texas Woman's University; and Bloomfield College.

Initially, my husband, Bob, and I had planned to work on the biography together. Shortly after the start of our research, Bob was offered a job that made his continuation on the project unfeasible. Although he discontinued his direct involvement, he has provided the constant support that made it possible to see this book through to its completion. He interviewed people and made a trip to Natchez with Eddie before he ceased his formal commitment to the project.

It was a joy to work with Eddie. He saw the interconnections between his personal biography and what was taking place in society. He understood the manuscript should not cover every minute detail of his life but rather tie in his story with history. He was a man who looked at the world from a sociological perspective, and this viewpoint guided his decisions on how a doctor should be involved in political and social issues.

Eddie's relatives accepted Bob and me with hospitality unmatched by any we have experienced. When Bob and I made separate trips to Natchez to do research, the Maziques welcomed us into their families as if we always belonged. Our relationship with Maude, Eddie's eldest sister, was special from the beginning. She and her daughter Dolores have remained part of our extended family. When I attended the Mazique family reunion in 1990, most of the people I did not know assumed I was the daughter of Eddie's brother Douglas. A writer has never received better treatment from her sources.

# ACKNOWLEDGMENTS

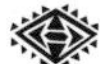

In a work involving this amount of research, it is impossible to acknowledge all those who assisted. However, there are many who have contributed so much; they do need to be thanked.

Each one of the individuals interviewed added something to my understanding of the life of Dr. Edward Craig Mazique, even though space limited the inclusion of material from all the interviews. The following people gave generously of their time to assist with this endeavor and deserve credit for many insights into Dr. Mazique and his special qualities: Archie Avedisian, Colley Rakestraw Bond, Thelma Beard, Brenda Boyd, Susie Boyd, Wilbur Boyd, Evelyn Brannon, Alice Boyd Burton, Mildred Burch, Judge Robert H. Campbell, Alma Carter, Hon. John Conyers, Dr. William H. Cooper, Dr. Paul B. Corneley, Hon. George Crockett, Kent Cushenberry, Michel Dumas, Dr. Halston Eagleson, Minnie Edwards, Dr. Ashraf El Khodary, Dr. Joyce Elmore, Jonathan Eugene, Reverand Albion H. Ferrell, Hon. Walter E. Fauntroy, Samuel Foggie, Baxter Gee, Dr. Hugh Gloster, Dick Gregory, Charlene (Sukari) Hardnett, Janie Haynes, Charles Hamilton Houston Jr., Charlene Drew Jarvis, Elaine Jenkins, Howard Jenkins, Larry Jenkins, Forest Johnson, Dr. Joseph L. Johnson, R. E. "Ike" Kendrick, Dr. John A. Kenney, Sister Carol Keehan, Hattie Key, Dr. Lewis Kurtz, Judge Marjorie McKenzie Lawson, Esther Mackel, Augustine Boyd Rogers Mackel, Anna Mazique, Dr. Edward Houston Mazique, Dr. Emory Mazique, Mamie Lee Mazique, Dr. Margurite Mazique, Maude Mazique, William Mazique, Lucille Banks Robinson Miller, Jerry Moore Jr., Judge Luke Moore, Judge H. Carl Moultrie, Father Patrick Nagle, Rip Naylor, Leo Nazdin, Sister Catherine Norton, Emmie W. Perkins, Dolores Pelham, Dr. Hildrus A. Poindexter, Dr. Joseph Quash, Dr. Raymond Scarletter, Gail Scott, Jerry Scott, Marcia Smith, Dr. Mitchell Wright Spellman, Dr. Herman Stamps, Reverand Robert L. Stanton, Larry Still, Dr. Warren J. Strudwick, John D. Sulton, Dr. Lionel Swann, Al Sweeney, Norman Taylor, Judge Mary Lee Davis Toles, P. Douglas Torrence, J. C. Turner, Ruby Van Croft, Cleopatra Charlotte Walton, Charles Wexler, Kay Wexler, Leon White, Dr. E. Y. Williams, Ernestine Williams, Larry Williams, and Dr. M. Wharton Young.

In addition to the interviews Bob Wheeler and I conducted, William A. Elwood, the associate dean and associate professor of English at the

Graduate School of Arts & Sciences at the University of Virginia, graciously provided me a copy of the transcript of a 1985 filmed interview he did with Dr. Mazique that was used for the documentary film *The Road to Brown.*

I have worked at numerous libraries during the lengthy process of completing this biography. Two of them especially deserve mention. Much of my research was done at the Library of Congress in Washington, D.C. As with any other work I have done there, reference librarian Dave Kelly was invaluable with his assistance, positive attitude, and incredible knowledge. At the Blagg-Huey Library at Texas Woman's University in Denton, Texas, Elizabeth Snapp and Dawn Letson created a space for me to work and, daily, provided me with friendship and an environment conducive to achieving my goal.

Merle Allshouse, the president of Bloomfield College, arranged for a wonderful place for me to write, and Bill Carey, Amy Geraghty, Julie Glosband, and Marian Lamin of Farleigh Dickinson University welcomed me into their office and heartened me each step along the way. Dr. Richard Wells of the Journalism Department of the University of North Texas provided me with an office, constant support, and colleagues and students with whom to interact. Many people have acted out of friendship to assist with this project. Susan Granai read every word of this manuscript many times. Her comments and critiques make it much better than it would have been. Marian and Gerry Batson provided me with a relaxing haven whenever I was in town doing research. The Averys—Wanda, Daryl, and Walden—solved all my emergency computer problems and did it cheerfully. Elaine French did everything possible to provide me with the time I needed to work on the manuscript.

Mimi and Ron Miller from the Historic Natchez Foundation have worked tirelessly to preserve the history of the African-American people of Natchez. I relied heavily on their knowledge of the history and expertise about local sources. They even provided a place to stay and work whenever Bob Wheeler or I were in town, and did it graciously.

The entire Mazique family gave generously of their time and resources. Every relative we met welcomed us and our project and extended every courtesy to assist us in our endeavors. Maude Mazique, the repository of much of the family history, and her daughter, Dolores Pelham, worked with us from the beginning of the research until its completion, doing whatever it took to secure information and access for us.

There were also those who helped to push the book to publication by emphasizing the need for a work on Dr. Mazique's life. Dr. Matthew

Guidry not only lent his personal support but also used his vast network of contacts to tell others about the project. Dolores Pelham organized everyone else! She made certain the publisher knew that Eddie's story needed to be told. Curtis Browder, Charles I. Cassell, Washington Davis, Amadou Dione, John Hammarley, Judith D. Hill, James P. Jasper, Dave Kelly, Alice L. Lloyd, Dr. Emory E. Mazique, Joseph H. Miller, Dr. Myron E. Moorehead, Dr. Debra C. Nichols, William H. Payne, Jean H. Peabody, Herman Saitz, Gail and Jerry Scott, Dolly and Gary Thomas, and Arthur Williams Jr. all wrote and explained the need for such a book. The National Medical Association lent their welcome support through the efforts of Executive Director Dr. James Barnes and Director of Communications Reese Stone. Dr. Louis Sullivan, former secretary of Health and Human Services and president of Morehouse Medical School, cared enough about the contributions made by Dr. Mazique to send a letter of recommendation for the book. His assistant, Shirley Dessaussuer, was not only helpful but expressive about how much Dr. Mazique meant to those at Morehouse. Luther Wilson, Director, University of New Mexico Press, has been supportive of this work from its early stages. Jill Root, my copy editor, was patient, pleasant, and helped to make this manuscript clearer and more precise.

Lastly, I need to thank my exceptional family. My husband, Bob Wheeler, and I started this venture together and he did many insightful interviews to start me on my way. He encouraged me during every phase of this long process and then edited and reedited at the last. The book would never have been completed without him. The project was begun in 1984 and my son, Rob, was born in 1989. He has been a wonderful blessing and, instead of slowing down my work, tends to make it more of a joy to do. He has been patient and understanding when my work takes time away from him and his cheerful disposition has lightened my load.

# INTRODUCTION 

> I'm very proud of my heritage. It may have been a bit rugged, but I am still proud of it.
> — *Dr. Edward C. Mazique*

Dr. Edward Craig Mazique, or Eddie, as he was always called, was a prominent physician in Washington, D.C.[1] He was well known for his wit, his humanitarianism, and his social and political involvement. Instrumental in the integration of the District Medical Society and the local hospitals, the passage of Medicare, the desegregation of many Washington organizations, and other numerous achievements, Eddie's life was exciting, interesting, and worthwhile. At a time when literature and the media present so few positive black male role models, the Mazique family history is full of strong men who provided for, loved, and guided their families.

When I interviewed him, he was a tall, robust man, quick to smile, with a vast knowledge that crossed many disciplines. His face was finely etched with lines and his hair was like a flowing white mane, much longer than he would have considered wearing it in the days of his youth. There was intelligence in the light brown face, which gave more than a hint of his Indian heritage. He treated everyone with the same courtesy and concern, whether they were famous or infamous, wealthy or poor, a Senator, a garage attendant, or a writer. His face, his demeanor, his intentness never changed as he spoke with different people.[2] Although his early years may have been "rugged," something about his Mississippi roots had made him feel secure, and his carriage reflected this assurance.

There have been drastic changes over the past one hundred years in the position of blacks in American society: from the slave cabins of Mississippi to the segregated world of the nation's capital, to the legally integrated world of the 1980s. During this time the Maziques went from slave status to one of the largest landowners in Adams County, Mississippi. Dr. Mazique moved from being denied front-door entry to deliver people's laundry to becoming a physician. He went from being refused access to practice in a District hospital to being its president of staff and from having urine dumped on his head at the YMCA to holding the position as its chairman of the board.

A month before his death on December 27, 1987, Eddie sent a tape answering more of my seemingly endless questions. In the thoughtful mood that having his biography written precipitated, he had decided at the end of the tape to sum up his life. His reflections showed a contented man who, despite difficulties, was pleased with what he had accomplished.

> During this Thanksgiving season, I reflect upon the fact that I should be thankful to know that I have really lived three lives: one life of poverty, one life as a second-class citizen, and a life as a first-class citizen.
>
> First, a life of poverty in which I was only a nonproductive farm worker. Finally chased by the boll weevils from the cotton fields of Mississippi to the high waters and levees of Louisiana, I felt the pangs of hunger and I have cringed from the cold drafts that resulted from being scantily clothed.
>
> I have lived the life of a second-class citizen. I lived with discrimination. I was threatened to be lynched in Mississippi. My sisters, brothers, and father died from inadequate and unavailable medical care in Mississippi and Louisiana and Memphis, Tennessee. I rode "Jim Crow" trains from Mississippi to Georgia and read Burma Shave signs traveling from Atlanta, Georgia, to Tuskegee, Alabama. I sat and listened to George Washington Carver in Tuskegee as he unraveled his experiments with the peanut. I climbed the fire escape of the Fox Theater in Atlanta in order to see a movie at Christmastime in the segregated balcony. I saw Lena Horne perform in *A Cat in the Sky* in a segregated pit called the "buzzards roost" in Griffith, Georgia.
>
> Yet I voted for President Jimmy Carter from Plains, Georgia. I saw *Raisin in the Sun* on Broadway in New York. I rode a "Jim Crow" train from Washington, D.C., to Detroit, Michigan, and our curtain was drawn to separate me from others in the dining car. I rode first class from Chicago to New Orleans and I sat upright in the dining car and was served. I was denied a room at a hotel in Cleveland, Ohio. I slept at the Waldorf Astoria on the thirty-ninth floor in a three-room suite with brass handles on the showers of the bathroom. I sat in the opera seats at

> the Schubert in New York and Josephine Baker threw me her garter. I heard Debbie Allen sing in *Sweet Charity* on Broadway. I stayed in the concierge exclusive quarters in Dallas, Texas, and my son practices medicine in Houston.

Eddie was justifiably proud of his family and the speed with which they overcame the impediments of their background. Unlike the famous novelist Richard Wright, who "preferred to have come out of nothing" than to come to terms with having slave grandparents, Eddie was anxious to speak of his past.[3] Always ready with a good story, Eddie would slip into the southern vernacular and recall with clarity both the joy and the pain of his early days in Mississippi.

The story of Dr. Edward Craig Mazique, however, is not just about an individual or a specific family. It is about the struggle of black men and women to achieve equality. It is about the conditions of slavery and the post–Civil War South. It is about the disgraceful treatment of blacks in our nation's capital in the first three-quarters of the twentieth century. It is about black professionals and their attempts to compete and succeed in a white-dominated society. It is about those who strove to integrate not only schools and restaurants but hospitals, clubs, and professional organizations. It is important to retell this story since, as Dr. Benjamin E. Mays said in the introduction to his autobiography, "Young people born just before and since World War II, and certainly since 1954, do not have the faintest idea what Negro-white relations were like in the South."[4] And the South included Washington, D.C., as Judge Carl Moultrie reminded me when I interviewed him:

> There were a lot of people, whose names you never hear, who contributed much to what my son and others enjoy now. They don't know how they got it. They walk into Hecht's and some other stores and are able to try on clothes without intimidation or to go where they want to go without intimidation. Somebody paid dearly for that.[5]

As a sociologist, I believe it is important that we do know about these people and understand how they were able bring about changes in society.

Dr. Mazique's story is also notable in that it gives us insight into the history of American medical societies and institutions. This is an often neglected aspect of our historical awareness. Although one of the most comprehensive books on race relations in the District of Columbia indicates that "the changes in attitude of the local medical profession were one of the most extraordinary features of the shifting pattern of the community in the 1950's,"[6] there is only one paragraph devoted to this issue in the entire book. Dr. Mazique was president of the Medico-Chirurgical Society and the National Medical Association at a time when blacks were being denied access into the American Medical Association and the staffs of many hospitals. The public and even many physicians are unaware of the pioneering efforts of Dr. Mazique and his colleagues. His work and the work of other black physicians on behalf of Medicare and Medicaid while the more conservative physicians, both black and white, opposed any type of federal health care is an important and habitually overlooked part of medical history. An understanding of the issues surrounding the passage of the Medicare Bill is especially important at this time when we are struggling as a nation to deal with the high cost of medical treatment and the consideration of a more comprehensive national health plan.

Through the telling of Eddie Mazique's story, we delve into the history of many African-Americans who, though oppressed by slavery, were able not only to come to terms with their history but to use it to strengthen their own sense of worth. Although it was clear that some of Dr. Mazique's past had caused him great pain, he showed no bitterness, harbored no resentments or grudges because of its "ruggedness." Instead he used his past as a way of measuring his achievements and as a sensitizing mechanism so that he would not forget the less fortunate.

The State of Mississippi }
Adams County } ss. The following is a true and perfect inventory and appraisement of the goods chattels & personal estate of James Railey, late of said County, deceased to wit:

(Schedule A.)

| | | | |
|---|---|---|---|
| 1 | August Mazique | aged 40 years Heart disease | 1,200.00 |
| 2 | Sarah " | aged 37 years Lungs affected | 1,200.00 |
| 3 | Jim — " — | aged 18 years | 1,600.00 |
| 4 | Alexr. — " — | " -15 — " — | 1,200.00 |
| 5 | Affy — " — | " 13 — " — | 800.00 |
| 6 | Isaac — " — | " -10 — " — | 600.00 |
| 7 | Rodolph — " — | " 8 — " — | 400.00 |
| 8 | Kavanaugh — " — | " 6 — " — | 300.00 |
| 9 | Celestine — " — | " 4 — " — | 300.00 |
| 10 | Adam Weams — | " 55 — " Diseased | 200.00 |
| 11 | Mary Virgin | " 60 years Broken Shoulder | 200.00 |
| 12 | Phil McAffee | aged 50 years Diseased | 500.00 |
| 13 | Holly McAffee | " 55 years Lumbago | 50.00 |
| 14 | Sam Bostwick | " 60 years | 400.00 |
| 15 | Mary — " — | " 60 — " — Diseased | 300.00 |
| 16 | Simon — " — | " 9 years | 600.00 |

**Fig. 1:** List of James Railey's slaves and their value from his will in 1861. Photo reproduced from records in the Natchez Courthouse.

# CHAPTER ONE

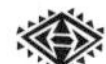

# Mississippi Roots

Where the magnolia blossom grows,
Where the muddy Mississippi River flows.
Where the mocking birds sing,
Where plantation bells ring,
In Mississippi.
Where boll weevils ruin the cotton,
Where black folks are forgotten.
Where pine trees grow tall,
There ain't no rights at all,
In Mississippi.
Where the rich delta land,
All owned by the White man.
The black man works and sweats,
He runs away, but never forgets.
Mississippi.
— *Edward C. Mazique, 1982*

Dr. Edward Craig Mazique's past began in an unpretentious home near Natchez, Mississippi. Today you must wind down a narrow dirt road and wade with your car across a driveway partially submerged by a shallow creek to finally come upon the small white house. Behind it you see nothing but tall woods and on the sides nothing but extensive fields ending in another forest in the distance. It is easy to visualize history passing by only outside the borders of this secluded area, but China Grove, as this plantation was named, saw more rapid changes in black history than many places in the heart of the metropolises. For in the 1850s this home was built for a highly favored slave whose total net worth as a human being could be written on paper as if he were no more than a valuable stock animal. Yet by 1871 the master was dead in the Civil War, the slave family was freed, and China Grove was owned by the former slave. Before the end of 1880, the slave's eldest surviving son had purchased Anchorage, a large plantation in the south of Adams County. By 1890 he had purchased Oakland, the plantation owned and inhabited by his master, and had initiated other purchases that were to make the Mazique family one of the largest landowners in Adams County. This meteoric rise is a story of a unique family, special circumstances, and the peculiar character of Natchez, Mississippi. But it is also the story of the South, of the meaningful black/white relationships that frequently developed there despite prejudice and racism, and of strong family ties, solid values, hard work, and painstakingly developed skills that enabled the survival of a people despite the prediction by the *Natchez Tri-Weekly Democrat* in 1866:

> The child is already born who will behold the last negro in the State of Mississippi. With no one to provide for the aged and the young, the sick and the helpless incompetent to provide for themselves, and brought unprepared into competition with the superior intelligence, tact, and muscle of free white labor, they must surely and speedily perish.[1]

By the outbreak of the Civil War, Natchez, Mississippi, was a thriving town. Agricultural production was booming and expansion into the Midwest kept its river traffic at an all-time high. On its bustling streets, merchants, planters, river men, and manufacturers vied for the money cotton was pouring into the local economy. The city could not expand rapidly enough to suit businessmen who clamored for "more room," "more stores," and "more houses." The foundation for this prosperity was the necessity for cheap labor, which was secured largely through the enslavement of black people: a foundation that was to rapidly crumble by the end of the decade.[2]

Natchez always was an unusual southern town. The xenophobia associated with many southern communities was not to be found there. Outside ideas and ways were of little threat to townspeople who were recently foreigners themselves. In 1850, 31 percent of the population of 4,680 was foreign-born. Many others (800) were Yankees and a significant number educated their children in New England. The river traffic also served as an avenue for nontraditional thoughts. Although the coarser elements of river gamblers and roustabouts congregated in the notorious dissipation of Natchez-under-the-Hill, new ideas could not help but be circulated from the more elegant passengers to the aristocratic part of Natchez sedately perched on the bluff overlooking the river. By 1835, the more reputable citizens of town were dominating and serious attempts were being made to civilize the disreputable area under-the-Hill. As an Englishman noted after his repeated visits to Natchez-under-the-Hill, "the most abandoned sink of iniquity in the West" was "much improved."[3]

Yet for all its cosmopolitanism, the frontier-town mentality was slow to die. In his diary of the times (1835–1851), a prominent Negro barber, William Johnson of Natchez, recorded street fights using everything from fists to canes to pistols among poor and wealthy alike. This situation did not change after the Civil War, and frequently a man's strength and gun were the only law to protect him.

Natchez boasted the largest slave market in the state of Mississippi. Despite this fact, Natchez and the surrounding area seemed to serve as a haven for free Negroes. The largest percentage of free Negroes living in any one locale in the Old South was in Natchez and Adams County. The 1840 census listed 1,336 free Negroes in the state, and 255 of these resided in Adams County.[4] Freeing one's slaves apparently elevated the owner in the eyes of his peers, much as "conspicuous consumption" was to be the mark of the wealthy at a later date. If a man could afford to give up something as valuable as one of his slaves, he must be very wealthy indeed. Although historians have written on the subject, many of us remain unacquainted with the relative success of some of the free Negroes, respected by both black and white, who amassed a great deal of property and had a sizable number of their own slaves.[5] Somehow these achievements cannot be made to comfortably fit into our image of the "Old South" and so we have tended to overlook them.

One of the best known of these free Negroes was the barber William Johnson. His mother was freed by her master when William was only five. Four years later in 1818, at age thirteen, his sister Delia was freed. In 1820, when Johnson was eleven, it was finally his turn to be freed by the man who was in all likelihood his father. Johnson built a sizable estate from the barber shop he purchased from his brother-in-law. By 1851, Johnson had fifteen slaves valued at more than $6,000 and a total estate in excess of $25,000. His home was in the middle of one of the better white neighborhoods. Respect among whites for Johnson was so great that he was allowed to engage in many activities that would normally be denied to free Negroes. His business transactions with whites included renting them rooms and buildings, lending them money, and even employing some of them to work his farm or erect his buildings.[6]

Other free Negro businessmen also fared well. Robert D. Smith operated a hack business in the 1850s in Natchez and was well accepted by the citizenry of Natchez, as his obituary in 1858 demonstrates:

> THE LATE ROBERT D. SMITH. All our old citizens—indeed we may say—all our citizens will regret to hear of the death of Robert D. Smith, a colored man of our city, but one who, by his industry, probity of life, correctness of demeanor and Christian-like character, had won the favor and respect of the entire community.[7]

The free Negroes were not all wealthy and respected. Just as with its white counterpart, the black community was marked by social divisions and economic diversity. Johnson was part of the aristocracy of the free people of color. The middle class was composed of those who had less chance for advancement, such as mulatto apprentices, stewards on steamboats, and hack drivers. The lower class consisted of the poor who were small farmers, day laborers, and peddlers. More than one-quarter of the free Negroes were in some kind of dependent relationship with a white family and were listed as attached to a white household.[8]

Then there were the slaves, the lowest class of the black population. However, even the conditions of slavery appeared to be moderated a bit by this sophisticated cosmopolitan community. Natchez boasted of a slave hospital, one of the few in the Old South. Frequently white preachers and physicians were hired to attend to the needs of slaves, and there is some evidence that two-thirds of the slaves in the Natchez area attended the church of their masters. In 1861, James Railey, the owner of the Mazique family, had the former rector of Trinity Episcopal Church, who was serving as the bishop of Mississippi, come to his plantation to baptize some slaves and to consecrate a burial ground. The slaves bestowed upon Bishop Green a beautiful silver private communion set, which James Railey must have given them to present. Doubtless, at this time, the Maziques were among those baptized if they had not already been.[9]

It has been argued that Natchez slave owners did everything to improve the lot of their labor force. Although such a wide-ranging generalization may be strongly overstated, there is evidence that the Natchez owners believed that temperate treatment was necessary if slaves were to continue working at their maximum potential.[10] The *Southern Galaxy,* a Natchez newspaper, ran an editorial in 1828 advocating more reasonable punishment for slaves.

> We have resided some years among slaves, and from often repeated inquiries, aided by personal observations we are justified in the remark, that the slave, to be useful, must not be barbarously treated. He must be well fed, well clothed, and humanely treated when sick; the master must not tamper with him—correction should not be often repeated, not done in anger.[11]

This attitude does not mean that life was easy if you were black and living in Natchez. There were many atrocities toward slaves recorded among the accounts of life in the Natchez area. The humane treatment of slaves advocated in the *Southern Galaxy* stemmed more from a business sense than a sense of justice. To ensure good work and nonthreatening relations with the large number of blacks in Natchez, reasonable treatment was a necessity. Given that one out of three inhabitants of Natchez just prior to the Civil War was a slave, it is no wonder the slave owners strove for harmony and a curtailment of racial friction.[12]

Although some impressive gains were made by free Negroes in Natchez, public sentiment turned against them as the white population began to feel threatened by the increasing number of freed slaves and the abolitionist philosophy. In the 1840s the lot of the free Negro in Natchez began to deteriorate during what Johnson, the respected barber, called "the Inquisition." The deeds records of Adams County tell of the changing times. In the 1830s, nearly a hundred emancipation papers were officially recorded. This number dropped to fewer than ten between 1840 and 1850. Although Johnson's position was reasonably secure from political maneuvering, the rights afforded the free Negroes were curtailed and some were actually deported. Johnson recorded with dismay the plight of the free Negroes during this time:

> Poor Andrew Leeper was, I understand, ordered off to day, and so was Dembo and Maryan Givson. They are as far as I Know innocent and Harmless People And Have never done a Crime....Oh what a Country we Live in.[13]

In 1851 William Johnson was murdered. The paper's account of the murder eulogized Johnson:

> It was ascertained that William Johnson, a free man of color, born and raised in Natchez, and holding a respected position on account of his character, intelligence and deportment, had been shot....This murder has created a great deal of excitement, as well from its atrocity, as from the peaceable character of Johnson and his excellent standing. His funeral services were conducted by the Rev. Mr. Watkins, who paid a just tribute to his memory, holding up his example as one well worthy of imitation by all his class. We observed very many of our most respected citizens at his funeral.[14]

The prosecution made a strong effort to convict Baylor Winn, who was doubtless guilty of the shooting. However, after two years in prison and three mistrials, Winn was released. The man who was with Johnson and witnessed the shooting was a mulatto. Mississippi law made no exception for William Johnson: a Negro witness could not testify against a white man. Despite the so-called respect in which Johnson was held, his murderer was allowed to go free by claiming to be a white man, thereby invalidating the testimony of the witness.

The ultimate worth of a black man in Natchez in the 1800s is perhaps best summarized by the results of this trial. No matter how much money he had accumulated, no matter how good a life he had led, a black man's life was not worth the life of a white man of dubious character.[15]

Despite the dehumanization of slavery, many other black/white relationships, obligations, and sometimes even friendships were formed throughout the South. William Johnson's diary gives ample evidence of his various interactions with whites that go against our stereotypes. In Natchez, the large number of single white male households composed of a black common-law wife and their mulatto children attests to the fact that black/white affiliations were far from the monolithic slave/master relationship.[16]

It is obvious that some blacks fared better than others under the rule of the "peculiar institution" of slavery. William Johnson's diary gives examples of slaves in Natchez who were treated almost as well as if they had been free. It was not unheard of for valued slaves to be plantation overseers for their masters and to be treated, if not equally, at least more humanely than most. Such was the case with August Mazique and his wife, Sarah. The Mazique family had their own small home on China Grove, a 625-acre plantation that adjoined Master James Railey's more opulent plantation of Oakland.

Approximately twelve miles south of Natchez, China Grove sat in virtual seclusion. To reach it from the Beverly Road that led from Natchez, a traveler had to go down a dirt road through another parcel of land known as White Apple Village past the Indian Mound, then wade across Second Creek. The next house was Oakland, which was three or four miles farther along the Beverly Road, separated from China Grove by thick forest. The Second Creek neighborhood in which China Grove and Oakland were located was considered one of the most desirable in the Natchez area. It rivaled the city of Natchez for elegance and a high social standard.[17]

The next town to the south was Woodville, another twenty-three miles past Oakland. A traveler in 1835 described the towns and villages in Mississippi as "located perfectly independent of each other, isolated among its forests, and often many leagues apart, leaving in the intervals large tracts of country covered with plantations."[18] Therefore, each plantation afforded its inhabitants a great deal of privacy.

The Mazique home was apparently built soon after James Railey purchased the land in 1854. It was a white two-room main house with tall windows and a wide porch set in the midst of chinaberry trees and dominated by a large oak. Separated from and behind the house stood the kitchen and dining room. A cotton gin, outhouse, barn, smokehouse, and slave quarters completed the property. The house was certainly modest by plantation standards, but compared to the shacks of the poor whites and many of the free blacks in the area it must have seemed like a mansion.

August's children were also treated well by Railey. At least one, Alexander, became a house servant, the most honored and valued position for a slave. "Originally chosen for their superior intelligence and attractive appearance, they [house servants] had the greatest opportunities for self-improvement, and often succeeded in handing their status down to their sons and daughters."[19] Planters liked to show them off, and in some cases even taught them to read and write, although this was not the case with the Maziques.

Just how special the Mazique family was to James Railey is evidenced by his last will and testament, written on February 1, 1860. Although he bequeathed "all the estate I own of *every* kind in the state of Mississippi" to his wife without restriction, he made an exception of the Mazique family. After his wife's death, August and Sarah and their children were to become the property of his brother, Logan, in Kentucky, who "will treat them with kindness and give them all the comfort they require and all the levity from hard work they may merit."[20]

Slavery for the Mazique family could not have been as traumatic as it was for some. They were given good housing and ample food, and their family was not separated or threatened by future separation. However, if one tends to doubt the loathsomeness of their lot, one only need look at James Railey's probate papers where the family is listed as property, and an account given of their illnesses and monetary worth.[21]

Natchez had no strategic value in the Civil War, so little destruction resulted from military battles. The plantation mansions and the town homes remained intact to serve as a reminder of a lost way of life. However, what war failed to do, peace achieved. After the loss by the South in the war, people abandoned their plantations en masse, leading to deterioration and decay.[22]

During the Civil War, the government leased plantations to men, generally white scavengers from the North, who frequently hired the recently freed slaves and treated them worse than their originals masters. By all accounts, the conditions in and around Natchez were abominable and continued to be so long after the war had ended. Quarrels between the military and the Treasury Department about how to run the leased plantations led to an inability and/or unwillingness of the troops to enforce law and order on the plantations. "Stock was stolen, houses were burned, and Negroes were abducted, driven off and murdered, as were the lessees."[23] The military proved to be totally ineffective in controlling the attacks. "Practically all the plantations in the vicinity of Natchez, Vicksburg, and Milliken's Bend were given up, while the Negroes who were not carried off by the raiders fled to the army camps for protection."[24] Conditions were especially harsh in town, where health conditions and vagrancy laws were used as excuses to round up recently freed blacks and forcibly remove them from Natchez.[25]

As if the man-made horrors were not enough to reduce all the Negroes to the wretched conditions of the federal camps,[26] the army worm invaded the cotton fields, leaving many areas completely devastated.

August and Sarah and their family stayed on China Grove during the war to take care of James Railey's son, Charles. James Railey, who had died during the Civil War (1861), provided for Charles but did not leave him the property outright. Charles had killed a man and was saved from the penalty of the law only because he was declared mentally unfit. He was known to drink and behave badly, as was reported in his divorce suit in 1866. When James's wife, Matilda, died (1869), she left the half of China Grove that contained the residence to Charles and the other half to her daughter.[27]

Despite the upheaval caused by the war, many of the slave owners managed to return and retain the rights to their property. The old elite were very much in control in the 1870s, and black ownership of land was discouraged in many areas. By the beginning of the 1900s, blacks still owned only 6 percent of the land in Adams County.[28]

August Mazique was one of those few blacks who prospered during this harsh time. In 1870, when China Grove came up for public auction after the impoverished Railey heirs lost their rights to the property in a chancery court suit, August Mazique had a white former plantation overseer named Wilmer Shields purchase the property for him. Shields promptly turned the land over to August, who completed paying for it by 1871, enabling him to own the plantation on which he had, less than a decade earlier, been a slave, albeit an honored and esteemed one.

# CHAPTER TWO

## A Country Boy

Just a country boy—a farmer's son,
Work in the cotton field ain't no fun.
Get up in the morning at the break of day,
Nothing but misery to live this way.
Hitch up that mule—go to the field.
Water Boy! Water Boy!
Bring that meal.
A bucket of grits with grease on top,
A glass of molasses and biscuits to sop.
Plow in the bright sun, hot as hell;
Listen for the toll of the dinner bell.
Eat greens and pot likker—corn bread on the side,
Back to the cotton field, just can't hide.
Skin boils in sweat, keep moving along;
'Til sun starts setting, I sing my song,
This kind of living is weary.
Going to leave this place one day.
Catch a freight train for Georgia—Make my getaway!

*— Edward C. Mazique, 1983*

Mississippi in the early 1900s was one of the most miserable places in this country for blacks. During Reconstruction there had been a vision of brighter days on the horizon. If they just worked hard, blacks could become mayors, congressman, senators, and successful farmers.[1] By the twentieth century, the life of the poor sharecropper, the long hours to end up with no more than they had as slaves, had dimmed, if not completely erased, the bright hopes of a quarter-century earlier.

Blacks were denied the vote, denied schooling past the elementary level, and expected to keep off Main Street in Natchez.

Despite all these difficulties, the Maziques fared well. There is no clear-cut explanation as to how their success was possible. August and Sarah Mazique could neither read nor write and their children, although favored slaves, were also illiterate. How August ever managed to put together the money to buy China Grove and how his children all came to own property is something that can only make us wonder. There can be no doubt that this was an exceptional family who, if not educated in reading and writing, certainly made up for it with extraordinary intelligence.

After the death of August, it was Alex, the next-to-the-oldest son, with his strong personality who was the unquestioned leader of the entire family. He was a tall, slender, coffee-skinned man who, when Eddie was growing up, sported a long white beard that fell down to almost touch his navel. All those who remember "Grandpa Alex" speak of him as a commanding figure despite the rather high pitch to his voice.

Eddie remembered his grandfather with respect and love:

> My grandfather was a very gentle man. He was relatively tall in stature although a little stooped when I knew him. He had keen features, brown skin, deeply sunken eyes, sharp nose, heavy eyebrows, and a tousle of hair on his head that was all over—it came right down to his neck. He had a long flowing beard that covered his face and came down at least five inches below his chin and it flushed out. It was black mingled with gray and white. He didn't drink or smoke. He was soft spoken. His eyes were sunken and piercing, making you know that he was firm in his commitments and decisions. He walked jauntily and pretty much erect. He had eight children. He decided he wanted all of his children educated and this he did.

On Sundays after church, all of the family would travel in their horse and buggy over the country roads to Oakland. As they turned up the long winding dirt and gravel drive they would just get a glimpse of the shining white of the house sitting in the midst of the leaves of the huge oak trees at the top of the hill. Near the main road they would pass Grandpa Alex's store, then the former slave quarters where sharecroppers now lived, past the old cemetery with the metal grate around the plot of land where the Railey family was buried. And apart from the Raileys, in death as in life, off to the side, outside of the fence were the headstones for August and Sarah Mazique.

The house itself was as majestic as when the Raileys owned it.[2] There was room after room—or so it seemed to the grandchildren. The main floor had five or six bedrooms and a living room, used only when they had company, with a piano and fine crystal. The kitchen had a huge wood-burning stove and the dining room had a table large enough to seat twenty people at once.[3] But what the children looked forward to, even more than the meals, was the large fan that hung from the ceiling over the table. This they were allowed to pull while Grandpa and his guests ate their meal. Grandpa Alex sat and enjoyed the cooling breeze much as James Railey's family had done when this was one of Alex's chores as Master Railey's slave. The lower floor contained another three bedrooms and this was where Grandpa Alex and Eddie slept. These rooms were underground on the front side and were especially cool during the hot Mississippi summer nights.

Going out through the kitchen door and down the large back steps would bring you to the original building on the plantation that Grandpa used for a livery stable and to store corn and hay on the second floor. Off to the right was a small two-room house that had served as a schoolhouse for the Railey children. There were a number of other buildings on Oakland: a huge barn, a gristmill, a gazebo, and an old church building. Oakland and the adjoining 836-acre plantation of White Apple Village that Grandpa owned seemed like a whole world to the grandchildren.

Grandpa Alex kept everything in perfect condition. The carriages were shiny and clean and the horses, a special love of the Maziques, were always slick and groomed. The lemon trees and wisteria grew in the front of the house and filled the air with their pungent smells. The front porch ran the whole length of the house and served as a natural place for the children to run up and down. The squeaks from the floorboards rang out as the children played and the adults sat, sipped lemonade or mint juleps, and talked over family business. Alex's brothers, Ike, Hubbard, Jim, and Rudolph, would be there. Jim was rather fat and brown and looked to the others a lot like an Indian. Rudolph, the youngest and handsomest of the brothers, always looked dapper on those Sundays, causing others to joke about his being the playboy of the family. The sisters would be there too: Celestine, who had married Haywood Roy, and

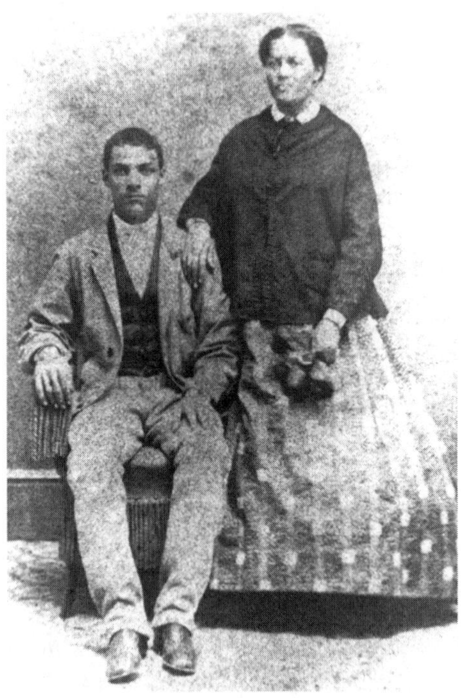

**Fig. 2:**
Eddie's grandparents, Alex Mazique I and Laura Craig Mazique. Photo courtesy of Maude Mazique and Dolores Pelham.

Affie, a fair-skinned girl with freckles, who married Lycurgus McMurtry. And at the center of it all would be Alex Mazique Sr.

Alex had amassed a great deal of property, had become a successful farmer and businessman, and yet could neither read nor write. Until near the end of his life, Grandpa Alex was still signing his name with just an *X*. But he didn't delude himself about the importance of an education. He often told the story of the unscrupulous whites who had tried to take away his land by saying he didn't pay his taxes or bank loans. Somehow he always managed to come out with his property intact but at times it was a close decision. On one occasion, a judge was about to rule against him when he attempted to explain that he had misplaced the receipt in one of his pockets. He began to demonstrate the way it occurred for the judge when, by accident, he discovered the long-lost piece of paper in the vest of his suit.[4] He knew being dependent on the goodwill and honesty of the white man to interpret contracts and deeds was no way for a black man to succeed. So he saw to it that all his children were educated. An elementary education was all that was provided for black youths in most of

Mississippi and Louisiana. In order to go beyond that, his children had to be sent to private schools, which meant there would be travel expenses along with the costs of education. All of Alex's children finished high school and he pushed others to go on even further.

Alex and Laura Craig were married when she was just fifteen. Laura's mother, Millie, was a slave whose two daughters, Laura and Lettie, were fathered by a white army officer. Millie moved in with Grandpa Alex and helped out around the plantation, as did Lettie, who never married. Millie was a lovely little woman who used to go out and ring the bell to call the men to work. Millie lived in the little house that used to be the Episcopal church in the back of Oakland.

Grandpa Alex ruled his eight children with a firm but loving grip. In turn, they all loved and respected their father and followed his wishes even when they were contrary to their own. James, the eldest, was sent to Howard University Medical School in Washington, D.C., and became a physician. Eddie's father, Alex Jr., went to Roger Williams in Tennessee to study to be a lawyer,[5] but was called back when his help was needed on the farm. An intelligent man who loved learning, Alex Jr. was to suffer disappointment the rest of his life for never finishing his degree. Robert and William (called "Uncle Bud" by the children) finished high school and went on to be successful farmers.

It was not just the boys who were educated. All of the daughters graduated from Roger Williams and married men that Grandpa Alex considered suitable, namely those who "would make something of themselves." Laura was a teacher and married Professor Washburn from Natchez College, who later went on to be the principal of a school in Memphis, Tennessee. Mary was a teacher and a singer with a beautiful contralto voice. She married James Boyd, a plantation manager and well-to-do entrepreneur who was the son of Judge Boyd and one of his slaves. Berta also was a teacher and married a contractor, C. S. Sims, who built one of the new buildings at Natchez College, the black high school that all the Maziques attended. Sarah, an educator who became the dean of women at Natchez College, married the man who would serve as its president for thirty years, S. H. C. Owen. This marriage was not Sarah's first choice, however.

She was in love with a handsome brown-skinned fellow but Grandpa Alex didn't think he was going to amount to much. Professor Owen, on the other hand, who was not a particularly handsome man by all family accounts, was an upstanding gentleman on the move and Grandpa Alex smiled kindly on their marriage. Grandpa was right about some things,

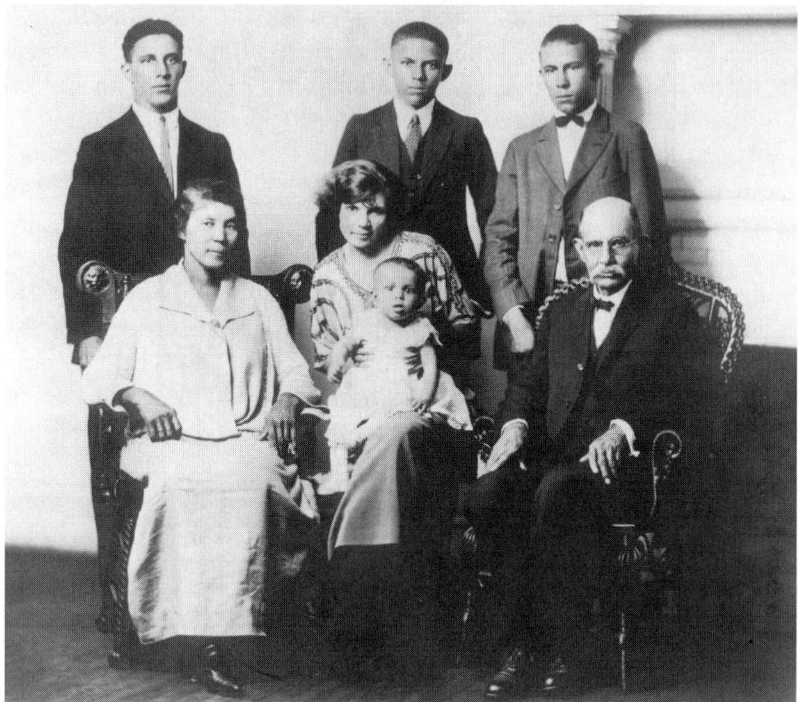

**Fig. 3:** The Boyd family. Seated, left to right: Mary Mazique Boyd, Alice Burton holding baby, and James Boyd. Standing, left to right: Wilbur Boyd, Seward Boyd, and James Boyd Jr. Photo courtesy of Maude Mazique and Dolores Pelham.

for S. H. C. Owen did well and their four sons who grew to manhood all became doctors, three physicians and one dentist.

The Mazique name was respected around town by both blacks and whites. Grandpa Alex had credit wherever he asked, Uncle Jim had an office in Natchez, and Eddie's father, Alex, kept a home in Natchez so that the children could go to school. Yet they seldom mixed in the political or economic affairs of the town and consequently their names were never mentioned in the newspapers of the day. They kept to themselves, and the center of their lives, the focus, where everyone "really lived," was on the plantations.

Grandpa Alex managed to set up all of his children on plantations. Eddie's father, Alex, owned China Grove. The Boyds ended up with Anchorage and Robert with Woodlands. James, or "Uncle Doc" as he was called, lived on Montrose.

There was a certain amount of security in owning nearby and contiguous properties. Being thirteen miles outside of Natchez and having family for neighbors served to provide the Maziques with a buffer against the vagaries of white malevolence. They grew up believing that people were people and all deserving of respect. Even though they were not treated as equals, many of the relationships they had with the whites they encountered were cordial. Grandpa Alex even let some white families sharecrop parts of his land.

All of the Maziques loved horses. Grandpa Alex raised horses and had a stud farm on his property. They all learned to ride well and cherished the sense of freedom they achieved while in the saddle. Eddie's sister Maude[6] once rode her horse right down the Main Street of Natchez. She rode as fast as she could, and it was hard to tell if the white faces were more startled by the black face that was invading their sacrosanct territory or the speed with which her horse was progressing. Many of the whites came to bet on the horses at the racetrack that Grandpa owned on the White Apple Village plantation. This seems more than a little ironic since one family story has it that August's wife, Sarah, was won by James Railey in a horse race on this very same White Apple Village track.

Grandpa Alex's plantation was a menagerie of people and animals. At various times there were former slaves, workers, aunts, great-grandparents, and grandchildren all dwelling at Oakland. And Grandpa was a stock farmer so he had sheep, cows, horses, chickens, and just about every other animal one could imagine. It must have looked wonderful to the kids. And some of them made a pretty permanent residence of the place.

Mary Mazique Boyd's daughter, Alice Boyd, was sent to Oakland to stay with her grandfather and console him after his wife, Laura Craig, died. Alice loved the genial grandfather who always had time to play with her, and she refused to leave when it was time for school. Her father threatened she would grow up to be an "ignoramus," a new word for her vocabulary, and finally her Uncle Bud had to haul her off to school on the back of his horse.

Eddie was another favorite of Grandpa Alex's and got to spend many of his summers at Oakland. Grandpa Alex would always ask Eddie's father if he could take "Buddy," as he called Eddie, with him after school was out. Alex Jr. idolized his father and would always agree even though it deprived him of Eddie's labor on the farm.

Grandpa Alex would tell Alice about how his father's slave ship originated on a tiny island, and he would ask her to get the geography book and name the smallest island in hopes that he would remember the name of the place. He would tell Eddie stories of what it was like when he was a slave. The grandchildren listened politely to the stories of their elders about the old days. As with most children, however, they were much more fascinated by the here and now. Although many of the details of the family beginnings and the slave days are lost, the remembrances of the people populating Oakland are as vivid as yesterday.

Stanley, a former slave at Oakland who stayed on after the war, was a special friend to Eddie.

> I never shall forget, one man there whose name was Stanley. Stanley and I became great friends. He was a bachelor and he was graying around the temples with a bald shiny head and dark complexion, very muscular and with great big deep-set brown eyes. He, at that time, must have been in his sixties.
>
> The slave quarters were still on Oakland. I used to go down to his quarters and sit and listen to him tell stories about slavery and I would watch him patch his pants.
>
> It was amazing to me how he would take and patch his pants from other cloth he had. It didn't make any difference about the color, whether it was polka dot going into a plaid or a plaid going into a plain. The point was, it was cloth. And then instead of just making this thing with small stitches one close behind the other, his stitches would be at least one inch long so that he'd get through the darn thing in a little while. But I loved to see him do that and he'd stitch his pants and put on his brogans.

Stanley and Eddie would sneak down to the watermelon patch in the morning when the cool dew had chilled the melons and would take their pick and start eating them right there. Grandpa often caught them but he never seemed to mind.

Grandpa Alex and Eddie had their own special breakfasts too. They would go to the livery stable with a long pole and knock the baby pigeons from the rafters and dine on squab to start their day.

Life at Oakland was different from the endless chores of Eddie's father's farm. Grandpa Alex gave the orders and being with him meant helping him supervise. In the mornings he would sit at the top of the steep steps leading from the kitchen down to the backyard. The rest of the men would sit under him on different steps. Grandpa Alex would tell what he wanted to be done in the various sections that day and his head man, Grant, would see that his orders were carried out.

Grandpa Alex would have old Queen hitched up to the buggy and Eddie would drive Grandpa all over his land to see how his tenants were doing. This was when Eddie and Grandpa Alex would have a chance to talk.

> He would talk to me then. Wouldn't it be wonderful if I had a recorder or been sensitive enough to write some of it down? But a nine- or ten-year-old kid doesn't care about history.
>
> A couple of things he told me, I do remember. He began to tell me about inequities and about difficulties he had in acquiring some of his land. He also began to tell me how on more than one occasion he had to go to court to defend himself. He would also tell me how there was no justice and no way to get justice. There was not a black lawyer in the whole county. It was time for black lawyers to become involved. He would tell me as we rode along that he wanted me to become a lawyer. I'm going to see that you go through law school. He did push me to become involved.

Traveling over all his property would take more than one day. Sometimes they would watch the horses being studded or see what was happening at the grist mill. There was a never-ending variety of things to do and yet the hard labor was all performed by others. This was definitely young Eddie's idea of a good way to spend his days. He wasn't fully aware of the luxury in which he was living, but he knew things were all right when he was on Grandpa Alex's plantation.

While Grandpa Alex was well-to-do and living in the Oakland mansion, some of his children were not faring as well. The year 1911 brought not only Eddie's birth but devastation to many farmers around Natchez. As early as 1860 a traveler could see that the constant planting of cotton and the method of plowing on hills was depleting the rich Mississippi soil. By 1874, excessive taxation on real estate that was decreasing in productivity due to the deteriorating soils was causing massive forfeitures of land around Natchez.[7] In 1899 cotton prices were finally starting to move

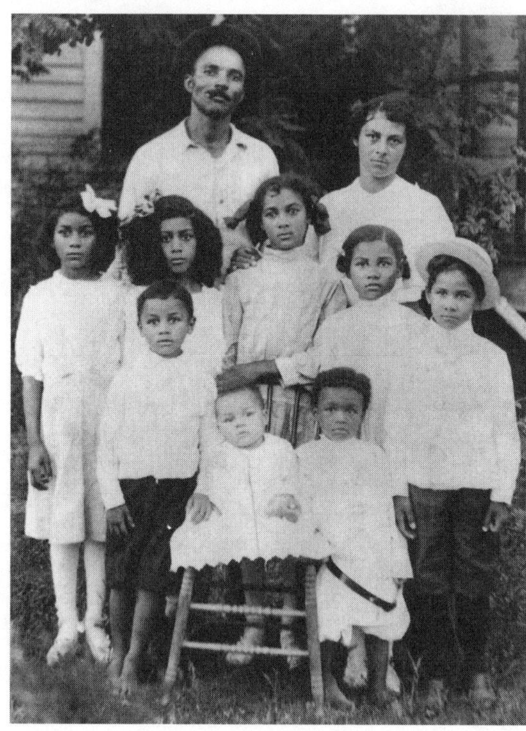

**Fig. 4:** The Mazique family: Front from left to right: Douglas, Jack (in chair), Eddie. Second row from left to right: Edna, Cousin Addie, Maude, Sadie, and Alex III ("Buddie"). Back row: Alex Mazique Jr.. and Addie Wilkerson Mazique. Photo courtesy of Maude Mazique and Dolores Pelham.

back up, after their post–Civil War slump, when the boll weevil made an appearance. The weevil devastated the cotton crop in the area and diminished the average yield to an all-time low.

Although the elements took their toll on Grandpa Alex's estate and he had to mortgage his property most years against the crops as did all but the wealthiest farmers, he was somewhat immune to the drastic slump caused by the cotton crop failure. His investments were diversified enough that his income came from several sources. He had the stock farm, the store, and a cotton gin, and was a landlord to numerous sharecroppers. Although his sharecroppers would not have been doing well during this time, farmers and other people would still need his animals and supplies. Grandpa Alex was always generous with his surplus. Eddie remembered how he would always assist his children:

> He was very thoughtful. In those days your house was heated by fireplaces. Every year he would send this man over with a wagon load of wood to be stacked for

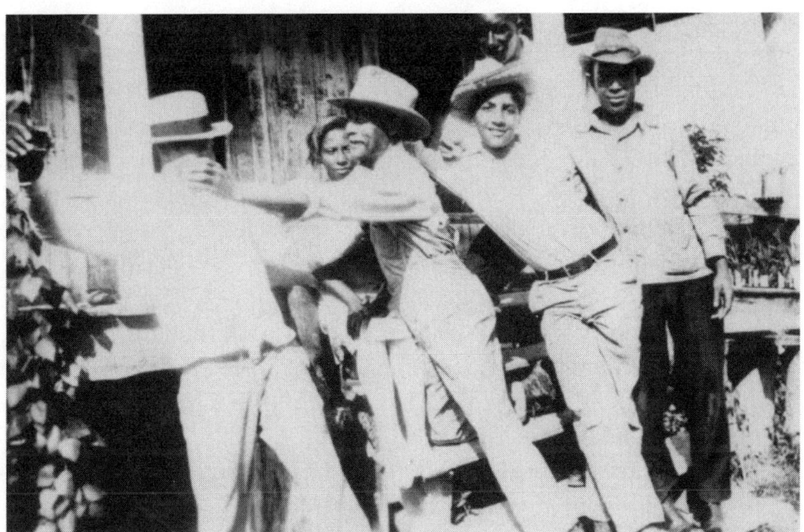

**Fig. 5:** The Maziques and Wilkersons in Wildsville, Louisiana. Left to right, Alex Mazique III ("Buddie," Eddie's oldest brother), Uncle Doug Mazique, Eddie, and Alex Wilkerson (Addie Wilkerson Mazique's brother). Photo courtesy of Maude Mazique and Dolores Pelham.

> fuel for the winter. Every time one of the animals was killed, he would always bring some of it.

The fall in cotton production led to an exodus in the area surrounding Natchez. Although born at China Grove, Eddie was never destined to spend much time at the family homestead. Alex Jr. moved his entire family to Wildsville, Louisiana, in 1911 to sharecrop land near his wife's relatives.[8] The soil was richer and, even though physically close to Natchez, the cotton and corn crop there had not been attacked by the boll weevil. By this time Alex and Addie Wilkerson Mazique (with five children older than Eddie: Maude, Edna, Sadie, Alex, and Douglas) had a growing family to support.

Wildsville was about forty miles from Natchez, and the Wilkerson family all lived on a spur off the main road. Eddie's maternal grandparents, Mama Caroline and Papa Doug Wilkerson, lived at the head of the road and all the relatives fell into place around them.[9] All of the land off this road was part of a big plantation and it extended even farther than this two-mile segment on which the Wilkersons lived. It was owned by "someone in the North" and managed by a Mr. Statom. Eddie's father, along with the Wilkersons, worked the land and gave one-quarter of what they produced to the landlord as his rent.

There were good things about this life. Being surrounded by family provided the children with security. Some of them cannot remember an incident of discrimination until they moved from the farmlands into the nearby towns.

The farm next to Alex's was inhabited by Charles Wexler, who moved there when he was twenty-seven and single. He always claimed that Eddie's father taught him how to farm. Mr. Wexler would get up early in the morning and begin work by 7:00 A.M. But when he looked over to Alex's farm, he found that Eddie's father had been out there with his boys since five o'clock in the morning. To compete with him he had to start keeping Alex's hours.

And those hours were long. Alex would get up at 4:00 A.M. and make a fire. Then he would check on the outside. When he came back in the family knew it was about time to get up. He would clear his throat loud enough for them to hear and then say, "The sun is up, everybody fall out." They would all sit down and have breakfast together before leaving for their various jobs. Maude and her sisters took care of the cows and chickens, and Eddie, when he was old enough, and his brothers went to the fields with Alex.

Eddie's father was a tall, thin man whose whole carriage spoke of pride and courage. A break in his leg that occurred when a horse fell on him had been set improperly and left him with a stiff leg. He still managed to ride horses and to work long days, but not to ride in the horse races that all the Maziques loved so well. He was the kind of man that others came to for advice and assistance. Many of the blacks in the area could neither read nor write, and Alex would explain and answer questions about current events and legal issues.

He was a perfectionist who wanted things done just so and believed that everything should be in its proper place. He always told the children, "Let all of your things have their places and each part of your business its time." Maude remembers one time when he was looking for the broom. He gave them "hell" because it was out of place. He felt he could have the job done in the time it was taking him to look for the broom and that his time had been wasted.

There is little doubt that Alex's frustration with being stuck as a sharecropper with no chance for advancement filtered down to his children and instilled in all of them a need to succeed. Believing strongly in education as Grandpa Alex did, Alex Jr. bought and maintained a house

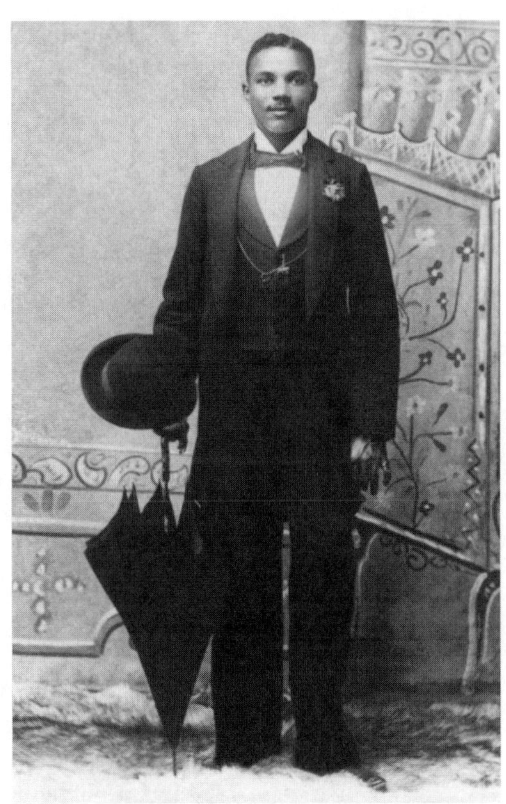

**Fig. 6:** Alex Mazique Jr., Eddie's father. Photo courtesy of Maude Mazique and Dolores Pelham.

in Natchez so that his children could go all the way through high school. Alex Jr.'s abilities far outweighed his opportunities, and this made him a bit of a perplexing person for the young Eddie to comprehend:

> My Daddy was a man who was built up of a multitude of complexities. If he were alive today, I don't know what kind of psychiatrist would be capable of analyzing him. His situation led to a sociological schizophrenia that is brought on as a result of conditions in which you have to live. He was a man who was denied the achieving of his potential.
>
> I really wish that you could see his writing and how he used to talk. He had an eloquent voice. He could sing, play the guitar, and dance—he had so much talent. He was aggressive.

I was never able to completely analyze him until later in life. I only saw him as a hard driver—an individual who would get up and work hard and sweat hard. He worked hard himself and the people around him worked hard, and the children, the same way.

He was born in 1880. His father, my granddaddy, had this sense of wanting to educate his children, and he wanted my father to become a lawyer. My father did finish high school. He was very learned, brilliant and very intellectual. He went to law school, at a place called Roger Williams Institute in Tennessee. After spending two years, my grandfather called him out to come and take over a plantation in Mississippi.

You could see the frustrations my father had. In spite of that, he had a great deal of character, strength and self-discipline. He was quite a disciplinarian and he preached that to you. He lived by hard work and honesty, and that was the way that it was. He lived in a segregated society and a place where most of the blacks in the area could neither read nor write.

In spite of the fact that my father felt cramped in on all sides and couldn't move much in society in the area in which he was living, he still made a decision that he wanted to educate all of his children. I heard him say more that once: "Look, I want to see that each and every one of my children gets a high school education." This was quite a feat for blacks in those days. So he went about doing just that.

In the twenties he bought a home in Natchez, 403 North Pine Street. That was the house that was used for the education of his children. We would go out to Louisiana and work on the farm during the farming season and go to school during the winter months.

Generally we only had the opportunity to go to school five months out of the year instead of nine. The cotton season began in February when you started clearing land and in March it was planted. Pa usually didn't bother us until the cotton was ready to be chopped or thinned out. That called for manpower. We were called out of school in March. We missed March,

> April, and May and went back to school in September. The principals of the schools understood this because black people had to live and this was the only way they could do it.

Since Eddie went to school in Natchez from the seventh grade on and spent many of his summers with his grandfather, the time he spent with his father was limited. Yet some of the events that played the largest part in shaping Eddie's life did not occur in the luxury of his grandfather's home but with his father in Wildsville.

Sharecropping could in many ways be a demeaning existence. The land was not your own. Goods were purchased through a commissary owned by the landowner, who had control over a man's total livelihood. Despite these conditions, Alex approached sharecropping with as much dignity and hard work as he brought to all his activities. His determination not to be taken advantage of despite his color and his impoverished circumstances made a lasting impression on Eddie.

> We were in Louisiana and Dad was a sharecropper at the time. Being young, just six or seven years old, I knew nothing of taking an active role in working hard but just went about with my father.
>
> We went to the commissary instead of the store to get what we wanted. Things were not packaged in those days. If you wanted five pounds of sugar you had to dig down and scoop it out. You would weigh it on a scale and put it in a brown bag. Same thing with lard and coffee. You got coffee green and you had to parch the coffee at home and then grind it.
>
> Most of the blacks had no education so when they would go to the commissary at the end of the year, they couldn't count so therefore they were always in debt. They just accepted it.
>
> For the most part, the boss on the properties would simply tell the blacks to come in and he'd say, "Hey, you did all right this time. Lookie here. You got your hat off? You made such and such number of bales of cotton this year and you been to the commissary. We look over your books here. By God, you almost paid off everything from the commissary, but

you got a whole lot left here. But give me your hat and hold it there."

And he would just take silver and throw it down until he filled the hat up with nickels and dimes and quarters, until it would flow over.

I was a little kid when my father went up there to settle one time, but I'll never forget. This guy's name was Joe Baker, and when my father went in there to settle, Mr. Baker began to do him that way and Dad said: "No, no, no. I got my books and you should have your books. So you're going to settle with me by me taking my books here and you taking your books there and seeing if we're together on this."

"No, Alex, we're not going to do it that way."

"I'll be back up here within the next hour and I want my settlement and you're going to give me my settlement."

I went back home with my father raising hell, cussing about Mr. Baker and the treatment and all this type of thing. He talked of what can happen and how people would do you when you're ignorant, not educated, and a Negro; and how whites take advantage of you. "This is why I want you to be educated," he said, "because you got to come out of this type thing and get into something else."

In those days there was no law. You made your own damn law. There was no sheriff or nobody else in the town. So the guy who packed the biggest pistol or biggest gun commanded the most respect and got what he wanted. My Dad always had his .38 handgun on his hip and he got a rifle that he had and took that in his hand and went back up to that store. All our black neighbors knew what was happening and were hiding under their houses for fear there was going to be big trouble. This was a very vivid thing and I'll never forget it.

The boss man said, "Look Alex, ain't no need of all that. We can go ahead and settle this thing without all that. You ain't got to worry about all them guns."

Dad said, "Well, I'll tell you, I'm going to deal with you in an honest way and I got my guns and I can use

> them. And you got yours and you can use yours. Now you may get me, but I'm going to get one of you too. So let's settle."
>
> And they sat there and settled.

Alex was not the kind of man who came to his children like a modern-day father giving them advice about how to lead their lives. He influenced them through the example of his life. And the lessons had to be repeated over and over if Alex were to maintain his dignity, for the whites were always there to challenge him or any other blacks who wished to get ahead. An incident with a fisherman made a deep impression on Eddie:

> At the base of Wildsville there are four rivers that come in together: Red River, Black River, Little River and Choctaw River. All these tributaries come together and then head into the Mississippi River. Where they converge is a center for fish, especially catfish.
>
> There is more than one kind of catfish. There are three kinds. One is called the black cat, then the blue cat and the white cat. They are all regarded as scavengers, but the black cat appears to go deeper down into the mud in the river, so he is blacker and the meat is a little tougher.
>
> My father sent me down to get fish. Well, in those days you got great big fish, two for a quarter. The fishermen lived on the boats on the side of the river. All they had to do was trap them in a net and put them in a box, sort of like a crate, and they could keep there in the water forever.
>
> Anyway, my father told me to be sure not to bring a black cat back—to bring either a blue or a white cat. Well, I told the man that and he paid me no mind except to call me names. He said: "Here Nigger, I give you what I want you to have." And I went back and told my father exactly what he said.
>
> My father got on his horse, said, "Swing in back of me," and put his rifle on one side and had his .38 on the other side. Dad was cussing and raising hell all the way down to the river. When we got there he got down

> and he told that man off. When he got through raking him over, that man gave him two white cats and we came home.

Many of Eddie's memories of Wildsville revolve around Mama Caroline. She was the mother of nine children, of which Addie Mazique, Eddie's mother, was third. She had married Douglas Wilkerson, for whom Eddie's brother Douglas was named. Eddie could remember just the way she was:

> She was an Indian woman and she was markedly pigeon-toed. But she was very fast afoot and always her voice was one of a song. It had a ring or a lyric to it when she would talk and it would carry a long ways. It was commanding, yet very respectful.

Mama Caroline represented the center and strength of the Wilkerson family as Grandpa Alex did of the Mazique family. She also represented the discipline of the family. When the children visited Mama Caroline's house they had to mind their p's and q's because Mama Caroline was the ruler of the roost. The children all knew that Mama Caroline had thrown a hatchet at her one son, Jim, and had never even paused in the tune she was humming at the time. No matter how old you were or how big you were, you were not immune from Mama Caroline's stick if you crossed her and nobody, not even Papa Doug, seemed to cross Mama Caroline.

Mama Caroline's house was known as a place to have a good time, especially during Prohibition. It was a place where one could acquire and consume spirits. Of course, you had to be of a certain class of people. Mama Caroline only let high-class white folks come to her house and drink. Fishermen were not respected by the family. They were considered poor white trash or rednecks and were not welcome.

Two of the frequent patrons of Mama Caroline's house were Mr. Statom, the plantation overseer, and Mr. Wilds, who was the manager of a nearby plantation. Apparently Mr. Statom and Mr. Wilds were not always popular among the other clientele since they were the managers or bosses and when the boss was around the "colored" folks didn't have quite as much fun. Eddie's remembrance of what took place at Mama Caroline's tells a lot about life in the South during the early 1900s and the inequities that blacks faced.

> Mr. Statom and Mr. Wilds would come in and by God they would stay pretty much all the day. They'd tell their wives goodbye. Mr. Wilds lived in a place called Cottonwood. He would leave that plantation in the morning and come on over and the first I'd know he'd be there until 5 or until evening time.
>
> Mama Caroline would say: "Come on back here, Mr. Wilds, get yourself some breakfast." She'd sit him there at the table, feed him and then he'd have a drink.
>
> Sister Amy was my mother's baby sister. She had hair growing down to her knees. A beautiful lady! Sister Amy had a room in that house—it was a big house—on the wing. When Mr. Wilds was there, he would go with her and the door would close. There was nothing said, nothing done but all I know was this would happen. It was not until I grew old enough to know about sexuality or any type of intimate experience to even realize what was happening. But this was going on in my grandmother's and my grandfather's house! Nothing was said about it, but it was done.
>
> There was a rivalry that came between the two white men—Richard Wilds and Statom. Statom hit town from Kankakee, Illinois. He was a northerner and Wilds was a southern rebel. And I could hear him round there talking "That damn Yankee done come up in here. Hell, I don't want to see him around this house." Statom had also fallen in love with my aunt, Sister Amy.

Although this situation didn't quite sit right with young Eddie, he could see it was accepted by the Wilkersons and it was something he too would have to learn to accept. It was his own experiences with Mr. Wilds and the double standard of it all that really hurt.

> I never shall forget it. I was coming from Natchez where I was going to school and on my way home to Wildsville. It was autumn, somewhere around November, and it was cold. Down there it don't get really too cold, but cold enough, and I didn't have an overcoat.

> I saw Mr. Wilds on the boat from Natchez to Vidalia. That was before the bridge. We were crossing on the boat, the Ollie K. Wilds, named for a member of his family. I had no way to get to Wildsville. I didn't have any money but I usually hitchhiked. So when I saw him I thought, "I know I'll get home now." So I walked up to him when I was getting off the boat. "Hi there, son." "Hi, Mr. Wilds. I sure wish I could ride home with you." He said "Hop on." He didn't say hop in, he said hop on. He had this Ford coupe. I hopped on and I stayed on. I couldn't sit by him; I had to stand up on that running board for that whole ride, which was 40 miles.
>
> He could have waited until he got out of Vidalia to stop the car and say, "Come on in and sit by me"—it was for two people. But even in that cold weather, he didn't. And I rode on that running board, knowing that he was going into my grandmother's home to drink, eat, and screw my aunt. Man, that just tore me up inside. I thought about it all night. And yet I said to myself, "What you gonna do about it?"

Many of Eddie's experiences in Wildsville made him question the way things were done in the South. While his father presented him an example of what it was like to be a strong-willed, independent man, his mother taught him not to challenge the system.

> I don't know what it was but somehow we were never taught to rebel against the system. I remember my mother always used to say, "You're not supposed to go to jail. Stay out of jail." I couldn't understand then. As I began to grow older, I understood what she meant. She wanted to tell me you can't win it. If anything happens how you gonna win? The best way to do it is not to go. How you gonna win when there is no law, no order. Never no blacks to practice law and no bail. The jury will all be a picked white jury. No black could ever sit on the jury then. So you were not taught to fight the system, but you were taught how to live within the system. I wasn't taught how to fight against

> the system until I left Mississippi and went to Georgia. That's when it started.

This was a common admonition for young blacks in the South. In his autobiography, Benjamin E. Mays, who served as president of Morehouse College from 1940 to 1968, tells about similar warnings from his parents when he was growing up in the South in the 1880s. There was a legitimate fear among blacks that they could not win in a dispute with whites.[10]

It was as if Eddie's father and the other strong, proud black men and women always walked a tightrope. They could not realistically challenge the system yet they could not allow themselves to be beaten by it. They fought for their dignity within very narrow limits. Eddie called it being "circumscribed." Alex stood up for himself and his family but in such a way that it was easier to let him get away with it than to challenge him. There were no sit-ins, or law breaking, or demands for equality. Eddie's father tried to show him how to be a man within an unjust system.

> They never taught me disturbances or uprisings as was done in the sixties. It was not considered wonderful to go to jail for a cause. We were living in a place with segregation and discrimination. They were teaching us how to exist but yet to be courageous and to keep walking and standing tall. You had to be tall even though you were circumscribed.
>
> I didn't get any tinge of joining groups for causes until I got to Morehouse. The only things that my father talked about in that area were individuals who were colored who had distinguished themselves.
>
> One man I remember him talking about was Roscoe Conklin Simmons who was a great orator. He would go around to different towns and speak on different issues regarding freedom and independence and the constitution. He was well educated and never was a slave. He and Fredrick Douglass were individualists.
>
> They did it alone, not through groups. Individual achievements rather than mass movements. It was not until I got out of Mississippi and went to Morehouse that I began to feel the impact of putting all this together. My colleagues and teachers at Morehouse would tell

> me about the percentage of money spent on the education of blacks and whites in Mississippi and how blacks were last on the totem pole.

Although his mother taught Eddie acceptance, this experience and similar ones in his young life could not help but raise questions of justice and fairness in the way blacks were treated. No experience made the young boy question the way things were done more than his observations of his Uncle Bud Wilkerson's family.

> Uncle Bud lived on this farm. His wife was named Aunt Hannah. They had the most beautiful daughters you ever saw. Every time one of their pretty daughters were plucking age—sixteen or seventeen—like my sister was, a white man would tap her and she would leave home and go across the railroad tracks and shack up. There he would keep her. He'd be married to the white woman but would spend all his day with this pretty little brown-skinned gal in Ferriday, Louisiana. White man would tap them and say, "Come on babe, I'm gonna put you up in a house," and he put her up in a house and next thing you know there would be a child.
>
> This particularly happened to Nettie, the oldest one that I remember so well. Nettie was beautiful and was taken away when she was just a teenager. I was just a little boy, but I remember this. She had a son by this white man.
>
> In other words they were snatched, early. The white man went right on through from Nettie to the next girl and to the next girl. There were three of them taken this way that I knew. Every time I look up one of his children gone! And by God, they robbed my Uncle Bud of almost all his children!
>
> I was ruffled by that. I was concerned about it. I'd say, "You know that don't sound right to me." There they were, in the blossoms of their life. Hell, they had no choice. What they gonna do? Those girls ain't gonna be picking cotton all their damn lives for nothing or washing dishes in no man's kitchen. How are you gonna live? You can't go to school. If you're lucky you

> get through the eighth grade. Beyond that there ain't no schools for you.
>
> They had in those days around there what they called the Julius Rosenwald schools.[11] But beyond the eighth grade there was nothing else. Not even a high school. In Louisiana, to finish high school you had to go to Mississippi. So while I did go to Louisiana elementary schools for several years, to get through high school, I had to go to Natchez.
>
> Here the white man can take them and say: "Babe I'm gonna put you up." It ain't gonna cost nothing to him but twenty dollars a month for everything he wants—beat her and screw her and have babies. And that's what they did. That's what happened in Ferriday.
>
> There were unspoken social rules: what was legal, what was right, what was moral, what was ethical. And once it was accepted no one thought anything about it. In order to make it, you had to accept it. In spite of this type of divisiveness, people managed to survive.

Ferriday was the kind of place for this type of behavior—a no-man's-land between Vidalia and Wildsville where gambling and cavorting were acceptable pastimes. Yet the double families of the white southern males were not limited to one town. Many of the stories of the freeing of slaves, as with William Johnson, took place because their white masters were also their fathers or husbands. This relationship did not end with the abolition of slavery. Maude Mazique remembers a Mr. Burns when she was growing up in Natchez. He owned Burns Shoe Store. Up on the corner of Pine Street he kept Mrs. Stampley. She was his "black woman," although she was as light as anyone—almost white. He had two children by her. He'd come there and take care of this "colored" family and then he would go home and take care of his white family. That was just the way things were.

Even closer to home was James Boyd, who was Eddie's cousin and Alice's father. He was the son of Judge Samuel S. Boyd and one of his slaves. The old judge was so fond of James's mother that his wife forced him to send her away to a property he owned up near Vicksburg. Although not treated as an equal to his half-sisters, James was given a favored position in the home. The complicated accommodations made to fit these black/white relationships stagger the imagination. The Boyds all sat in the dining room for meals. The servants had to wait on James too, but he didn't sit at the main table. Instead, he was at another little table near it. James Boyd lived with the family, after the judge died, until he was twenty-two years old. His half-sister, Catherine Boyd Suzette, was so fond of him that she eventually hired him to manage her husband's estate at Suzette Ashley, a job he held when he met and married Mary Mazique. James Boyd held himself so aloof from everyone that even his wife, Mary, called him Mr. Boyd.

In the early 1920s, Alex Jr. again moved his family. This time he tried Wisner, Louisiana, where the soil was better suited for farming. Eddie was just beginning his teenage years, approaching the time that he should be doing strenuous farm labor. However, his few years in Wisner taught him once and for all that he was not cut out for the rigors of farm life. Eddie's memories of it are vivid and mostly oppressive.

> My Dad decided to go to Wisner to farm because the land was more fertile. There was no town. There was nothing but country—just sparse houses here and there. I was about twelve or thirteen years old.
>
> My father had as many as seven men plowing for him on a big farm. He must have tended seventy or one hundred acres of land. He would be responsible for paying them. But in those days the wage for a plowboy to work from sunup to sundown was only one dollar per day. He had twenty-one women hoeing who were paid only fifty cents a day. All these plow hands would sing about "Sundown Let Tomorrow Come" and all those things. "If I feel tomorrow like I feel today, I'm going to pack my suitcase and get away." Songs of sorrow and meaning.
>
> It was in this setting that I really learned that I was not made for the farm. I didn't want no part of it. I learned I hated it. It was nothing but hot weather. The sun! Because of the intensification of the heat and the condensation, configurations were created that you could look and see. It would get so hot you would see these little things dancing up and down in the air and we would call them "haints."
>
> In coming up, the boys in my family were much more rugged, stalwart, muscular, and much bigger than

I was. For some reason my real growth and development didn't take place until a few years later when I left Mississippi and went to Morehouse. They were stronger, more vibrant, and more outgoing. My older brother, Alex, and Douglas next to him, oh man they were terrific. And then I came along. I was not a total weakling but one that could not compete as far as the physical type of thing was concerned, although I attempted to do it. Yet I think my father expected me to compete in some way. So he threw the work at me. They would go out in the morning and hitch the mules up and go plow the cotton and the corn and all that stuff. He probably felt that I wasn't able physically or capable to do that kind of work so he relegated me to the water boy.

I had quite a time as water boy! I remember that very well. We had to pump the water, fill the buckets and take them out into the fields and walk all this way. On your way it was nothing to run across a water moccasin or some other snake. We would use the gallon molasses cans which they would put the syrup in and there was a top that you push down on them and that made a gallon pail. You would pump the water out of the well into one and then another. You had to find a place to bury it because there was no refrigeration.

I was relegated to these kinds of chores as well as the chore of taking breakfast buckets to them in the morning. When they left for the fields in the morning the sun was not up and there was no breakfast that early in the morning, like five o'clock. So I would take breakfast and then water to them around ten o'clock and then around twelve the bell would ring for them to come in for dinner.

I would go through the same thing again in the afternoon around four o'clock. And the hands would be hollering and screaming, "Water boy!" All you did was carry these two gallon buckets of water, one in each hand, and a simple gourd or a dipper that was made out of aluminum or tin.

Cotton picking time would come and you would go through all this and your back would ache. I did so

> well performing that task; no one knew that I didn't like it except me. But when I bent over and would hear a whistle blow on the train, I was wondering when I could catch a train and get the hell out of there. It was a deplorable place and I got out of there as quick as I could.
>
> The landlord was Mr. Pennybaker. I would look at this fellow coming around from day to day riding on a horse: the white man. And I would look at my Dad sweating, with a hoe in his hand and with an ankylosed right leg. Mr. Pennybaker would come on his horse every morning and drop by and say, "Hi there, Alex, how are things going?" My father would stop and they would talk awhile. He would never get down off his horse. First thing I know he would jog along and go somewhere else just looking over the land to see how it was going. This is what happened. I saw all that and then I would ask myself as a boy, "Why?" You know I couldn't understand that. I never saw anybody else ride that horse looking over fields but the landlord.

The bleakness and drudgery of this life were enough to convince Eddie that he would never be able to do this work for his living. One of the most painful experiences of Eddie's young life also managed to convince his father.

> There came a time when my father decided that OK, I guess it's time that Eddie should get out there and start plowing. I was being moved into the next advanced stage, which means I got to drive a mule. I will never forget the first mule that he gave me was one I couldn't do anything with. He was slow, would take a step at a time when he wanted to. I was anxious to do a good job. My brother would teach me all the time. I wanted to please my father. The mule's name was Trim, and I would say all the time "Get up Trim. If you don't get up for me and start walking I'm going to tell my Papa on you." My brothers would tease me all the time about that. Anyway, I did pretty well with that. And that was with a cultivator. I had not been given a plow yet.

From the cultivator you moved to a plow and from that you were gone.

Getting me ready for the plowing, Father finally decided he could give me a faster mule. So he gave me this other mule, Ollie, who was a very fine animal. So I got out that day and I started cultivating and she went right along. I was doing very well until about five o'clock in the afternoon. The cultivator has sort of concave teeth. It sinks its teeth down into the ground about one to two inches deep and as it goes along it loosens the soil. But in going along it can very easily strike an object like a rock or a root of a tree and can disturb you when you are holding it. It so happened this day, it struck a root and one of the teeth got caught in it. The impact of it caused it to jerk back and it turned the cultivator over so that the teeth were exposed. At the same time the hands of the cultivator struck me in my groin. And I don't know when I have had such pain in my life. Man, it was really painful! It threw me down in the row and I just simply could hardly stand it. The impact was such that it pulled the mule back and one of the leaders in the hind leg, the Achilles tendon, was cut in two by the tooth of the cultivator.

Well I tell you, I don't know anything I was more disturbed about than that accident because I had to face my father. Not with the fact that I was injured, that was secondary. What bothered me was the fact that the mule was cut. What could I do about that? How could I face him with this kind of a problem? Well, I was done for the day—five o'clock, which is unusual. I started home with the mule limping and bleeding and me in tears.

My father hadn't come in but my mother was there getting dinner ready. I told her what had happened and she was concerned, number one about me first. I guess that's the way a mother would be. And I showed her the bruise that I had sustained in my groin and she began to patch it up and put something cold on it. I kept in tears for quite a while because I was really frightful of what my Dad would do and how to face him. I told

> Mother that. She told me: "Well that's all right, you just have to face him and tell him exactly what happened." When he came in, I just went to him and faced him in tears and told him exactly what happened. I had expected him to really tear into me; I knew that was the end of it. But it wasn't. He looked at me. He stood me up and turned me around and then he looked at me again and he said: "I have my doubts about you ever being cut out for the farm. Look at you, you just won't grow. Look at your bothers, how strong they are, how big they are, and look at you."

Even though doubts about being cut out for farm life had long ago formed in Eddie's mind, this experience served the purpose of convincing his father that he was never going to make him into a farmer. Instead of displeasing Alex, it was instrumental in developing a certain comradeship between the would-be lawyer and his son. Realizing Eddie would not succeed on the farm, Alex took more of an interest in his intellectual progress.

> After that my father had a warmer concept of me and my capabilities. My father and I were close despite his firmness. He never put his arm around me and rocked me on his knee but at the same time we talked a hell of a lot. He encouraged me to get an education. He was aware of his father telling me to go to law school and he let me know I should pursue it. He had several sayings that let me know that he wanted me educated. One was: "Don't be hidden by the bushes in the cotton field. Sometimes they grow so tall you can't look over them to see the lilies of the field nor the watermelons on the ground in the watermelon patch." He meant if you stay in the cotton field all your life, you are not going to be able to see what is happening on the other side. Get the hell out of there. Another was "When the wall of discrimination becomes so tall that you can't climb over it, then you must devise a way to go under it or around it."
>
> If he wanted something done that was more academic he would call me to do it. Like to print a sign that said "No Hunting" or "No Trespassing" or a sign to be

> hung on the property that said "Posted." When the time would come for newspapers on the weekends, he would call me to gather the newspapers and he would encourage me to read them. He also began to spend a lot of time with me talking about affairs of the world that would appear in the paper and then we would discuss them. When I became relegated to the state of partial academia I was very pleased about the whole thing.

In 1924, when the farming in Wisner was bad, Alex took up logging to supplement the family's income. Eddie sometimes went with his dad on these trips.

> My father went into logging, cutting down trees and putting them on a log wagon and taking them to the mill to sell. He was not cutting them from his own property. If anyone had timber to sell, you would go out there and cut that timber down. I don't know what kind of financial deal he made.
>
> In those days you had nothing to work with but sweat, blood, and a cross saw. A log wagon had wheels but the diameters of the wheels were smaller than that of a car. There were eight wheels on the front and then the bottom of the wagon had four wheels in the back. The logs would go on it and be chained. They would be driven by mules. The fellow who was driving it would be called a skinner.
>
> I would go out and stay with him sometimes when he was logging. They would pitch tents and live in the tents. The tents would be by marshes and we had to fight water moccasins and, even worse, mosquitoes. My father had a cot he slept on with a mosquito net. I would see him get up at four o'clock in the morning.
>
> Gag Scales would sit up there with the mules and drive them and pull them up out of the bogs. The secret was getting them to pull in unison. Gag could get them to do that. That whip popped loudly and you would see the hair fly from one of the mules.
>
> I contracted malaria but it didn't bother me too much because Mama always gave us quinine anyway

> during the spring of each year. Two things you had to have: quinine and cream of tartar. My father always made me take a dose of "black draw" every Saturday night. It was a laxative with all those greens I was eating, but he insisted that was one way to stay healthy.
>
> That summer I spent with him I learned a lot about the courage of my father and his determination and what he was doing to make it economically. I didn't do a thing to help him except take care of the mules and his horse. I helped Margaret, the cook, bring in the wood and start the fire.

The bond between Eddie and his father grew as Eddie matured, and Alex chose to have him participate in some of the more private parts of his life.

> When I got older and learned to drive an automobile, he would choose to have me drive him where he wanted to go even though I would spend the whole day. My father sat in the back because, having a stiff leg, he could do better sitting in the back, crosswise.
>
> There was a time when my Dad liked to booze a little bit, especially on weekends. You think about a fellow who's gonna spend all that time with roadblocks and all that hot summer heat and all the inequities out there. What you got to look forward to anymore? I think you need a drink, you know, to stick with it or you need something. So, it didn't bother me. I justified it on the basis that if you got to live this kind of life, you can get some kind of temporary relief, some type of euphoria, from a bit of alcohol consumption... you can't afford much of it anyhow... you enjoy every damn bit of it. It was always concealed. He never told me not to go back home and tell Mama this, but he expected me to be able to hold secrets. I would never talk of his activities or where he had been and what he had been doing.
>
> The matter of play and extra activities were almost out of the question because they didn't have anything to do. What could you do as a man, working that way five and one-half days a week (half-days on Saturday) and

then go into town once a week on Saturday and then come back Saturday night. You're supposed to get drunk to live with it. There was nothing else to do. I know of no planned activities except on Sunday, you go to church; nothing else. So when you really objectively look at it like that, I wonder how I could have made it as an adult.

I would drive him from Wildsville to Ferriday. I remember he had a friend in Ferriday, named Alex Hanks. He never worked in the fields but he was a hustler. He was pretty much of a gambler and stayed around town and would smoke his big cigar and drink good whiskey. He didn't have to drink no white lightning. He always wore a tie and a vest and had a watch and chain that fitted on his vest. He was a big, tall, brown-skinned fellow. He was quite a character. The two of them would get together and they were really good buddies. They were in this little place where they would have a few drinks and play cards for a little while. The little money they had...hell, they couldn't have had over five dollars to lose anyhow. I think in retrospect that Alex Hanks waited for him to come to town with that five or six dollars that he had, which in those days was worth like fifty dollars, in order to do him in.

So my father would come in to see Alex Hanks and I would drive there and wait. Sit in the car. "OK Boy, you just wait here" and I'd sit and wait. He'd go in and Alex would receive him and the first thing I knew I would peep through the keyhole and they'd be holding the cards, playing poker. Then I'd notice on the side there was this jug. He and Alex Hanks and two or three more round this table.

I'd set out there. Sometimes, I'd be too scared to leave to go to pee. I stood right there and waited in that car for two, three, four, five, six hours 'cause my father was in there. I saw the gambling, but I never saw a relationship with another woman. But at least he knew one thing when I got back home; my lips were sealed. I would never say anything to Mama. I would always find a way to evade any issue that was directly involved with my father's concerns. I just walked away from it. I never

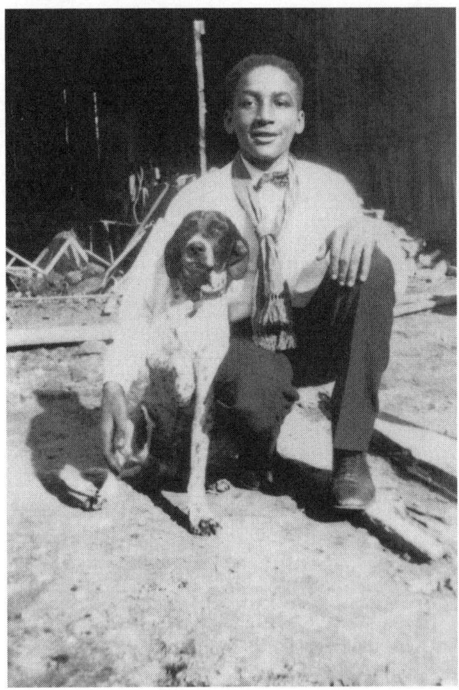

**Fig. 7:** Eddie with his dog at China Grove. Photo courtesy of Maude Mazique and Dolores Pelham.

> did tell her, but I knew what my Dad was doing and I knew then that he couldn't afford it. Five or six dollars, that was a lot then. But, how are you going to live if you don't do it? What else you gonna do?

In 1923 Grandpa Alex died at the age of eighty-two. The boll weevil and the depleted soil had finally caught up with Grandpa Alex's finances too. Even though he still owned Oakland, White Apple Village, and parts of Kilmarnock plantation, there was not enough money after the sale of goods and property to pay the bills he still owed. With over eight hundred acres, he had become land poor. Eddie's uncles, Dr. James Mazique and Robert Mazique, went together to buy Oakland and managed to preserve it for the Mazique family for several more generations before it was to return to white hands.

Getting out of working on the farm was one of Eddie's specialties. He was smart and a family favorite and they chose to let him elude most of the arduous tasks. It wasn't that he didn't want to work. Actually, he was very industrious. He just did not want to do that farm work! After Grandpa Alex died, he tackled all kinds of jobs to make up for the work he avoided doing on the farm.

Although options were limited for black youths, he always found some way in which he could make money, like selling "pop" on the excursion boat or train from Natchez to New Orleans.

> I did most of my hard work in Wisner. I got enough of those cotton rows to know that it was not my field and I did what I could to stay away from it. You might call me a modern-day house boy. I had the means of getting away and I used them.
>
> I used to go on excursions from Natchez to New Orleans and I would handle the confectionery stuff, selling goods. I would sell cold drinks. In the bucket with the pop there would always be bootleg whiskey with a corncob as a cork. We had a bucket of ice with strawberry pop, Coca Cola, raspberry, and whatever else you sell for a nickel and dime. And the brothers knew what was happening. They would reach down and get them a Coca Cola and get a whiskey and give you seventy-five cents and you just keep on moving.

In 1926 Alex again moved his family to Wildsville in time for them to experience the high waters of 1927. Wildsville sat on a low, flat stretch of land. When the rivers rose, the high waters would flood Wildsville, while Natchez, sitting on its high bluff, would remain dry. Although Eddie was spending most of his time in Natchez attending school, he still managed to be in Wildsville for the flood. If his resolve to get out of the farming life needed any strengthening, the flood took care of that.

> This was the first time I was in a flood. In order to survive, the animals would run up on the levees. I saw the levees break and come in.
>
> The houses in Louisiana in those days were always built on a lift. The lift was brick or logs that held the houses up about four feet off the ground knowing that water would come. We had to move up from the first story to the second story and finally to the attic. We would find the water twenty-five or thirty feet deep and we had to stay up there in the attic and live. And it was

> nothing in the morning when you woke up to find a huge water moccasin up on the rafters, flicking his tongue out and looking down on you. One sucker was about six feet long. Really that big! I saw my Daddy take a shotgun and shoot him and he tumbled right down in the water. That was a rough way to live. I decided again that I didn't want that kind of life.

After the 1927 flood, the city life of Natchez seemed even more appealing. It was not a large city, but in relation to Wisner and Wildsville, it looked immense. And compared to the life offered by the farm, it looked like a utopia to the young Eddie.

Since Louisiana did not offer a high school education for blacks, Alex Jr. maintained a home in Natchez on North Pine Street specifically so that his children would have a place to stay while they were going to school. Over the summer and other vacations most of the children would return to the farm to work with their father and mother. Maude had wanted to go to Rock Castle to become a nun but, as the eldest, she was needed in Natchez all year round to take care of the house and the children who were living in it. From the time she was thirteen, this was her full-time responsibility.

Natchez in the early 1900s was not the bustling town of pre–Civil War days. The southern economy had not recovered from the withdrawal of the cheap labor force provided by slaves and the destruction and disruptions caused by the war. The decreasing importance of the river as a mode of transportation for people and goods, coupled with the setback in the economy, turned Natchez into the proverbial slow-moving southern town. Cows, pigs, and chickens could be seen in the dooryards. And up the street from the Maziques' Pine Street home were several acres of empty land owned by the Catholic Church. After the morning milking, the Maziques and their neighbors could be seen leading their cows up the street to munch on the hallowed grass.

As long as the blacks knew their place, there was little racial friction. If a black man saw a white woman coming, he would have to get off the street and not look at her. There were just some things they couldn't do and there was no pretending otherwise.[12] As Eddie remembered:

> We were never taught about slavery as such or the Civil War. We were taught not to be belligerent because it would end only in one thing, death.

> I would pass by and see the old antebellum estates. No teachers ever took us on a tour or said let's talk about the significance of it. Those were things that were off limits. You were supposed to accept. To challenge means you are going to end up in a struggle. We were taught not to be combative or hostile.
>
> Natchez was a funny kind of town, a paradoxical place, blacks and whites together.

Provided their position was understood and they kept mostly to themselves and avoided Main Street, which was off limits to blacks, there was fairly peaceable coexistence. The housing was not segregated into black and white neighborhoods as in the North, but blacks did not mingle with the whites under normal circumstances.[13] Pine Street was such an integrated neighborhood. The Maziques had white people living on each side of their home. A wrestler, Jack Humberto, was on one side. He would give them tickets to come to his wrestling matches and he would always talk with them when they met on the street. They would never visit each other's homes—that would be considered improper.

Of course this protocol did not prevent a white man from having a black mistress and family, and at times integrating them into his white family. Mrs. Brannon, the cleaning lady at the Natchez post office, who lived across the street from the Maziques,[14] had a mother who was raised with a white family. Her grandfather was a white man who, when he married, kept his daughter by a black woman with him and had her raised right along with his other children. Her white kin came up to visit her when she was ill, but they could not stay with her. They had to go on to the Natchez Hotel.[15]

The whites had their special section of businesses and stores on Main Street. The blacks had Franklin Street, the Bourbon Street of Natchez. Here they gathered and here local musical talent flourished. The bands would wander from the area to serenade local black families in the wee hours of the morning. Bud Scott and his orchestra would play beneath a window and all the neighbors would come out to hear his melodious voice and the children to see how his big belly bounced as he sang. Bud played for the white folks for all their events and became quite the popular figure in town. The blacks had their own hotel, the Blue Goose, owned by Eddie's cousin Wilbur Boyd, and their own theater, the Hamilton. There were several stores owned by blacks like Montgomery Market and Mann Davis Butcher Shop, but they were free to patronize the national stores like Woolworth and Kresge and they were generally treated with courtesy while they spent their money, although, of course, they were not allowed to try on clothes or hats or anything else that might someday be purchased by white patrons.

Every now and then there would be a mean white man who would demand, "Nigger! Get off the sidewalk!" to let him pass, but this was not a common occurrence. There were no organizations to fight discrimination. Black people just accommodated themselves as best they could to their situation and the years passed quietly. The black residents considered themselves lucky because, in general, there was a high class of white folks in Natchez. They knew it wasn't the worst place in the world, even though it was certainly bad enough.[16]

One of Eddie's schemes to get away from the farm life was to work for a cleaners in Natchez. Picking up and delivering laundry was one of the few jobs available to black youths in the southern states in the early 1900s.[17] Despite the fact that the task was defined as menial by whites, Eddie learned lessons of courage and dignity from his encounters with the white people the cleaners serviced. Eddie's boss encouraged him to stand his ground as his father's example had taught him earlier. Once he was "adopted" by his white boss, he found her to be an ally who believed in his right to challenge *some* of the mores of southern life. Eddie was willing to contribute to the family's income by working in Natchez and in this way made up for his lack of work on the farm.

> Another way I got away from farming was the Day's Cleaners job. In 1927, I was sixteen years old. I decided to get a job in Natchez while Pa was waiting for the water to go down. I would work Monday morning through Saturday noon driving and soliciting clothes for the cleaners. I never shall forget I was making $7.50 a week of which I gave my father $5 for permission to get away from the damn farm so I could stay in Natchez. Then he was living in Wildsville. Every week when he would come to town, he got that $5.00 and I kept $2.50. And with that $2.50 I survived and ate at Professor Lang's up the railroad tracks.
>
> I was soliciting clothes and driving this truck. I would go and pick up clothes and then take 'em back. There was a fellow in the car with me who was an elderly man who would sit there to tell me where to go

when I was driving. He was one armed. We called him "Tip." Tip Frazier loved what he was doing and took great pride in it. But then he was brought up in a different school than I was.

On this particular occasion, I went to the front door of this home and the lady in the house, an Italian woman named Mrs. Passavanti, told me that I should come to the back to get clothes.

When I mentioned to Tip about going to the back door, he said: "Well, you just go to the back." And I told him, "I had never been to nobody's back door to get clothes. I was going to take it up with the boss." The boss's name was Mrs. Day but down south, we don't call people by their last name. We call them by their first name. So it was Miss Sadie. I said, "Miss Sadie, I want to see you." She said, "Come on, Eddie." Once the white folks decided they liked you, they sort of adopted you. They had a feeling that as long as you were working for them and as long as you do what they called "right," then you belong to me and nobody else is going to bother you. So I went and told her. She said, "Look, you're right. Don't you dare be caught going to anybody's back door."

The next time around I went to get the clothes. I had them in my arms getting ready to go out and she came in there and Mrs. Passavanti says to me, "Boy, I thought I told you not to come to the front door. You're supposed to come to the back door to get the clothes." I told her I was not going to the back door and rather than to do that we just didn't want her business and with that I simply dropped the clothes right down on the floor and turned to walk out. At that point she screamed and she walked upstairs angrily and she screamed again. "Boy, I'm going to call my husband and I'm going to have you lynched." Well, that was the first time I really heard the word, *lynch*.

When I walked out to the car, Tip asked me what had happened. And I related it to him. He told me I should never have done that. I said, "Well, let's go on." And he said, "No, let's go back to the shop; I'm going to report you."

The minute I walked into the shop, Miss Sadie says to me: "You don't have to tell me what happened. That woman has already called up here and told me what happened. Eddie, you did exactly right. Now her husband wants to see you and I want you to go up there and see him. You are growing up now and it is time for you to learn." I don't mind telling you, I walked reluctantly up that street.

He was a tailor and he had a shop right on the corner of Franklin and Rankin Street in Natchez. I walked there and when I walked in, there was someone in the front who was like a secretary and she said he was in the back waiting for me. So I reluctantly walked into the back. And there he was.

His name was Sam Passavanti. He was small of stature and had a heavy Italian accent. He had a tape around his neck, you know, like tailors do, and scissors in his hand. He said to me, "Eddie my wife she just called and she told me what it was all about. Now I'm gonna tella you something. There is such a thing as these kind of racial problems that you going to be having. You just beginning to grow up now and this is the beginning of what you gonna see and you gonna have to be careful because if you don't be careful you gonna get in mucha trouble. But I know you. I know of your family and I know Alex. He's a good man and you a good family, so I'ma not gonna do anything to you. I'm only gonna tella you that as long as you stay around here you are gonna have to be a good fellow and listen to what the white man say and do what he say. Otherwise you get into mucha trouble. You can go back, but I say to you from now on, when you get ready to go to my house to pick the clothes up, you sit in the truck and you let Tip go get the clothes." I said, "That's fine."

And that was how their laundry route continued with Tip Frazier, the old-generation southern black, giving in to convention and Eddie questioning and testing the boundaries of acceptability, discovering what he could get away with and changing things where he could.

At times the Pine Street house was crowded when a lot of the children were in Natchez for school. After Maude, Edna and then Sadie were the next oldest children. They along with Maude finished Natchez College and then went on to study teaching and business in college. All the sisters continued to live in the Pine Street home when they began their teaching careers. Alex was the oldest son in the family. He was a fun-loving guy who hated the farm life as much as Eddie. When his father found he was playing hooky from Natchez College, he sent Alex to Tuskegee to study. Once he decided on the trade of brick mason, he became a perfectionist at his craft. Alex built many of the houses around Tuskegee and came to share with his father the belief that if you worked for him, you had better do it right. Douglas was the next in line and was always known as the most patient one in the family. Only a year older than Eddie, they went through Natchez College in the same grades. Walter, or "Jack," came after Eddie. He and Eddie were always together. Addie Birdie was next, but only lived to be a few years old. And then came the youngest, Theodore.

Sometimes Eddie's mother, Addie, would be there to help Maude with the house and the children. Addie was a perfect housekeeper and homemaker. She had to be to keep track of her children and keep a house going in Louisiana and in Natchez at the same time. Addie was strict, but mild in comparison to Alex. When Alex was not around, the young boys would get with their friends and "cut up." The house was a two-story house with a kind of apartment to it and the children would go upstairs and "raise sand" as they called their mischief.

When Alex was in town, he remained the same strong personality and the lessons that Eddie learned in Wildsville and Wisner were reinforced.

> Although blacks were not expected to challenge the system, within limits my father would let you know what he thought was right and what was wrong. He taught that you had to fight to survive in spite of the circumstances and you could live courageously within them.
>
> Once we were home on a Sunday morning. My father was reading the paper, the *Natchez Democrat*. He had a Crook cigar in his mouth that cost a nickel and he was on the porch in his rocker. We were out on the sidewalk, skating.
>
> There was a place on the street called the Salvation Army Home; it was for white boys. Some kids from the

> Salvation Army came out and were skating. Pretty soon the master of the Salvation Army came out and got on me and brother. He said, "Look, you boys get off the sidewalk, don't you see my boys up here skating?" My father heard that and immediately came off the porch and walked around to the man and put his finger right in his eyes and said: "Let me tell you one God damn thing. I pay as much taxes on this sidewalk as you do and I am a citizen. My boys have the right to skate on this sidewalk as much as yours. Dammit they're not going to leave." Dad told us: "Go on out there and skate."
>
> That guy turned as red as a beet but he spun around and went back and sat down and everything went along all right. My father didn't tell me what to do; he showed me what to do.

There wasn't much money to go around and sometimes Eddie would get teased about his clothing.

> Being poor, my mother had to do all the sewing. She made shirts; they were called "mammy-made" shirts. We had patches on our knees. We couldn't afford anything more. I went to elementary school and I came home in tears and told her that the boys were teasing me about the patches. My first cousin, who was the doctor's son, was wealthy and teased me. My mother said to me, "That don't matter none. You should be proud of your patches because that makes you different. There is nothing wrong with wearing patches as long as you are clean. If no one wears patches but you, then you stand out from the others. Your job is to make yourself distinguished and you are distinguished if you wear patches. Remember, only when you do something different and distinct will you make progress and you should be proud when others criticize you as long as you are right. That is when you are beginning to amount to something."

The comparison of their town life with the life they lived on the farms was striking. Despite its hardships, there was something to be said for the country life. There the Mazique children didn't really consider themselves poor. They had racehorses and horses to ride. They had a lot of fun among themselves. If they wanted something, they had to work for it but considered this natural. The boys all had odd jobs and Eddie's brother Alex built Maude a henhouse so she could raise chickens and sell them. Everybody around them was a relative. They always had clothes to wear and plenty to eat. They didn't know anything about being poor. They thought everyone lived as they did except someone like Grandpa Alex who was special. And after all he was their relative. It was not only that they felt poorer in town; they also experienced more racially motivated rebuffs. In the country they did not feel the full brunt of prejudice. It was the wife of a white tenant on her father's China Grove property who taught Maude to cook chickens and to bake pies out of berries.

As the oldest, it was Maude who first learned the lessons of town, and she talked things over with the younger children. One day on her way to school at Natchez College, a white girl passing her deliberately came close and knocked the books out of her hand. When she got home, she talked to her brothers and sisters in an attempt to prepare them for similar situations.

At times Eddie and Maude were the only two living in Natchez while other children helped out on the farm. Eddie recalls how at times it was not easy being the little brother.

> One summer there was nobody but the two of us living together in the Pine Street house in Natchez. Maude had a way with people. They all loved her—the way she did things and she was beautiful. The boys were around after her one after the other. There was nobody in charge of her. I was the only one, and I was like her son.
>
> She got a job working at the Baker Grand Theater, which was a white theater down on Pearl Street. She's the only girl I know who was colored working in that theater. She'd walk down that street and she'd look good all the time. She'd smile and everybody would make passes. One day there was a white guy who made a pass at her that I didn't like. It riled me up. He owned a jewelry store on the way to the theater and Maude was standing there looking at the jewelry and he came out there and made some remarks to Maude

> about what he wanted to do to her. He invited her to come in and he would give her something. I was trailing along on the side and Maude just walked away. All she could do was to walk away. There was nobody to report nothing to. The law and the order was your long gun, your pistol, whatever you could do or whomever you knew in the town.

Some of the memories of town are the saddest memories of Eddie's life. It was in the Pine Street house in Natchez that two of his sisters and one brother died. Eddie and Jack were like twins: always together and always up to good or bad together. Maude compared them to the Katzenjammer kids. She would never think of calling one without the other. It was always "Eddie and Jack" when you wanted either one of them to come. At nine years old Jack became ill. Eddie remembered:

> My brother Jack was a year younger than me. The two of us were just about inseparable. One of the reasons I went into medicine was because of what happened to Jack. I remember when he got sick with a fever and it turned out to be typhoid. As far as I was concerned there was nobody doing any damn thing for him. There were only two black doctors in Natchez and one of them was my uncle, my father's brother, James C. Mazique. The other doctor there was Dr. Dumas. Those were the two largest black families in Natchez, both well respected.
>
> Jack's death really hurt me. That was the first serious thing that I ever remember that shook me up. It was one thing that spurred on my desire to be a doctor.

Edna and Sadie also died as young women. Eddie recalled:

> There were three sisters in the family and they were the first three children. There was Maude, Edna, and then Sadie. They were very beautiful girls. The family being large, they were sort of set up to be role models and mothers for the boys. My father stressed education so they all went to high school and then on to a normal school about two years above high school. When a poor

man like that could send somebody away to Memphis, it was a big thing. Most of the people lived and died in their county. He sacrificed for it.

My sister Sadie was described as a bookworm. She loved reading and she loved clerical work. She decided she wanted to become a stenographer. Maude and Edna both got jobs teaching school when they got out.

The conditions under which they had to teach were horrible. They had to hitch up the buggy and drive in the rain and in the cold winter months it would be five or ten miles to the schoolhouse. When they got there, there would be no heat and they would have to heat it up. There were cracks in the wall and all this stuff. Their jobs made them highly subject to exposure. It is difficult to live or survive in a situation like that.

Maude survived it but Edna did not. She came down with pneumonia—this was about 1926. She became ill and came home to Natchez from Louisiana where she was teaching and was put under the care of my uncle. I saw my uncle, Uncle Doc, come in to take care of her. White doctors weren't prone to do much for you. I would see him come in and there was nothing except aspirin and spirits of nitrate to give her and have her wash it down with warm tepid water. But that was not to fight the bug and she died with pneumonia. That kind of tore me up.

Then only about a year later, my sister Sadie suffered the same thing but she got hers in a different way because she was going to school in Memphis, Tennessee, in Henderson Business College to take up the secretarial course. Through overexposure and overwork she got pneumonia too. I remember well seeing Uncle Doc come in. I remember she had what we called then water on the lungs. They had to draw the fluid off. They both died in Maude's arms.

I was about a senior or junior in high school. I can see Professor Henderson now walking into the house when he heard of the death. He was all decked out. He had his striped pants on, a long coat cut away and a black tie and collar that came way out.

> After these three episodes of losing Jack to typhoid fever and two sisters to pneumonia, I felt that those lives could have well been saved. All I wanted to do after that was to be a doctor. That was all I could think of. I never thought of anything else.

Death was faced directly in those days and conditions were such that not all the members of a black family were expected to reach a ripe old age. The children died at home and each member of the family had to come to terms with it at a young age. Maude was like a second mother to all the children and when death was near she was there to comfort both those who were living and those who were dying. It was she to whom the young Eddie turned in frustration that nothing could prevent the deaths of his beloved brother and sisters. It was Maude who first heard Eddie vow when he looked in there and saw them drawing that fluid from Sadie's lungs that he was going to be a doctor and "do all he could for young people who were sick and didn't have nobody to do nothing for them."[18]

But Eddie did not spend all his time in Natchez thinking about social injustice or the need for qualified black doctors. He was a cheerful person and certainly had a way with the ladies. Children from other black families found themselves pushed by their parents to "keep up with the Maziques." But Eddie was not always industrious. He was known by the ladies as a "white-doodle-dandy." He was good looking with a red mustache and black hair and could really "talk that talk" that made girls' heads go round. But somehow he still managed to get his lessons.[19]

While Eddie was jolly and full of fun, his older brother Douglas was more on the serious side. They were both very popular with the ladies, but Eddie was the cut-up and managed to get away with most anything. Despite their different natures, after their brother Jack's death, Eddie and Douglas became a team, doing everything together, including going to Natchez College for their high school education.

The campus of Natchez College was located on a large plot of land near the outskirts of town. It was here that all of Grandpa Alex's children and the fourth generation of Maziques in this country were educated. Natchez College was "an advanced institution, for the colored people" that was located in the suburbs of the city and "successfully managed."[20] So states an 1897 promotional pamphlet that was designed in an attempt to attract people and business to the city of Natchez.

Comprised of four separate buildings and appearing much like a small college, Natchez College, despite its name, functioned mostly as a

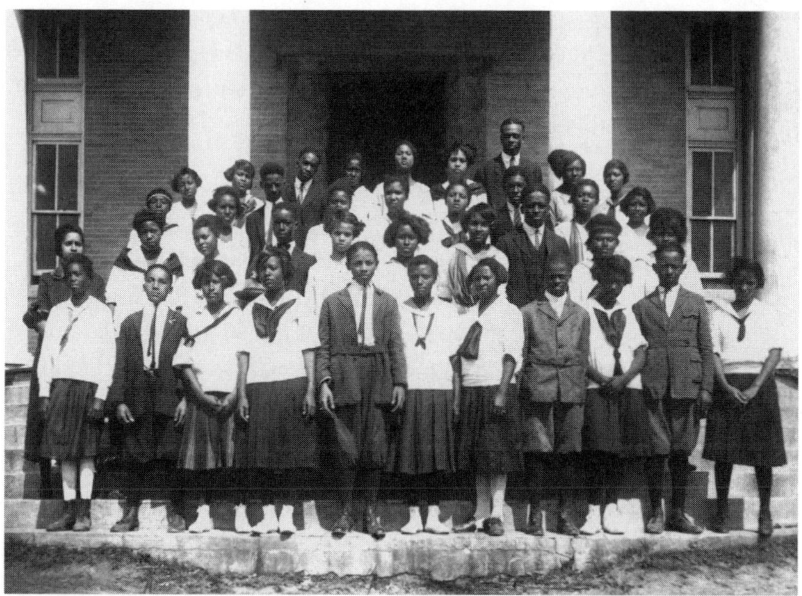

**Fig. 8:** Eddie (second from left, front row) and Douglas (fifth from left, front row) graduate from Natchez College in 1929. Photo courtesy of Maude Mazique and Dolores Pelham.

high school. The front of the campus was an athletic field where the boys played basketball and baseball. A large edifice with four concrete pillars dominated the campus. It served as a home for the principal and his family and also contained a small library and a huge auditorium. The basement of this building was used as a dining room and kitchen. The adjoining building contained the administrative offices, classrooms, and a boys' dormitory on the top floor. Opposite was the girls' dormitory and classrooms for the domestic sciences. To the right was a smaller building designated for science and biology.

During Eddie and Douglas's enrollment, the principal of the high school was S. H. C. Owen, the husband of Eddie's aunt Sarah Mazique. He was a pale, immaculate, and profound black man and a strong disciplinarian. He possessed all the characteristics that the students commonly associated with whites: keen, sharp features and the airs of a man in control. It was he who set the tone for Natchez College.

In 1929, Eddie graduated from Natchez College as the valedictorian; Douglas was the salutatorian. Educating his sons to this extent was the maximum that Alex could accomplish given his financial situation.

If Grandpa Alex had lived and pulled through financially, there is little doubt that he would have assisted, but Eddie and Douglas were instead left to their own devices. Eddie's conversation with his father upon graduation was still clear in his mind:

> My father said: "I have kept my promise to you. I told you I would see you through high school. What you do with your life now is up to you. I can't do no more. I'm poor. I have lots of land, but land don't make money. If you are going to do it, you are going to have to get out of here and do it yourself."
>
> He was helping to send my oldest brother, Alex, through Tuskegee and he gave the little money he had to him. That was all the family could do. So everyone put their weight behind the eldest son to get him educated. My brother Alex was a chauffeur for Robert R. Moten, who at that time was the principal of Tuskegee Institute in Alabama.
>
> My father and mother always did say to get the hell out of Natchez. Mama used to tell me all the time, get out of here, and I didn't know why she'd tell me. And Miss Mary Henry who lived across the street in Natchez would tell me, "Boy, a man can gain no honor in his own country." I didn't know what she meant. I couldn't understand it at the time, being young. I had some experiences which were not the best but for the most part I was making out all right. I was enjoying it and had a lot of fellowship, a lot of friends, and a lot of things that were very pleasant to me.

An English teacher at Natchez College, Ben Blackburn, was an important role model to the young men. It was he who recognized the potential in the Mazique brothers and encouraged them to go on with their education.

> Benjamin Blackburn was my English teacher. Ben was my ideal of a man. I liked the way he carried himself. I liked the way he dressed. I liked the way he was respected. I liked the way he walked. Something about him just represented culture and development. He had

the kind of qualities I thought a man should have. He realized I kind of idolized him.

He was a graduate of Morehouse College in Atlanta, Georgia. He obviously saw something in the two of us and he called us in one day and sat us down and said, "Look, what do you guys plan to do?" We thought, hell, what can we do? Ain't got no money. Can't go to school. Ben said, "You should go to Morehouse. You sit down and I'll write a letter." He wrote it right away regarding both of us. He opened the doors of Morehouse for us by getting both of us a scholarship.

We left home in September of 1929 for Morehouse College. We did not see Natchez again until July of 1933 when we graduated. It didn't cost but $9.50 by train but that was a lot then.

# CHAPTER THREE 

# Shedding the Shackles of Natchez

A Soul with an over-mastering desire for a higher life will not remain shackled. It will live life in all its fullness, anxious to make the best of its powers.
— *Edward C. Mazique, valedictorian speech, Natchez College, 1929*

Even the lack of screens in the segregated seats that allowed the cinders to blow in their faces didn't dampen the Mazique brothers' spirits as they boarded a train and pulled out of Natchez on a warm September day in 1929. Eddie and Douglas each had one pair of shoes, which they seldom wore. Now they were sitting, dressed up, wearing those tight shoes, and anticipating their future at Morehouse. It wasn't long before Eddie could be seen slipping out of his shoes and walking up and down the aisle to take away the pain from those pinching demons. Douglas, always the more reserved of the two, suffered the whole trip with his still on.

It was quite an experience for two young men who had never ventured farther than Natchez and the surrounding rural areas of Mississippi and Louisiana. Once Eddie had seen a postcard his aunt sent to his mother of the capitol building in Jackson, Mississippi. At the time he thought that was something from a fantasy world. Soon he was to see such wonders for himself.

As the train progressed, Eddie and Douglas both had settled into a state of excessive quietness. The thrill of the adventure had begun to wear off and the apprehension of what they would encounter was mounting.

Just about that time, a young man boarded the train in Birmingham, Alabama. Guessing their destination, he approached Eddie and Douglas and introduced himself as a junior at Morehouse. He began to extol the glories of the college and regaled them with stories about the wonders of Morehouse. They knew very little about the school except that they each had a forty-five-dollar scholarship, it was Ben Blackburn's alma mater, and it was their chance to get out of Natchez. As they listened to the stories, they began to realize there was something very special about Morehouse.[1]

Upon arriving, they found the campus as impressive as imagined, and not just the Morehouse campus. Spelman, its sister college, was within sight and Atlanta University was only a few blocks away. It was a real center for black culture and learning. Near the campus was a corner called Conn's Corner. On it was a store owned by a black man that supplied all the amenities for the Morehouse students. There were pens, ink, pencils, paper, and ice cream sodas. The students would meet there and talk about all the campus gossip.[2]

The Maziques were assigned a dormitory room in Graves Hall, which had served as the entire campus when it was completed in 1889. The building was an imposing four-story, red brick structure with a huge bell tower in its center. In 1929, Graves Hall served as a dormitory for freshmen and sophomores. Eddie and Douglas along with the other lowly freshmen were assigned rooms on the upper floors, a placement that undoubtedly assisted in building stamina along with character.

Graves Hall meant many new experiences for the Mazique brothers. At home the boys had always worn long drawers, never seeing the necessity for something different in which to sleep. However, Maude had made sure each of them had a pair of pajamas before they left for Morehouse. Graves Hall boasted a shower big enough for sixteen men at a time. This was the first time the Maziques had ever used a shower. Each morning, Eddie would come trudging down the hall in his blue pajamas with his P&G white Naptha soap in hand, always a few minutes behind Douglas, to be awakened by that invigorating shower.

Quarles Hall had been erected in 1898 after the collegiate department had been formally recognized at Morehouse. It was a square-looking, three-story brick structure that contained classrooms, lecture halls, and science laboratories. It was placed in a location that would also be accessible to the female students of Spelman. It had served as the main academic building until Sale Hall was erected in 1910.

At its completion, Sale Hall took over as the administrative center of the college. The large, rectangular, brick structure had three stories above the basement level. Most of the classrooms were housed in this building as was the library during the 1920s. It was to Sale Hall that Eddie and the other students would come every morning to attend the mandatory chapel and to be stirred by the inspirational speeches and the sound of the men's voices lifted in song.

The president's residence was also a part of the campus when Eddie arrived. It was a two-story brick house erected in 1902.

The junior and senior men at Morehouse were lucky enough to be housed in Robert Hall. This was a modern dormitory completed in 1916 that offered spacious rooms, electric lighting, central heating, and suites for the professors. The basement housed the dining room with the kitchen in a one-story annex in the rear.

Perhaps the most impressive building on campus, more for its purpose than its looks, was the new science building completed in 1920. This was the first building on any Negro college campus to be devoted completely to science, a clear indication of the seriousness with which Morehouse approached the education of its students. For Eddie and Douglas, both of whom were interested in medicine, it was an inspiration. It was this orientation of Morehouse, more than its buildings, that made Morehouse stand out as exceptional among southern Negro colleges.

In the early 1900s the southern states offered blacks little in the way of education. Eddie and his brothers and sisters had to leave their home in Louisiana and travel to a private high school in Natchez to progress beyond the eighth grade. Louisiana was not alone in its backwardness. Prior to World War I almost no high schools existed for black youngsters in the South. In the late 1920s blacks were rather reluctantly beginning to be offered a high school education. Yet in the academic year of 1926–1927 there were only 251 high schools open to blacks in all of the southern states combined.[3]

When it came to education beyond high school, even less was available. That which was, such as Tuskegee, headed by Booker T. Washington, was manual in orientation and geared to making blacks better fit to work for white folks. Blacks were considered intellectually inferior and the wisest course for a college, it was believed, was to accept this limitation and to train young people in professions where there were jobs available.

Morehouse stood as an anomaly in this southern educational system. At its founding in 1867, the Augusta Institute, which was to become Morehouse College, not only provided a Baptist seminary education, but completed the high school education for many of its students, most of whom were adults. But by 1906, John Hope, the new acting president of Morehouse, had other ideas. He was not willing to accept the premise that blacks should be given training instead of a true liberal arts education.

A rift between two theories of black education was starting to become evident when Hope ascended to the helm of Morehouse College. Booker T. Washington's orientation toward training for manual jobs seemed particularly acceptable to the white philanthropists who heavily funded Tuskegee. However, many of the blacks who initially supported Washington and the Tuskegee Movement with a belief that elementary and industrial training were a first step on the road to equality had become disillusioned. A strong spokesman against the dominance of the thinking of Booker T. Washington came on the scene in the person of a close friend of Hope's, the eloquent W. E. B. DuBois. DuBois spoke out for an equal education for blacks as well as for full equality in all areas of life.

At their first open conference at Storer College in 1906, the Niagara Movement, headed by DuBois, promoted educational and civil rights.[4] The fifth resolution in DuBois's "Address to the Country" called for education for black children:

> We want our children educated. . . . And when we call for education, we mean real education. . . . Education is the development of power and ideal. We want our children trained as intelligent human beings should be, and we will fight for all time against any proposal to educate black boys and girls simply as servants and underlings, or simply for the use of other people. They have a right to know, to think, to aspire.[5]

In 1906, John Hope was in his first year as acting president of Morehouse College. Despite the tenuousness of his position, Hope went to the conference at Storer College. He was the only college president to attend and ally himself with the Niagara Movement as it strongly stated its opposition to Booker T. Washington and his theories of education. Challenging him was an especially courageous move for Hope since Washington was the only black educator who seemed able to succeed in securing large donations from philanthropists such as Carnegie and Rockefeller's General Education Board. It was not a practical commitment for a college president, but Hope obviously considered it necessary to take a stand in favor of the complete equality of blacks as opposed to the freedom for them to make only limited gains.

John Hope was a well-educated man. He was white-looking, and white in fact by all but the strictest definition. His father was Scottish and his mother was a very pale brown. Of moderate stature, with red hair and gray eyes, Hope could easily have "passed" for white, but instead chose to identify with the problems and concerns of African-Americans and set about to improve conditions.

He first began by teaching at what was to become Morehouse College in 1898. Eight years later he assumed the presidency. Under his leadership, the school grew from a secondary school and college for teachers and preachers into a first-rate academic institution. It was his character, demeanor, and moral beliefs that were to mold what it would mean to be a "Morehouse Man." He was a pragmatist who took much-needed assistance in fundraising from Booker T. Washington even though he vehemently disagreed with his idea of training Negroes only with technical skills. John Hope was also an idealist who firmly believed in the expansion of the Negro mind through a liberal arts education, a belief that was at best frowned upon by southern whites and many of the northern philanthropists as well. He was not a radical who advocated the overthrow of the southern system. Instead he worked patiently to change it through his long-time membership in and tireless work with the Atlanta Interracial Council. Despite the system, he never believed in the inferiority of his race. One of his popular sayings sums up his philosophy: "I will ride in the back of the streetcar because a law (however unjust) forces me to, but my spirit rides up front." It was this philosophy that he imparted to his men.

Eddie's first encounter with John Hope shows the kind of impact he had on the young black students.

> It takes more than just books to make a man. It takes knocks and bruises and falling down and getting up and holding your head high. As a freshman when I went to Morehouse, I didn't have any money to pay for tuition. The scholarship I was given didn't go very far. I was called in by the Bursar, Skipper Gasset, to see about fees and monies and how I could manage to pay. I told him Douglas and I had a scholarship. He said, "Well, young man, forty-five dollars isn't even going to pay for your tuition for the year."
>
> I was outside the Bursar's office. He had a little hole cut in it shaped like a half moon so you could talk to him. I had my head down because I didn't know how to answer Mr. Gasset when he was talking about money and finances. I saw another man standing back there.

> The man stepped from behind Mr. Gasset and I looked to see who it was. There was the president of the school, John Hope. He looked like a white man passing for black. He talked very softly. He said, "Mr. Gasset, who is that young man there talking to you?" Mr. Gasset said, "This is Eddie Mazique from Natchez, Mississippi." President Hope said: "Tell him to come in here." Mr. Gasset called me into the office.
>
> I walked in and the president said, "Young man, put your head up." I held my head up. "Mr. Gasset, don't listen to him any more. Don't give him any considerations about anything. As a matter of fact, Mr. Gasset, we don't want a man at Morehouse who can't hold his head up. Young man, when you learn how to hold your head up and look Mr. Gasset in both of his eyes, then he will be able to listen to you. You've got to understand there is nothing to be ashamed of if you are poor. Most of the people at this institution are poor. But if you show that you have some courage, you will manage and make it in spite of being poor."
>
> I held my head up from then on and looked him in the eye when I talked to him. That was my first big lesson from the likes of the president of the college, John Hope. He was known to have a deep sense of understanding for the poor, so the boys loved him.[6]

The early 1930s was a time when John Hope's and his successor Samuel H. Archer's compassion for the poor were sorely needed. Eddie was at Morehouse during the Great Depression years. There was no Social Security system. People were hungry and unemployed, and bread lines were not an uncommon sight. Blacks, who were always the last hired and the first fired, tended to suffer even more. The boll weevil had hit Mississippi again and the farmers were no better off than the city residents. Banks were failing and people were losing any savings they might have had. Charles Evans Hughes, a staunch conservative, was the chief justice of the Supreme Court. All the societal difficulties were mirrored on the Morehouse campus. People could not afford the luxury of college. Enrollments were drastically reduced: in 1929–1930 there were 561 students; 1931–1932 enrollments were 470; and in 1932–1933 there were only 296. Many of those who did attend were as likely to be unable to pay their bills as Eddie and Douglas. Faculty salaries were seldom paid on time, frequently reduced, and sometimes even went unpaid. President Hope was quoted as saying: "Morehouse is poor, but we live in respectable poverty." Societal problems were never used as an excuse at Morehouse for the diminishment of academic standards or a lack of responsibility of the student to excel, and this was not to change with the Depression.[7]

John Hope had an impact on every Morehouse man. His biography is full of anecdotes of his encounters with students and the lasting effect he had on their lives. In 1931, he left the presidency of Morehouse to assume the role of president of the new Atlanta University Affiliation, which had been created through his efforts. It was his dream to have Atlanta be a center for Negro colleges, a haven in the South. In 1930, Morehouse College and its sister Spelman College joined with the new combined Atlanta University (Atlanta University and Clark and Morris Brown Colleges). Atlanta University provided graduate work and Spelman and Morehouse handled the undergraduate education of females and males respectively, to form an affiliation that would create an intellectual center for black students.

Although absent from the helm of Morehouse, Hope's influence was still felt. His dictate that a "Morehouse Man" was not to be beaten by the injustices perpetrated against him remained the basic philosophy of the college. At the 1965 commencement, President Benjamin E. Mays eloquently summed up the values that Hope had instituted and that still guided the college:

> For ninety-eight years this institution has striven to make men free and responsible. Born and nurtured in a segregated economy which cramps the mind, stifles the soul, and circumscribes the heart, Morehouse has always taught that the mind can be free in a tightly segregated society; that a man's body could ride, sleep, eat, worship, and work in a segregated society without ever being segregated. Our philosophy has been, and is now, that no man is a slave, no man is in prison, and no man is segregated until he accepts it in his mind. The minds of Paul, John Bunyan, Nehru, Frederick Douglass, and Martin Luther King, Jr. were never in bondage. For ninety-eight years this has been our philosophy.
>
> We want Morehouse men to enter a desegregated society standing erect on their feet, accepting the rights,

> privileges, and responsibilities inherent in a free society. And wherever you go... whatever you do, whatever you say, never forget you are a Morehouse Man, and that the College will never release you from the obligation to strive to do whatever you do so well that no man living, no man dead, and no man yet to be born could do the work better than you.[8]

Although colleges are often described as ivory towers, to its dismay Morehouse could not escape the racist environment in which it was created and somehow managed not only to survive but to succeed. Morehouse was located only about two miles from the hub of Atlanta. Streetcars ran nearby for a dime, and it was within walking distance for the poorer students. With its location, it is no wonder that the students and faculty of Morehouse were not exempt from the demeaning experiences common to blacks throughout the South. Despite these social barriers, however, President Hope would accept nothing less than academic excellence, character, and courage from his students. This was no easy task for the men of Morehouse.

In Atlanta, as in the rest of the South, Negroes were subject to constant insult and humiliation. Segregation was a way of life. "White" and "Colored" signs could be seen at bus and railroad stations, drinking fountains, bathrooms, and most any other public facility. On railroad trains, blacks were crowded into the Jim Crow car, nearest the locomotive, where they were sure to get most of the soot produced during the ride. The term "boy" was used to address all black males, despite their age and community standing, while they had to call white men "mister." In the 1920s, when Benjamin E. Mays, the future president of the college, was teaching at Morehouse, two white men forced him out of a Pullman berth at gunpoint for daring to locate in quarters normally reserved for whites.

In the late 1920s and early 1930s, there were two incidents that were even more threatening to the students at Morehouse and to President Hope's ideals. In 1928, a student named Barnes who delivered papers to earn money for school went into a cafe to request payment of an overdue bill. The proprietor did not like the way the student spoke to him and proceeded to shoot him in the head to "teach him how to act when talking to a white man." Young Barnes died as he tried to reach the exit. Much to Hope's dismay, the incident was pretty much ignored since the youth was poor and from an obscure background. A grand jury refused to indict the murderer because his actions were considered "justified."[9]

A second student, named Dennis Hubert, the son of a prominent Baptist minister who was also a Morehouse graduate, was shot and killed by white men as he sat in a public park in Atlanta on a Sunday in 1930. Two inebriated men and two women emerged from a thicket adjacent to the park. A youth playing in the park apparently remarked: "They'd better take those women home." The men left but returned with four others and a shotgun. Dennis Hubert was sitting on a nearby bench. One man, upon seeing him, shouted, "That's the s.o.b." The other shot and killed him. This shooting nearly precipitated a riot. The college was successful in acquiring the services of Georgia's most famous white criminal lawyer, William Schley Howard, who managed to get a conviction with fifteen years for one defendant and five years for the other. This was the first time a white man had been convicted for the murder of a Negro in Georgia.[10]

The incidents of harassment of Morehouse men did not end with the 1930s. A future president of Morehouse, Dr. Hugh Gloster, was a 1931 graduate of Morehouse who had just come back to start teaching in the fall of 1941. One Saturday he was on a train going from Atlanta to visit his mother in Memphis. The train stopped along the way in Birmingham and then in a small town called Amory, Mississippi. While in Amory, the train picked up a number of farmers, some of whom were very old. The farmers would go on to the next stop, Tupelo, to do their shopping on Saturdays. Two white men occupied seats in the middle of the coach on one side and another white man on the other side: one was the conductor and another was the railway mail clerk. There were seats on each side behind them but the black passengers did not dare to take those seats and instead stood in the aisles in great numbers. Professor Gloster asked the conductor if he and the other two men could move so these people could sit down. He was promptly told: "Nigger, you have a seat. That's what is wrong now, too many niggers trying to run the train."[11] When the train arrived in Tupelo, the conductor got off the train and called the police. The police came and yanked Hugh Gloster off the train, saying he was under arrest for violating the segregation laws on the train and for causing trouble. He was placed in the back seat of a car between two policeman who proceeded to hit him in the head, the body, and especially the genital area as a third officer drove them to the jail. Once they looked in his bags and found that he was a teacher at Morehouse, they treated him better but still locked him up and kept him in jail all night. He was beaten so badly that he required medical treatment when he was released.[12]

Despite the hostile environment in Atlanta, Eddie and Douglas were made to feel welcome by the staff at Morehouse. Of more personal, if not greater, impact on Eddie's life than President Hope was the dean at Morehouse, Samuel H. Archer. Archer had taught at Roger Williams College with Hope before coming to Morehouse. He, along with Benjamin G. Brawley and John Hope, is viewed today as one of the main founders of the prestigious liberal arts college that Morehouse has become. Archer became president of Morehouse in 1931 when John Hope took on the presidency of the new Atlanta University. It was the Archers who welcomed the Mazique brothers into their family and provided them with odd jobs that would enable them to meet the financial requirements of college.

Samuel Archer was a large, vigorous, and dynamic individual. Although not the intellectual equal of Hope, his folksy humor and philosophy provided the young men with inspiration and his honesty and integrity with a role model. He was very approachable and, unlike Hope, who had a rather distant and aristocratic demeanor, Archer provided an open and welcoming personality. His gangling six-foot-plus frame could be seen all over campus, including on the football field where he coached. It was known that his principles did not change to suit different occasions. He took one of his football players out of a game for what he considered a dirty play. When the player protested he was just trying to win the game, Archer reportedly replied with impatience and disgust: "Ah, son, I'd rather lose the game through clean playing than to win it through dirty playing."

The Archer family provided the support and love that the Mazique brothers missed when they left their own family behind for their four years at Morehouse. Eddie recalled:

> Had it not been for the kind people at Morehouse—the officials, the administrators, and the Archers, particularly—Douglas and I would not have been able to last at Morehouse. Dean Archer gave my brother and me a chance to develop our potential by letting us stay there and work. It made me believe in myself. I knew I had a friend there. I learned about sharing and discipline.
>
> We couldn't afford to go back home for four years. On Christmas and Thanksgiving and at the end of the school year when the other men would leave, we would still be there. The administrators would allow us to stay in the dormitory with no one living there but my brother and me. The Dean accepted us into his family and his

> son, Leonard Archer, "Josh," became like my own brother. He was an English major and in drama. He became an educator and taught school at Tennessee A&I and at Wilberforce. The whole family fell in love with my brother and me and carried us along.

Morehouse was a very conservative school during the 1920s.[13] The emphasis was on daily chapel where the students would hear outstanding and frequently inspirational speakers. On Sunday, compulsory religious services were held at nine o'clock in order that the students remain free to attend church at eleven. Some students complained about chapel and yet much of their intellectual development was fostered by the speakers they heard and the issues to which they were introduced during these chapel lectures.

Even though Spelman stood nearby, social contacts were limited. The men of Morehouse were forbidden to go on the Spelman campus except for certain assignments on designated days. On Sunday afternoons, they were allowed to attend the Spelman vesper service. This was the main opportunity for the Morehouse men to see their girlfriends and to dress up and stroll with them. Socializing was limited to about an hour after vespers, and there would be someone on security duty to make sure they left the campus. Failure to adhere to this strict routine meant expulsion.

There was even a ten-o'clock dormitory curfew for the young men. However, it was not unheard of that some of the students would sneak out and visit their girlfriends at Spelman and climb through the windows to get back into their rooms. Some of the younger and more liberal faculty also objected to all the restrictions; they left the institution and went elsewhere.

Naturally there were ways around the regulations and college students were bound to test the rules. The typical escapades associated with life as a college freshman brought a smile when they were recollected by Eddie:

> As you may guess there were always manners in which the students would find a way to somehow get around this rule. Many romances, courtships, and marriages were the result. It was considered a coup for a Morehouse man to marry a Spelman woman because she was well educated and well trained in etiquette and discipline as well as in morals. I had many

> good experiences emanating from there. They were not always entirely intellectual, educational, and cultural but they were social and this is a part of man too. You learn a lot of good things from it.
>
> There were also ways of sneaking out after curfew. On the same floor in the room adjoining us was an athlete from the state of Kentucky. He was tall, handsome, and brusque. The very essence of strength was portrayed in his walk. He became an All American in football. There were various episodes where he would stay out at night. One of his favorite exercises when he came home, if he were imbibing a bit, was to drag us and our beds out of our room and leave them in the hall. He would say, "Let me see you get the hell out of those beds and get those beds back in there."

Eddie's first year at Morehouse turned out to be especially difficult. Not only did he have all the normal adjustments of a freshman to make, but he was also very ill.

> The first year at Morehouse I got malaria and developed phlebitis in my left leg from it and a massive fungus infection. I went to the hospital at Morehouse for two or three weeks. Antibiotics were not known then and so infectious diseases like pneumonia were the leading cause of death.
>
> We only had one doctor, Dr. Raymond Carter, at Morehouse. He did everything. When things only got worse, Dean Archer spoke to his wife about it and they both decided I should see their doctor. They got me to go to their white doctor in Atlanta and he did tests and diagnosed the malaria. That is how I knew what I had. Every spring, it would act up again.

Despite setbacks, Eddie and Douglas always managed to have a job.

> We had all sorts of odd jobs to get us by. At Morehouse, I progressively became the head waiter, the teacher's waiter and, finally, I was moved into the kitchen and became a chef and a baker and had the keys

to the commissary. We would haul over the juices that would come from the peaches, pears and plums and would put them in one pot and would make our own wine to take to the fellows. I also worked at the post office every year during Christmas season. That really paid well. One day I worked from five in the morning 'til midnight and I made twelve dollars and something.

When school was out we didn't have anybody to wait tables for or make bread for, so we had to find another job. Dean Archer called Mr. Carson, the superintendent of buildings and grounds, and said, "You find work for these boys." We went over and the project was to paint every dormitory at Spelman College. In those days, we had to scrape off the old paint. We would get a brush and soften it up with water and use the scraper to peel the paint off. I got $14.25 a week and that was good money. In addition to that we lived free in the dormitory and we had a key to the pantry down at Morehouse and we always had a big, forty-five-pound can of peanut butter and jelly and syrup and that was our meals.

I would say to Douglas: "Damn, I sure am tired of eating this." He would say to me: "Use your imagination. Just imagine that this is a steak and it will be steak." Then we would talk about the nutrients of peanuts and George Washington Carver and about all the products that he had made from them. Then we would come to the conclusion that this had to be an elegant dish that we were having. This man Carver had made over two hundred things out of the lowly peanut. That was how we got by.

When we finally got through scraping, Mr. Carson said to us, "You guys did all right. I believe I can teach you to paint." He put a Sherwin Williams cap on our heads and put brushes in our hands and showed us how to paint. For the next three years that was what we did. We painted every damn building at Spelman College and at Morehouse and the last one we painted was the gymnasium at Morehouse. I never shall forget we painted it maroon and white, the colors of Morehouse. It looked like an old barn. That was the last thing we did before we left there. But when we left, we didn't owe one penny.

Atlanta and Morehouse taught Eddie more than the value of hard work. It opened up intellectual vistas that he had never imagined and widened his horizons beyond Mississippi and Georgia to global issues.

Atlanta had its poor black sections. To get downtown, the Morehouse students would have to go down Westfair Street through a slum area nicknamed "Beaver Slide." Here there was drink, anger, and resentment. What the students saw once they successfully maneuvered their way through this section, however, were thriving black businesses. These were not small ones like those in Natchez, but prosperous major companies.

> We would frequently go downtown to see Auburn Avenue and to watch blacks, called Negroes then, who just about owned Auburn Avenue. There were some great edifices and black men had established them. Places like Milton and Yates drug stores and one of the first black banks, Citizens Bank and Trust Company, which still survives. This area was the epitome of black culture. This is where Ebenezer Baptist Church and one of the first black daily newspapers, the *Atlanta World*, were located. We didn't learn much about black accomplishments in Natchez even though there was black history being made there. In Atlanta we could see it and at Morehouse we learned about it.

Morehouse was a small college and its size allowed the faculty to take a personal interest in the students. Emphasis was placed on individual effort and the students were constantly challenged to reach their full potential. Extra attention from faculty was common and frequently stands out in the memories of alumni reminiscing about those early days at Morehouse. George Crockett was a colleague of Eddie's who graduated from Morehouse in 1931. He became a lawyer, a judge, and later a congressman. What he recalled most about Morehouse were the informal contacts he had with his teachers.[14] Many of the faculty lived in the dorms and were very accessible to students who wished to socialize. Eddie was also impressed by this student-faculty interaction, as was evident as he discussed his professors.

> After work, I spent the evening down at the corner room where Professor Dansby lived. He was our mathematics professor. For some reason I loved symphonies. Professor Dansby had a radio and he would play that classical music and I would listen. I was a little weak in calculus and while I was there, he would teach me. Later when I didn't have a tuxedo to wear for the debating team, he lent me his for every occasion.

It was not only Professor Dansby who entertained the students in his room. Great thinkers such as Howard W. Thurman made Eddie and the other students aware of the responsibility they had to better themselves despite the hardships they might suffer.[15] Eddie remembered well what he learned from Professor Thurman:

> One of the most profound teachers I had was a great philosopher and minister by the name of Howard Thurman. He was a well-known theologian who just died a few years ago. He wrote many books and articles. Professor Thurman taught more about character and what religion really means and stands for than any man that I have ever known.
>
> His special gift was that he would make it so easy. He was humble, yet you knew that he was great. We would go to his home after hours and just sit down and crack peanuts and listen to him talk about situations that existed all over the world. I had never been to India but from him I learned about it. He taught us how to think and to philosophize. He showed us how our own society was inconsistent and yet explained how we had to live with it, how we had rights that are all written down and that have been documented and constitutionalized. Yet blacks were in no position to partake of these rights. Yet as a people and as individuals we had to survive. But surviving was not enough for him or for Morehouse. You not only had to survive, you had to make a contribution. That was the challenge.
>
> He told us that "the greed of man is like fish that swim in the water, yet can never quench their thirst." He said: "Over the heads of Morehouse students there

> is a crown that is so bright and so great and so remarkable that it challenges every Morehouse man to grow tall enough to wear it." He talked about discrimination and segregation. He talked about how we were held back in American society and yet we still had to try to wear that crown.
>
> Morehouse was concerned with developing the individual. It put it all on you. You were supposed to know all about the subject—our job was to develop ourselves academically. We were given an awareness of the problems we would face but we were not taught to be crusaders. Yet Morehouse gave us the equipment to crusade. We were supposed to go out of Morehouse displaying scholastic and academic excellence.

The faculty also remembered Eddie. Mildred Burch was on the staff at Morehouse when Eddie arrived. She still recollected her first sight of him:

> When Eddie came to Morehouse College, we had a reception, as we did for all freshmen. We got them together and sort of talked with them and told them a bit about what was expected and how we hoped they would develop. We asked each one of them to say something about why they came to Morehouse. Most of them said a polite but curt, ordinary thing. When it was Ed's turn, he said: "I came to Morehouse to make it what it should be." I turned to a faculty member next to me and I said: "Gee. We've got a live one here." He has done just that all through his affiliation with the school—as a student and alumnus. Working with Morehouse College in mind first; his own achievement was secondary to the college.[16]

George Crockett remembers Eddie as a brash young freshman when he arrived during George's junior year. He was studious but also gregarious and made friends very easily. Eddie did not have the same educational background as some of the young men who came from city schools in states where blacks were not subject to as much discrimination. "He came out of Mississippi and he needed quite a bit of Morehouse polishing," George remembers. But he promptly acquired

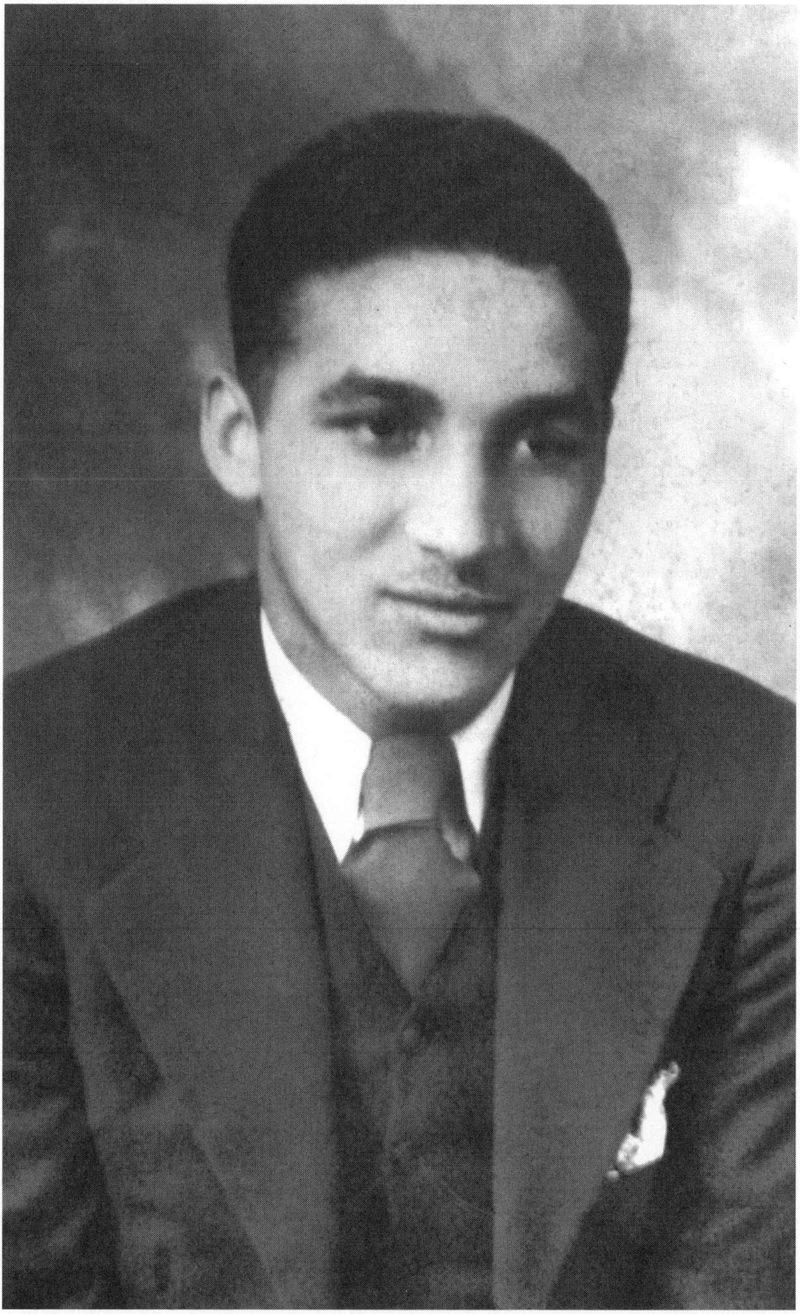

**Fig. 9:** Eddie as an undergraduate at Morehouse College. Photo courtesy of Maude Mazique and Dolores Pelham.

that refinement and George claims that "Eddie is now one of the most polished graduates of Morehouse!"[17]

A large part of that acculturation process was supplied by the debating team. Debating was considered one of the major intellectual challenges at Morehouse. It was most successful in the decade between 1920 and 1930, during which time the team was coached by Benjamin Mays, Nathaniel P. Tillman, and Brailsford R. Brazael. Much of this enthusiasm and expertise carried on into the 1930s. It was the men on the debating team, like George Crockett, to whom Eddie looked up. As Eddie recalled, becoming a member of the debating team played an important part in his education:

> I became a member of the debating team, for which I had to do a lot of reading. We would take on issues such as "Should the caste system in India be abolished?" and other issues that would be dealing with worldwide situations that took us beyond where we were. We debated at Alabama State and Tuskegee. For the first time, I realized there was more to the world than Adams County. My periphery began to expand and broaden as far as my thinking was concerned.

This experience of broadening horizons was not limited to the debating team. Eddie found constant challenges to his thinking no matter with what he was involved at Morehouse, including the baseball team.

> When I got to Morehouse I experienced a greater feeling of freedom and mobility. I was the baseball manager and I was chasing a baseball down the street off the baseball field. A store was on the corner. When I stooped to pick the ball up, a little Jewish girl came out of the store, smiled and said, "Hello," and asked my name. A white girl speaking to me! Then another one came out and she said, "Come in and meet my father." I went in the store and I met him. He said: "Aren't you a student at Morehouse? Well, we have studies and discussions over here." It was some kind of student labor group. He asked me to come over and listen. Well, I had never been invited by a white man to come, to sit, and to listen.

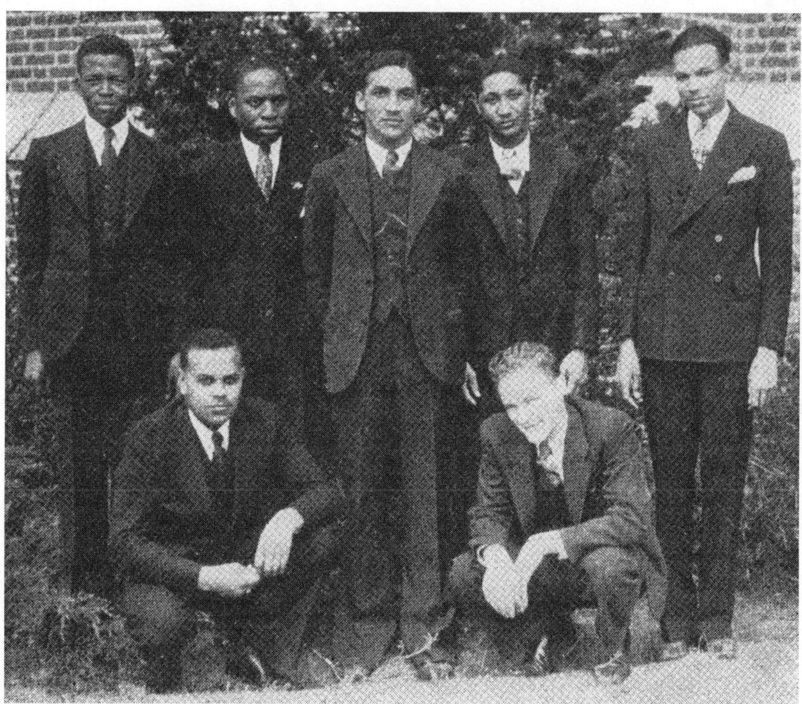

**Fig. 10:** The officers of the senior class from Morehouse College in 1933 with Edward C. Mazique (center) serving as class president. Photo courtesy of Maude Mazique and Dolores Pelham.

I was thirsty for knowledge so I went over and sat there. As I listened, I found out about labor groups, their trials and how they were fighting for jobs and for freedom and equality. This was during the Republican administration of Hoover. FDR came in 1932, so this must have been 1930.

It occurred to me that maybe somebody else out there was having a problem with discrimination other than me because I was colored. Here was a group inviting me to come in to join with them to do something. I thought, maybe they will come with me to help me fight mine. I expressed myself this way and the answer was, "Most assuredly, yes." It didn't take me long to disseminate this information to my colleagues. We began to talk about it. One of the guys who

> was high in the echelon of the debating club said: "Eddie, I don't know about that; I think that's a communist group." At that time I didn't know what a communist was. However, since he advised me not to bother with it, I respected him and took his advice and did not follow through with it. But at least it gave me something to let me know that things were happening to other people.

When graduation came in 1933, Douglas and Eddie both graduated with honors. After a four-year absence from Natchez and their family, they were ready to head home. They realized there would be few opportunities for black men in Natchez with bachelor's degrees, so they talked to some friends about starting up a business before they left.

> Douglas and I hadn't seen any of our family in those four years at Morehouse. When we graduated from Morehouse my brother and I were very homesick but we didn't know what we would do with our degrees in Natchez. We had no job to go to. We had a degree but that was all we did have. What could we do? What was available? What the hell could you do as a black man in Mississippi? You could either teach or you could preach. And if you were lucky enough you could become a doctor or dentist if you had enough financing. There were no other areas. If you had any other forms of education you couldn't do a damn thing with them. You can forget about becoming an engineer or electrician, or holding a job as a bookkeeper. There were no black businesses or firms to hire you.
>
> While at Morehouse, we had come to know some people in the news and publicity business. One of them was Lucias Jones. Lucias carried us down to meet a Miss Scott who talked with us about starting up a paper when we got home to Natchez. That is how we entered the newspaper business.
>
> They showed us how to be reporters. In the morning, we would go to Butler Street in Atlanta and Lucias would show us how to get the news. First, we would go to the jail house and the courthouse. Then we did the

> social side of it, the parties and who was getting married. The format of the paper was all fixed.
>
> When we got to Natchez, we used the same format but instead of calling it the *Atlanta World*, we named it the *Mississippi World*. On the front page of the paper was the local news of Natchez—that would sell like the devil. It was the first black newspaper in Natchez.[18]

After paying their expenses at Morehouse, Eddie and Douglas had just enough money left over from their odd jobs to get them back to Natchez. Instead of taking the train, they decided to buy a car.

> From painting the gymnasium, we got enough money to get us home. We wanted to buy a 1925 Ford coupe. In those days, the coupe had the rumble seat in the back. It cost $25. I had $8, my brother had $8, and we couldn't figure out where to get the rest. A friend named "Woo" Foster chipped in and helped us buy the car and headed with us to Natchez. Of course we had a lot of flats on the way, but we had a hell of a time driving it.
>
> When we got to Natchez, Woo Foster was not too far from his home near Monroe. He said: "Take me to the bus station and if you all can buy my ticket to Monroe, I'll give you my share in the car." The fare to Monroe, LA, was $2.30 so we scraped around and were still a little short. We went home and got 50 cents from my mother and we gave Woo the $2.30 and put him on the bus to Monroe, LA, and we inherited the car.
>
> We started the newspaper business and used the car to get around peddling the papers. That was in July. We didn't make enough money for both of us to be living off that paper. So we went to see about getting jobs as teachers.

Eddie stayed with his parents on China Grove for a few days before starting up the newspaper route in Natchez. Things were still pretty much the same on the farm, with his father working hard for very little income. Eddie could tell that his father was not well, and yet he was to give Eddie a piece of advice that Eddie considered his most important gift from his father.

In 1933 I spent three nights with my mother and father on China Grove. They were the only two left at home. My daddy was still sweating, still working and laboring in the fields and living in the same home at China Grove. Every time I looked, he would be getting up. He was sick.

He sat there in his chair and I sat down beside him and Mama was in the middle of us shelling corn to feed the chickens. We were sitting down out on the porch in the evening just about twilight time. I can see him now with the sweat on the shoulders of his shirt and his brow wet and damp with sweat. He lit up his corncob pipe and for the first time in my life, I'm twenty-one now, I decide to light up a cigarette in his presence. He said "Damn, I guess you think you are a man now don't you?" I said, "I guess I am." "Well, now you got your education what are you going to do with it?" I said, "I'm going to look for a job and go to work." "How are you going to find a job? It's going to be real rough and if you do, I don't see how you could be satisfied with it."

He got up from his rocking chair and said, "Get up and come here." I got up out of my chair to follow him. We walked out in front of the house to the east. He said, "I want you to look over there as far as you can see. See all that land? You see all those trees; you see that creek down there? That's mine." He turned me west then and said, "Look there. As far as you can see, that is mine. Now you can go and work for somebody if you want to, but let me tell you something. You will never be a man unless you become your own boss. I own every damn bit of this land and even though I am poor, I have the freedom of knowing that it is mine. And that feeling is worth more than anything else you can get." Telling me this was the biggest thing that he ever did for me.

Eddie's father was right. There weren't many jobs available for an educated black man in Natchez. Eddie ended up going back to the stand-by of teaching.

> I started out that Monday searching for a job. Finally, I went to the superintendent of schools in Natchez, a Mr. Brady, and got a job as a teacher in Natchez College. School was opening the next Monday. I went to one teacher's meeting. That Friday I got a special delivery letter from Morehouse stating they had recommended me for a scholarship at Atlanta University and asking if I would come back. I contacted them right away. They said they were offering me a one-year scholarship to come back and study towards a Master's degree in education. I didn't want education, I wanted science. But then, education was better than nothing.
>
> Now, I had a job and a scholarship. My brother Douglas, on the other hand, only had the newspaper business. I thought if he took the teaching job and the newspaper business he could live. So we went up to see Mr. Brady. I figured no one knew me anyway. I had only been to one teacher's meeting. I explained to him what happened and asked if he would have any objection to my brother taking over the job that I had. He was pleased that I was going to get a further degree and readily agreed. I got on a train and went back to Atlanta to spend one more year there from 1933 to 1934.

The graduate school of Atlanta University was beginning to flourish in 1933. New dormitories had just opened for men and women graduate students and John Hope had begun to put together a faculty, including W. E. B. DuBois, that equaled that of any school in the country. John Hope's health was greatly diminished by a heart attack he had suffered in June. Despite his attempts to work, he had to delegate many of his duties to other members of the administration. Florence Read, the president of Spelman since 1929 and the treasurer of Morehouse during the Archer presidency, was a close friend to John Hope.[19] It was to her that many of his duties fell during the last years of President Hope's life. Following Dr. Hope's death in 1936 until they elected his successor in 1937, Mrs. Read acted as president of Atlanta University. It was Florence Read whom Eddie recalled when he remembered his year at Atlanta University:

> I just sailed through education like nothing and wrote a thesis: "A Comparative Study of Negro Students

in Rural and Urban Schools." The urban scores were higher due to environmental differences and the opportunity for further education of the urban blacks. Many of the kids were born in the country and never left their county. The chance for expansion of their minds was limited. I studied under Dr. Whiting, who was a psychologist at Morehouse and Atlanta University. He was a beautiful friend. I worked hard in the library and I completed the courses and the thesis in one year.

When I went for the defense of my thesis, my orals, I had to confront the head of the department, a Dr. Nathan, who was from the Isles and had a Jamaican accent. Dr. Whiting and Mrs. Ferguson, who was in secondary education, highly recommended me and said that I was ready for the degree and had satisfied the requirements. Dr. Nathan said: "We can't give you a master's degree for one year of work." He was very adamant. We don't want to lose the caliber of student that you are in one year. We want you around another year and extra credits you earn can be put towards a Ph.D. The others said they would take it to Florence Read. So we did. She said: "Why shouldn't he get the degree if he is qualified?" But then she opened her book and said, financially, I would not be able to graduate because I still owed $425. All that time, I had been working scrubbing and polishing the floors. That was how I kept my expenses down.

In the meantime, my sister and brothers had gotten together and chipped in to give Mama a trip up to see me graduate. All my colleagues heard about it. They were upset, especially Charles Beckett, who is a CPA now. The word began to get around. The students went in as a delegation to see Florence Read to complain about it. She finally gave in and told Charles to bring me to her office.

Everyone had their caps and gowns on getting ready to march. Beckett came up to me laughing. I was in the lavatory, really disappointed. He used to call me Colonel all the time. He said: "Colonel, come with me, Miss Read wants to see you." I had a brown suit on. I had on my

> one white shirt that I could take the collar off and wash it and put it back on so I always looked clean. I would wash that collar every night. I had the tie in my hand. We ran down the street and everybody was in the march line waiting to go in. We went to Miss Read's office. She was waiting for me and had papers there. She said: "Mazique, your colleagues are disturbed because you're not marching. If you are willing to sign this document that says you agree to pay me a certain number of dollars each month until the full amount is paid back, you can march." I smiled and I signed it. When I walked across to get that degree you should have heard the thunderous applause. My mother was there. It was the first time she had ever been on a train.

With a master's degree in education, Eddie was promptly offered a job teaching for the state education system of Georgia at Forsyth State Teacher's and Agricultural College. There was a reorganization going on in the schools as the Board of Regents slowly began to realize the state needed to offer blacks some sort of a high school education. The emphasis, however, had not changed: education was still to be mainly in agricultural and industrial subjects—something relevant to the kinds of jobs available. All the teachers and the administrators at the college were black but still the white Board of Regents maintained control.

Forsyth, Georgia, was a small country village located some seventy miles southeast of Atlanta on the way to Macon. The bank, shoe store, restaurant, doctors' offices, food market, haberdashery, and upstairs dentist all inhabited buildings that were clustered near a monument that let you know you were in the center of town. Everyone knew everyone else; the whites knew the blacks and vice versa. They all knew where everyone worked and the teachers at the college were treated with respect by the residents and addressed as "professor." Relationships were generally courteous. Blacks were welcome to consult a white doctor in town or a husband-and-wife team of black doctors named Boddie who had both graduated from Meharry Medical College. If illness necessitated surgery, there was a basement in the hospital in Macon where blacks could be operated on by white surgeons, black physicians not being allowed to practice in the hospital.

Eddie and his colleagues could go into the restaurants to get something to eat as long as they went through the back door. Blacks couldn't sit down anywhere to eat; they had to take it out. As a matter of course, the blacks removed their hats when they walked out with their dinner. There were no black businesses right in the town of Forsyth. There was one prominent black family named Bush. Mr. Bush was noted throughout the area as having one of the best barbecues in the county. He would dig a pit on his own farm and build a huge fire. He would spend the whole day Friday and Friday night barbecuing pigs. He made it quite a ritual. There would be people around enjoying themselves and eating when he was carving. You could always see cars, including some belonging to whites, driving up to get their barbecue. That was it for black enterprise in Forsyth.

The college was located a few miles from the town in the countryside. There wasn't much in the way of entertainment in Forsyth. Fifteen miles away in Griffin, Georgia, there was a movie theater that was segregated. Blacks were allowed to go upstairs and sit in what they called the "buzzards' roost." Most of the entertainment for the faculty and students was provided by athletics and camaraderie with others from the college. The people at the college were very dedicated, grateful, and proud. They were proud of themselves and proud of what they were doing. It gave them a lift in self-esteem despite their poverty. There never seemed to be a dull moment. With the athletic programs, the teaching, the social programs, and the escapades with the females around the area, Eddie and his friends managed to have a lot of fun.

Eddie and his fellow faculty members initially lived in rooms on the campus. It was not a glamorous place. Eddie had a little back room that had no plaster and no heat. There were cracks all over the ceilings and walls. Their mattresses were made out of corn shucks and when the wind blew, it would blow through the cracks and shake the shucks. They tried to improve their conditions with oil heaters but they were of little avail against the winds that whistled through their quarters. The food was not much better than the accommodations. The main ingredient in every dish seemed to be kale and not much else.

It wasn't long before Eddie and several of his colleagues figured out that there were certain advantages to living off campus. There was a lady who lived up the street named Mrs. Gordon, whom they affectionately called "Hookey." For a fee of twenty-one dollars per month they were treated to a cozy room, three meals a day, and clean laundry. The faculty was paid eighty dollars per month so they were able to manage well. Soon there were three other young professors living at Hookey's house: Josh Archer, Samuel Archer's son and Eddie's good friend from Morehouse; Shipwreck Kelly, also from Morehouse; and

Iris Glover, who had been a football star at Hampton. They congregated together with G. M. Sampson, the elder statesman of the group, and had a wonderful time.

As with most black colleges of the day, Forsyth served mainly as a high school for blacks whose education had ended abruptly after the eighth grade. The majority of the students were teachers who had taught for years and yet had never obtained a high school education. The main goal of the college was to test and upgrade the quality of black teachers in the state.

In the summer of 1934, at twenty-two, Eddie was hired as the head of the science department. The fall found him moved to director of the Department of Education. Although continuing to teach mostly science courses, he was also responsible for administering the program for the testing and upgrading of the teachers.

These were still the Depression years but they were also the time of Franklin Delano Roosevelt's "alphabetized" programs to reach and assist the downtrodden and underprivileged. Under the National Youth Administration (NYA), Forsyth would seek out worthy students all over the state of Georgia and give them scholarships. During the summer of 1935, it was Eddie's job to travel the state to interview and recruit students who wanted to come to college to study to be teachers. Eddie remembered this part of his summer fondly:

> I would go all over the whole state to high schools and interview students whom the principals would recommend and give them scholarships with an emphasis on teacher training. This was enjoyable for me. I got paid extra for each mile I drove in my car. The recruitment raised my salary. I got to see all the different cities in Georgia and the different kinds of people. It gave me the best course in humanities that I could ever want to have. When I look back I know that that experience taught me more about dealing with people than anything I have ever had to do in my life. I had to visit the homes of the prospective students. I had to have a knowledge of families: what they were going through, their relationships, their domestic problems, and their social problems. It was a very rich experience.

One can imagine the impression Eddie made during those trips. A young, good-looking man, smartly dressed, sparkling with that Morehouse polish and his own special sense of humor. What student would not want to go to Forsyth?

Eddie's joy in his job and his academic life at Forsyth were dampened by the telegram he received notifying him of his father's death in the summer of 1935. His mother had written several letters letting Eddie know that Alex was ill and had been taken to New Orleans for surgery. There was only one old hospital in Natchez and that had meager facilities, but even what was there was generally not available to blacks. If blacks were taken into the hospital they were taken to a little basement room. In New Orleans, Alex was able to get into a hospital that treated people who were too poor to pay. He had surgery and died of cancer of the colon at the relatively young age of fifty-seven.

The long train trip from Georgia to Natchez gave Eddie time to think. He was deeply shaken by his father's death—a world without Alex would not be the same. And what was to become of Addie with all the family away from Natchez except Douglas, who was planning on leaving to go to medical school as soon as he saved enough money?

Everyone made it home for the funeral. Uncle Doc still owned Oakland and so Alex Jr. was able to be buried with his father, his mother, and his two daughters near the Railey family plot.

The possibility that his father might still be living if he had had adequate medical care haunted Eddie. He returned to Forsyth more determined than ever to go into medicine.

By 1936 Eddie had become the dean of instruction, second only to the president. In his new capacity he had more input on policy issues and the formation of curricula. One of Eddie's favorite duties was the supervision of the exchange teacher training program, an innovative system sponsored by the Board of Regents. When students were ready to do their practice teaching, they were sent to rural schools in the surrounding counties and the teachers from the rural schools went to Forsyth, enabling them to further their education while the student teachers gained practical experience. The rural schools all had one-room classrooms where the student teacher would have to plan lessons and teach as many as thirty or forty students who ranged from the third to the eighth grades. During their exchange experience, the student teachers would live in the community where they were teaching and handle all the responsibilities of the regular teacher.

The student teachers and the pupils and their families held a special place in Eddie's memory. Each of them seemed to have a history that was already rich in experiences, like the poor young student who had polio whom Eddie saw coming to school each day on a go-cart pulled by a goat, much like the Porgy character in the 1959 movie *Porgy and Bess.* And there was Colley Rakestraw, a sharp young lady who became one of Eddie's favorites. Colley's story is unique and yet representative of the hardships faced and overcome by the students of Forsyth.[20]

Colley had come from a family that had been well-to-do. Her father, Lafayette Rakestraw, was a retired teacher who had gone into farming. He was so successful that his farm became one of the model farms for the University of Georgia. Lafayette was well respected in the community and frequently was asked to sign notes so sharecroppers could borrow money from the bank. Things went well until the boll weevil hit Georgia. The sharecroppers could not pay back their loans and Lafayette became responsible for their debts. It took all his savings and would have taken his home as well had not one of his sons, who had done well in Detroit, stepped in to pay off the mortgage.

At age twenty, Colley decided she wanted to finish her high school education. She had already completed the seventh grade, which was all the schooling offered to blacks by her small town. There was no money in the Rakestraw family available for education so she typed a letter to the college asking if they could give her a scholarship. In less than a week she had a letter back saying if she could type, they would be happy to offer her a scholarship for room and board and she would only have to pay three dollars per month tuition. In order to decide in what grade to put students, Forsyth tested them when they entered the school. Colley scored the highest, surpassing even the seniors. She was placed in the tenth grade and began catching up.

Colley started off in Eddie's biology class and remembers well the impression he made on the students. Eddie was a handsome young man who naturally made a hit with the young females in the class. However, he seemed to be just as popular with the male students. Professor Mazique was a wonderful teacher—demanding, yet full of fun. One day the students were told to draw amoebas on the board. Everyone had completed their task except a diminutive student named Jimmy Rodgers. Professor Mazique continued with his lecture and would turn around periodically to find that Jimmy was still standing there and had not drawn anything on the board. Finally Eddie asked Jimmy where his amoeba was. Jimmy pointed to the board and said, "Here it is." Eddie looked at the blank board and said, "I don't see it." Jimmy calmly replied, "It's microscopic, you can't see it." The class and the teacher broke into peals of laughter that could be heard throughout the other classrooms.

According to Colley, it was not just the students who loved Eddie; all the staff seemed to feel the same. She said they all thought of him as ethereal—just a little too good to be walking on the earth.

Colley was one of those student teachers who were sent to a small rural town to live and to teach. She boarded with a local family and handled all the responsibilities associated with teaching. The school where she taught had never seen the likes of her. She coaxed the parents into spending their hard-earned leisure time in planting shrubs and landscaping the schoolyard. The white superintendent who was in charge of both the "Nigra" (as they were called then in Georgia) and the white schools was invited by Colley to come to see the students' exhibits. Much to everyone's surprise he came, explaining he had never attended before because he was never invited.

As the supervisor of the program, Professor Mazique visited Colley and the other student teachers twice a week to hold conferences and make suggestions. Getting around to the communities was not always easy, but what Eddie learned about human nature and the plight of the poor and elderly was to stay with him and influence his decisions throughout his career.

> I had purchased a Chevrolet for my travel and that was how I got around. Going through the winter months of Georgia with the muddy roads was quite an ordeal. Many times I would go down there with an automobile and get stuck in that red mud. Once you got in a ditch with slipping and sliding there was no way you could get out. More than once I sought help from nearby farmers to bring some mules to pull me out of the ditch.
>
> I learned a lot from the people I taught. The individuals were much older than I and had lots of experiences. I respected those experiences. I spent a lot of time, not only teaching them, but also visiting their homes and learning of their trials and tribulations, meeting their sons and daughters and coming to understand about their lives.
>
> I would visit our student teachers in the country schools where they were teaching. They would have all the way up to eighth grade in one room heated only with a potbellied stove. There was a lot of poverty in this area. Most people had only the bare necessities of life—very

> little in the way of comfort. In the eyes of many of the family members you could see resignation and only a few dim rays of hope for the future. Yet they carried on.
>
> I would listen to debates in the school building at night: What is more important, the plow or the cultivator? Then on Sunday I would go to church there and sometimes even do the preaching.
>
> Out of my conversations with them, I gained a lot of information on the needs of the elderly and the poor. I considered this an invaluable learning experience for me.

One of the homes Eddie visited was the Crawford home in Forsyth. Two of the boys and one girl were in Eddie's classes. It just happened that during one of his visits their sister Jewell, who was a student at Spelman, Morehouse's sister college, was home for a visit. Eddie remembered her from when he was a student at Atlanta University. How could he forget? Jewell was beautiful and intelligent and sure to catch any young man's eye. They had only spoken in passing when Eddie was in Atlanta, but her home in Forsyth gave him an excellent opportunity to get to know her better. Their relationship blossomed.

Jewell was not only very bright but also very ambitious. After receiving her bachelor's degree from Spelman, she applied to Howard University in Washington, D.C., and proceeded to obtain a master's degree in history while working at the Library of Congress. During all this time, she and Eddie continued to communicate through letters, and the distance did not dampen their ardor.

The governor of Georgia during Eddie's stay at Forsyth was Eugene Talmadge. He and the president of Forsyth, Mr. Hubbard, were on good terms, and this relationship was especially helpful in securing funding for projects at the school. As Eddie recalls, Governor Talmadge was an easy man to remember:

> The governor of Georgia was Eugene Talmadge. Characteristically, old Gene wore red suspenders. In the summertime, he would take his coat off and walk around popping those red suspenders. It was known that he was not afraid to take a drink from a jug with an old corn cob stuck in it. He was a very popular man.
>
> The political dynasty continued—Herman Talmadge carried on as a senator from Georgia. If you went into

> Herman's office you would see his daddy's suspenders hanging right up there. On the side there was a brass spittoon where his father had spit his tobacco. Herman continued the family tradition of aiding black education by serving on the board of the medical school at Morehouse College.
>
> If President Hubbard wanted anything for the school, he would talk to Gene, the governor, and he would come away with it. One time when the governor was called to Kentucky to make a speech for a black agricultural conference, he told the people that he couldn't make it but he would send the black governor of Georgia to make the speech. He pulled up to the campus in a car with two motorcycles around it in a flare of dust. Mr. Hubbard called me in and said in his nasal voice, "Professor Mazique, the governor has invited me to take his place at an educational conference. I will be introduced as the black governor of Georgia. While I am gone, I want you to serve as acting president of the institution." He stayed away for two or three weeks once he found out that I was doing all right.

Eddie's relationship with the members of the Board of Regents for the Georgia school system was amenable. However, despite their assistance to Forsyth and the updating of the black educational system, the board still had a limited idea of what education for blacks should entail. They would come to the school and discuss how they wanted to ensure the "Nigras" a better chance of learning. Yet they maintained their own opinions of the learning they considered important and the proper place of blacks in society. Black education should be centered on agricultural and teaching skills. They insisted the students be trained to be good Christians while at the same time convincing them that any attempt to change the system would be an abuse to their religion and Christianity in general. In 1936, Eddie agreed to take over the principalship of a school in Athens, Georgia, for the summer. However, Eddie's ideas of education and theirs were so at variance that he could not see his way clear to accepting a permanent high school position when they offered it. Besides, Eddie's goal was still medicine, and by the summer of 1937 Eddie had saved enough money to at least enter Howard University in Washington, D.C., to begin his medical career. As Eddie recalled,

> As I was in the process of making a decision to do this, there were several people with whom I consulted. One was my brother Douglas, who was in Natchez teaching. We both made the decision that we should go to medical school. Douglas decided he would go to Meharry. I in turn made an application to go to Howard.
>
> Another factor that prompted me to move forward into medical school was a letter I had received from a very dear classmate of mine at Morehouse named Charles Beckett, who was a CPA. By that time, he was working in Chicago and doing well. As I was advising him of my proposed change and that financially I was at very low ebb, he stated: "So what do you have to lose—you never had any money, anyhow? You had no money to begin with and you made it through Morehouse with a B.S. and Atlanta University with a M.E." With that advice, I made a definite decision to leave Georgia.

Eddie was sad to leave his old friends at Forsyth, but the timing was propitious. The spirits and enthusiasm of the faculty had been dampened by a scandal about the misuse of funds. One of the men who had been secretary to the president had inflated the number of students who were attending in order to increase the funding. A Board of Regents investigation showed there were students listed who were never enrolled in the college. They never did figure out exactly where the money went. The entire atmosphere of the college changed. There was a severe decay in morale, and the faculty never again would approach their tasks at Forsyth with the same joie de vivre. Also, at this juncture, Douglas had just been accepted at Meharry Medical College and would be entering in the fall. Naturally, Washington had the additional appeal for Eddie of being the current residence of Jewell Crawford.

Eddie made the trip to Washington with a friend and, as usual, made an adventure out of it.

> Before heading out, I had only one material possession and that was an automobile, a 1936 Chevrolet. I decided to stop over in Atlanta and sell the vehicle because I would need the funding for school. I sold it for $250. When this was done, I felt I had entered the realm of richness.

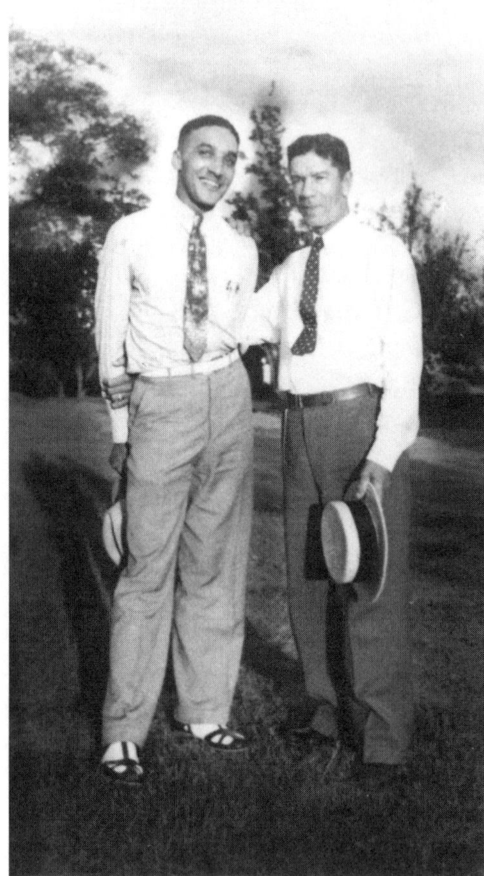

**Fig. 11:**
Dr. Mazique (left) with G. M. Sampson, mathematics teacher at State Teachers College, Forsyth, Georgia, in 1937. Photo courtesy of Maude Mazique and Dolores Pelham.

Mr. Sampson, who headed the department of mathematics at the school, was going up for a vacation. I got in with him and we began to drive in his Ford automobile called "Tilly" through the various states. It represented a great transformation for me. Every mile of the way was sheer excitement. We passed through Georgia, South Carolina, North Carolina, and headed into Virginia. Finally, when we got to the Potomac, Mr. Sampson said to me, "Look, there is the Washington Monument," and he began to explain to me about the buildings and the nation's capital. I was simply enchanted by these things that at one time I felt I would never be able to see.

We had little or no difficulty on the road as far as discrimination was concerned because we knew that we were forbidden to go into the front of places to secure food and had to go to the back. We were thoughtful enough to have our food packed into a shoebox and we munched on cold chicken and bread throughout the trip.

We crossed the Potomac and headed into Washington, D.C., and headed directly for the YMCA on 12th Street. After spending one night there, Mr. Sampson left me alone and cut me loose and said, "You are on your own." That was the last time I saw him.

# CHAPTER FOUR 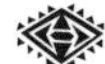

# The Nation's Capital

## A City of Inconsistencies

> There is a time to do everything. There is a time for striking, a time when you don't strike. There is a time when you move forward, there is a time when you retreat and think and decide, refurbish your forces and make new plans and go out again. When I came up to Washington and walked into church and found they would tell me to come back here to sit, the timing was then. I just kept walking and walked out of the church.
>
> — *Edward C. Mazique, interview with author, 1984*

Over the years, race relations in Washington, D.C., were anything but consistent. At times, blacks and whites peacefully coexisted. At other times, there was animosity and hostility between the races. During some eras, whites even commingled and socialized with blacks with ease and grace. It is impossible to understand what Washington was like when Eddie arrived without knowing a bit of the history of these race relations.[1]

Washington, D.C., and the then-adjacent municipality of Georgetown were centers of liberalism in the pre–Civil War South. With the exception of New Orleans, they offered their black residents a more cohesive community and greater opportunities than were provided by any other southern city. By the outbreak of the Civil War, blacks in the District owned $650,000 worth of real estate and supported their own churches and schools.[2]

The Civil War found blacks streaming into Washington, threatening to upset the fragile social relationships between the long-time black and white residents. Housing and food were insufficient and the resulting health conditions were deplorable. This increase in poor, unemployed blacks brought with it an increase in white hostility.

However, from the conclusion of the Civil War through the 1870s there was a rapid growth of civil rights for the District's black residents. Washington served as a showcase for laws the various legislators believed should be enacted to protect and extend the rights of black citizens, laws that, since their jobs were dependent on voters in their own states, at times they would hesitate to propose in their home locales. As a result, antidiscrimination laws were tougher in Washington than in the rest of the country. Blacks were allowed to serve on juries. Racial discrimination was forbidden in most places of entertainment, barber shops, bars, bathing houses, and ice cream parlors, and the word *white* was removed from the District charter wherever it appeared. Education was viewed as an important means of upgrading the quality of life for black residents and, in 1867, Howard University, including a medical department, was chartered to serve as a model for biracial education. In 1869 and 1870, there was even talk in Congress of abrogating the charter of the District Medical Society after they refused to admit to membership three qualified physicians of African descent. Race relations seemed to be improving so much that when a stronger antidiscrimination law was proposed by a black councilman, two of his fellow black councilmen argued it was unnecessary since racial prejudice was rapidly disappearing.[3]

By the late 1870s, however, such optimism was gone as conditions for blacks began to worsen again. The gulf between the blacks who had succeeded and those who remained in poverty increased, taking away any sense of oneness in the black community. Supreme Court decisions started working against integration. In 1883, the Waite Court declared the Civil Rights Act unconstitutional in the states, and in *Plessy v. Ferguson* (1896) it was determined that if facilities were "separate but equal" they met the requirements of the Fourteenth Amendment. Segregated housing began to be the norm in D.C. and, by the end of the century, equality under the law had pretty much disappeared. In 1884, in the midst of these worsening racial conditions, black physicians, prohibited from joining the District Medical Society (the local organization sanctioned by the American Medical Association) because of race, founded their own medical society, the Medico-Chirurgical Society, to further professional improvement, with functions paralleling its white counterpart.[4]

By the early 1900s the living conditions for the very poor blacks had somewhat improved while the middle- and upper-class blacks became subject to greater and greater humiliations and defeats. The genial relations that had existed between the upper classes of people of different races had all but disappeared. A social worker observed, in 1908 in Washington, "the separation of the races is more nearly complete than in any other city of the Union. The better class of white and colored people know absolutely nothing of each other."[6]

It was not only the interaction between races that was disappearing. More importantly, it was the hard-won rights of the black residents that were eroding at a fast pace. Soon after the turn of the century came attempts in the District and in the federal government to force the segregation of the races in public places with the imposition of what were termed "Jim Crow" laws. Changes in presidential administrations did little to correct the injustices. The inauguration of Woodrow Wilson in 1912 brought even fewer appointments for blacks to federal positions, and throughout his administration discrimination increased in the federal workplace. Separate work areas, lunch tables, and toilet facilities became the standard in federal departments. During this time, the Supreme Court decided the Civil Rights Act of 1875 was unconstitutional not only in the states but also in federal territories, which included the District. Although blacks had already begun to be barred or separated from whites in theaters, restaurants, hotels, and places where they had previously been guaranteed access, the removal of the final barricade of protection, no matter how flimsy, made it even easier for the legislators to proceed along the path toward complete segregation.[6]

The one positive factor that seemed to come out of this diminution of black rights was that it forced blacks into a more cohesive group. The elites began to see they had something in common with their poorer brothers and sisters. It was no longer that well-to-do blacks were acceptable and poor blacks were discriminated against. They were all faced with discrimination, no matter how lofty their position. When the black Register of the Treasury and a black companion dared to lunch in the House Office Building restaurant, something that in the past would not have caused a stir, five congressmen protested and threatened a boycott.[7]

The 1906 Niagara Movement claimed four prominent Washingtonians among its ranks. The District residents, like educated blacks around the country, were turning away from the apolitical tactics of Booker T. Washington. The National Association for the Advancement of Colored People (NAACP) was founded in New York in 1909, and by 1916 the Washington branch, headed largely by black leaders, boasted the largest (1,164 members) and arguably the most active branch.[8] Blacks began a more concerted effort to patronize black establishments rather than those that practiced Jim Crowism. A black YMCA was built with black labor and this is where the Medico-Chirurgical Society along with other black community groups held their meetings. While far from a totally unified community, blacks were showing more racial spirit or at least less divisiveness than had been in evidence for the past thirty years. Along with protest, a new sense of racial pride seemed to be in the offing.

The hope was that with their courageous participation in World War I, black servicemen would have proven themselves worthy of equal rights. Instead, their achievements went unrecognized and the gulf between the races increased. Race riots erupted in Washington in 1919 as a result of attacks on black men by white servicemen. When the riots were over, thirty-nine men, black and white, had lost their lives due to injuries incurred during the riots. Yet Congress failed to investigate.

Conditions for blacks improved very little under the Harding and Coolidge administrations, and by the end of the late 1920s parks and beaches were closed to blacks; the only places where segregation did not reign were on trolleys and buses, at Griffith Stadium, the public library, and the reading rooms of the Library of Congress. With the 1926 Supreme Court decision upholding the legality of voluntary covenants, segregated housing patterns became institutionalized and upper-class blacks lost what was left of their mobility.[9]

Perhaps one of the most blatant indications of worsening race relations was the lack of attention and concern expressed by the white press and Congress when, in 1922, the District Ku Klux Klan was formed. But it was the dedication of the Lincoln Memorial on Decoration Day in 1922 that made the position of blacks in Washington all too clear. One of the featured speakers, Robert Moten, president of Tuskegee Institute, and other "honored" black guests were grudgingly shown their seats by a surly marine who obviously did not approve of seating the "niggers" even if it was in an all-Negro section separated from the rest of the audience by a road.

There were a few bright spots for blacks during these years: the appointment of the first black president of Howard University, Mordecai Johnson, and the election of the first black congressman in the twentieth century, Oscar De Priest of Chicago, to the House. However, the promise of a unified black community was far from realized. Petty jealousies continued to divide blacks at all levels, even at Howard University, where a verbal attack on Mordecai Johnson by a black professor at a trustees' dinner undercut an increase in congressional appropriations to the institution. "Passing" as white became common among the lighter-skinned, upper-class blacks. Highland Beach, the summer colony for blacks that had been founded by Frederick Douglass's son, banned darker-skinned blacks. And the taste in literature and the arts among the upper-crust blacks was not supportive of the work of young artists who were proud of their black heritage. This lack of support led to an exodus of young black talent to cities like New York, where the "Harlem Renaissance" was welcoming the skills of black writers, artists, and musicians.

As the decade of the 1920s neared its end, forward progress in race relations was made when the soon-to-be-formed Community Chest of Washington chose as a fundraiser Elwood Street, a man who insisted that residents and community organizations be included as part of the Community Chest regardless of race. At his insistence, black and white Washingtonians again began meeting and discussing common problems. Although far from a panacea for race relations, it was an opening, at last, in the wall that had separated the two communities, clearing the way for contacts in other areas.

With the crash of the stock market in 1929 and the following Depression, many Americans began to question the old assumption that if blacks were not so lazy and would just work harder they could pull themselves out of poverty. For the first time they began to understand that there were aspects of a person's life over which the individual had no control.

With Roosevelt's New Deal, less was done for blacks than had been anticipated. Ninety percent of the federal government jobs held by blacks remained custodial in nature. Racial segregation in housing actually increased. The formation of the Civilian Conservation Corps in 1933 evidenced the amount of discrimination still considered tolerable during Roosevelt's administration: Southern states insisted on and were allowed to have separate camps for black and white recruits, and the number of blacks actually admitted to the integrated camps in the North was very small. Racial discrimination also was in evidence under the U.S. Employment Service at the District Center. White and black applicants were made to go to separate buildings to seek employment. However, this insult to their egos was far overshadowed by the discriminatory practice in job listings in the two different buildings: the whites were offered every category of work opportunities while the job listings for blacks were largely confined to domestic work and common labor.[10]

Despite these setbacks, there were some positive strides made during the Roosevelt administration. Mrs. Roosevelt's interest in and concern for "colored people" and the institution of fair and color-blind policies by Harold Ickes, the secretary of the interior, and Harry Hopkins of the Works

Progress Administration made for some advances. Especially impressive was the addition of a clause by Secretary Ickes requiring any company contracting with the Interior Department to follow nondiscriminatory policies in their employment practices. When the new Department of the Interior building opened in 1937, it housed a completely nonsegregated cafeteria.

There were also some heartening signs within the black community indicating they would finally unite to challenge injustices. In an attempt to persuade the new federal agencies to institute nondiscriminatory policies, a group of national Negro organizations banded together as the Joint Committee on National Recovery. At the same time a group of young Washington activists, including William Hastie, who was soon to be appointed the federal judge for the Virgin Islands; Robert C. Weaver, the first black who would be appointed a member of the president's cabinet; and Charles Hamilton Houston, a brilliant young lawyer who was later to become a special counsel of the NAACP as well as Eddie's lawyer and friend, formed the New Negro Alliance. Many of the stores within black neighborhoods were owned and manned by whites. The Alliance advocated a policy of "Buy where you work," advocating that blacks should not patronize stores that refused to hire blacks. They suggested picketing and boycotting businesses that refused to supply jobs to black workers. Some of the black community, including many Howard professors, criticized this strategy, arguing that it was racist and would make matters worse, but when three hundred jobs were filled by black workers as a result of these boycotts, criticism by local blacks died and blacks in other cities started emulating the Alliance technique. The boycott was ineffective against some of the larger companies that could absorb the loss, but a Supreme Court decision in 1938 upheld the legality of the boycott and strengthened confidence in the Supreme Court as a means of correcting racial injustices.[11]

Those who came to Howard University in the 1930s found themselves facing contradictory social cues: the university with all its black luminaries on the faculty evidencing all that blacks could achieve, and a city with backward southern racial ideas. Many of those arriving were prepared by their own background in southern cites. Dr. Hildrus A. Poindexter, one of the country's foremost bacteriologists with a medical degree from Dartmouth, was one of Eddie's professors at Howard. Born and raised in Tennessee, when he came to Washington he felt he was already conditioned to the type of treatment he was to receive there; as he said, "You survived."[12]

On the other hand, Dr. Paul Cornely, who was Eddie's public health teacher and came to Howard to teach in 1934, had more difficulty adjusting. Originally from the West Indies, he had lived in Puerto Rico, New York, and Detroit. Although realizing beforehand that D.C. was "like any other southern town," he found it difficult to accept some of the restrictions, especially in the churches. When blacks attended predominately white churches, they were made to sit in the back or on the side. During communion, blacks had to wait until all the whites had received communion before they were served. When his wife went to shop for clothing, she found she was not allowed to try on dresses or other articles of clothing in the department stores. At one point, when the president of the University of Michigan Medical School, the school from which he had received his degree, came to visit, he realized there was no place to take him for a dinner except the train station, Union Station, the only nonsegregated restaurant in D.C.[13]

It was into this highly segregated, racially prejudiced, frequently humiliating, yet constantly changing city that Eddie brought his high aspirations and dreams. He was nervous about leaving the South and the world he understood, if not accepted, to head north. He promptly found he had not escaped the degrading effects of southern segregation by his move; yet once he saw Howard University and realized what it had to offer, he knew he had chosen correctly, despite his reservations.

Although small in comparison to some of the major universities (less than three thousand students), Howard looked huge to Eddie. All the edifices and all the students were more than he could take in with one look. The buildings were embellished with finery and a decor that Eddie had been unable to envision from his experiences at Morehouse or Forsyth.[14]

It was not just the physical aspects of Howard that made a strong first impression on Eddie, but the intellectual atmosphere and the inhabitation by famous black scholars that went beyond impressive to downright intimidating. It would be easier to discuss who among the black intelligentsia was not at Howard during the thirties than those who were. There were very few opportunities at major universities for black scholars, and so many of the best took refuge at Howard. To name but a few: in sociology there was E. Franklin Frazier; Dean of the Law School William Hastie; Ralph Bunche in political science; Charles Drew in pathology; Howard Thurman and James L. Farmer in religion; and perhaps most impressive of all, Howard's first black president, Mordecai W. Johnson. The tall, pale, robust man came to Howard University in 1926 as a second-choice, compromise candidate, but he was to rule

Howard University as if his presidency had been ordained by God. There was little doubt he thought it was. Johnson was a strong-willed man, one toward whom few people held moderate opinions.

There is little argument that it was he who built Howard into a fully accredited university with a cosmopolitan community of scholars. He secured money for new buildings and more and better faculty. With two appointments in 1929, he ensured the legitimacy of the medical school under the direction of Dr. Numa P. G. Adams and the Law School with Charles Hamilton Houston as vice-dean.

Johnson had received his early education at Roger Williams University in Nashville, Tennessee, the school that Eddie's father and aunts had all attended. He was a man who evidenced great control. He seldom lost his temper, except perhaps in Board of Trustees meetings, but his ability to convey "controlled anger" was itself intimidating. Speaking from brief notes or completely off the cuff, he was an impressive orator with a phenomenal memory and a resonant voice.

President Johnson provided the faculty with a great deal of latitude in what was acceptable material to present to students. He was considered "one of the most fearless critics of American democracy in modern times."[15] As such, the faculty was guaranteed the freedom to teach and write pretty much what they wanted within reason. However, when it came to their relationship to the university, the faculty had little real control. Johnson maintained a tight grip on the power and they had little say in how the university was run. This lack of control led to many disputes, including arguments with some of the more prominent faculty such as Ernest Just and Kelly Miller. Johnson's disagreements were not limited to faculty but extended to alumni and sometimes to Congress. Yet through it all, Johnson was able to secure federal funding for Howard that assured its future as a major university.

Dr. Cornely was the medical director of Freedman's Hospital in the early Johnson years, and he remembered vividly President Johnson's presentations before the House Committee on Labor and Education.[16] Johnson gave such a masterful presentation that people would come just to hear him. The committee members showed a great deal of respect and would listen with rapt attention as Johnson presented his case for more funding for Howard.

What Johnson had done for the college, Dr. Numa P. G. Adams did for the medical school.[17] Initially, the school was held together by physicians who taught part time. The faculty received what the students paid and they split the money at the end of the school year. With the arrival of

Adams under the auspices of the Rockefeller Foundation, the medical school was promptly turned into a professionally accredited institution. With the further assistance of the Rockefeller Foundation, fellowships were offered to individuals to earn degrees in their specialties and then come back to teach at Howard. Drs. Paul Cornely, Montague Cobb, Charles Drew, Robert Jason, and Joseph L. Johnson were among those who came in under this special fellowship program. Salaries were still low, $3,500, when Dr. Cornely started at Howard in 1934, but at least they were consistent, allowing the faculty to teach full time.

When Eddie initially arrived in Washington, it was not Howard University or race relations that were the first thing on his mind—it was Jewell. Eddie had begun his stay in Washington at the YMCA, but he recalled that it was not to be his residence for long:

> My stay at the YMCA was short-lived. I was only there one or two weeks when I had had enough of the Y. Jewell was living in a room that could easily be shared. It was near the end of July and it didn't take long before I proposed marriage.
>
> On August 28th, 1937, we had a not-so-formal marriage ceremony. A former schoolmate at Morehouse named Brooks was also staying at the Y and I asked him if he were doing anything for the next fifteen or twenty minutes and he said, "No." So I asked him to come with me and be my best man and he did. While walking along the street, I saw a gentleman with his collar on backwards and assumed he was a minister. I stopped him and asked him if he would mind performing the marriage ceremony. I had two dollars in my pocket at the time and I offered to give it to him. He smiled and agreed and turned around and walked with us as we proceeded to go up to where Jewell was living on Fairmont Street. We were married and the ceremony hardly took ten minutes and it was all over. I walked in with the minister and the best man and that was all at the wedding except the landlord and the landlord's daughter.
>
> After the wedding, in the afternoon, Jewell's landlord, Jerome Osborn, asked where we were going on our honeymoon. This was August and I had already enrolled in medical school for September and we had very little

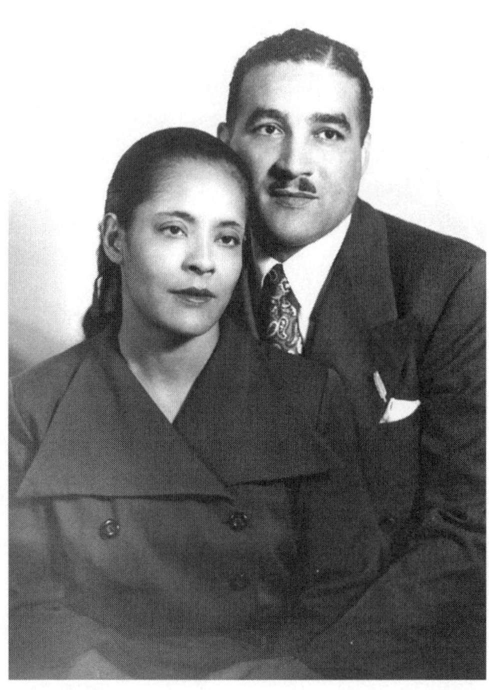

**Fig. 12:**
Jewell and Eddie in their early years together. Photo courtesy of Maude Mazique and Dolores Pelham.

money. Naturally, we weren't planning on going anywhere. So he said, "Okay, get in the car and I'll take you on your honeymoon." He drove us out to Arlington Cemetery and drove us all around in the late afternoon and showed us all the graves, the Tomb of the Unknown Soldier, the marchers and the tombstones. I don't know why he got the idea of taking us to a cemetery unless he wanted to give an opportunity to bury all that had gone before in our lives and have our wedding as a new beginning. We ended up staying in there a bit too long and the gates were locked so we couldn't get out. We were stuck there a little while until we got a guard to unlock it and let us out. Soon we got home and that was the end of our honeymoon.

Once things were settled with Jewell, Eddie was ready to get started at Howard. Eddie remembered Jewell during his time at Howard as being very encouraging of his studies:

> Her relationship with me during the entire time I was in medical school was indeed very supportive and she proved to be warm, affectionate, and beautiful. Intellectually, she had no peers as far as the promulgation of new ideas and her interests in advancement as far as education was concerned.

From their apartment it was an easy four-block walk to campus. The medical school had a small enrollment: only twenty-one in Eddie's class. They were warned, however, that even from this select group not all of them would graduate, and Eddie's yearbook shows that the warning was justified since only nineteen finished in 1941. Yet with classes this size, Howard Medical School was producing 48 percent of all Negro physicians and surgeons.[18]

Eddie found that Howard was very different from the colleges with which he was familiar. It did not have the southern hospitality and friendliness that he had grown accustomed to at Morehouse or Forsyth. And it was difficult for Eddie, who was older than most of his colleagues, to adjust to being a student once again. He remembered how difficult those first few months were:

> For the most part, the professors in the school of medicine were very cold and their mannerisms were entirely different from those which I experienced at Morehouse. Many times, a professor would be coming down the sidewalk and as he would be nearing me, he would hold his head high and turn so that he did not have to see me even for a moment to give me a cordial "Hello." I remember on one occasion when a question was asked in the class and I raised my hand to answer it, the professor said to me, "No. Let the other student answer the question because he has experience, he was born with a stethoscope around his neck and of course you just got out of the cornfield so there is no way for you to compete in this manner." So I quietly took a swallow and a big gasp and said nothing. This experience stayed with me.
>
> I didn't get too much encouragement or a feeling of warmth until I got to the department of parasitology. After spending some time with Dr. Poindexter, he stated

> to me: "Mazique, you are ready to go into clinical medicine and you are going to be a good doctor." This was the first time I had ever received any encouragement.
>
> Most of the students were several years younger. I was the only one in the class who was married. I was also the only one who had been out of school for three years and taught and was returning. I don't mind stating that it was difficult to get back in the habit of studying again. Once my mind settled on it, however, I did all right.

Eddie was impressed by many of the intellectual greats at Howard. He heard lectures by E. Franklin Frazier, Ralph Bunche, and Howard Thurman, but it was the professors of the medical school who were to have the biggest impact on him. Eventually, Eddie did become close to several of the professors and formed friendships that were to last throughout his life. Drs. Paul B. Cornely, Halston Eagleson, Joseph L. Johnson, Hildrus A. Poindexter, and M. Wharton Young all had a deservedly strong influence on Eddie. Each one of these physicians had his own impressive background and history. They had each met the massive challenges faced by blacks who wanted to enter medicine and they had succeeded. Each had fond memories of Eddie in his student days.[19] Eddie was an industrious student whom all of the other students liked and respected. He was always questioning, always wanting to understand more about what he was studying, traits that professors were bound to find endearing. Dr. Poindexter summed up the general consensus about Eddie by saying that he was "a good student, his assignments were always well done and he was very highly respected by his colleagues. He didn't wear anything which was antisocial on his shoulders. He seemed to have a good, wholesome philosophy of life: respect for mankind in general and politically active but not violent."[20]

It was not only the black professors who had a dramatic impact on him. Dr. Benjamin Karpman, a white psychiatrist who was to become well known in the late 1940s for his work on female alcoholics, made the students aware of their environment and their responses to it. Eddie recalled their dinner outing:

> Dr. Karpman said he was going to take the whole class out to dinner. I was nervous with anticipation. For the first time I was really about to visit a restaurant that the law stated had to serve blacks. It was at Union

> Station, the train depot in Washington, D.C. I think it was called Harvey's. The law in regard to transportation was that in facilities where the train stopped, everybody had to be served. This was the first time any of us had been there. Imagine how I felt and how the rest of the class felt to be going to a place in Washington that was integrated!
>
> Benny Karpman took this opportunity to pull out from his students how they felt on this occasion. The reactions were amazing. Some of the guys said, "I don't think I can eat here. I don't think it's right." Others thought they would not be able to keep their food down, they were so nervous. It just didn't seem right to many of them that they could sit down at a table and eat with white people in Washington, D.C.
>
> Psychiatry was not all that advanced at that point. You were either OK or you were crazy. Yet Benny Karpman showed us how to examine our own feelings about an issue that would be important to us throughout our lives. He was a great guy.

Eddie's arriving at Howard as an older student had both advantages and disadvantages. Since he had been away from studying for several years, his academic achievements were not as great as they would have been had he gone straight to medical school. Eddie was a better than average student, but not at the top of the class as was his custom. On the positive side, Eddie was more seasoned than the other students. Dr. Cornely remembered how he already had a deep maturity that made him conscious of problems of the disadvantaged of all races. The field of public health in which Dr. Cornely specialized was generally not appealing to the medical students who were not experienced enough to see the larger picture. Most of them did not realize the importance of immunization and prevention; they looked at it as some kind of social work. Dr. Cornely believed that "Mazique was sensitive enough, knew enough, to see that this was an important approach to the sort of problems that faced us."[21]

Financially, medical school was difficult but, as always, Eddie found a way to make money while he was going to school.

> The matter of survival was a great factor in my life because I was without finances, so being able to stay in school was a problem—working as well as studying.

> On weekends, I began working at the Olney Inn in Maryland as a waiter. This was attained as a result of meeting a dear friend, Eugene Robertson, who had been working there as a waiter and began to carry me out to wait tables.

By far his most successful venture was the bookstore. The manager of the bookstore was responsible for selling a wide variety of items to the medical students. After all expenses were paid, the profits were his. Eddie remembered when he started there, it was considered a way to work your way through medical school:

> There was one doctor who had started the bookstore whom I befriended and very soon I joined him in selling books and medical instruments (such as microscopes) to the medical students. It was his senior year and my freshman year. When he graduated I inherited the bookstore from him. When I took over, I was called into the dean's office of the School of Medicine, who told me forthrightly that Howard University was not going to assume any part of the bookstore and the responsibility was entirely mine. They did not want Howard University's name on it. If I failed to pay my bills or if there was a failure to maintain the proper ethics or moral concepts, he said I would be put out of school. With that challenge and that understanding, I continued to develop the bookstore and I ran it for the whole time that I was a student.

Dr. Numa P. G. Adams was the dean when Eddie started at the bookstore. Adams died before Eddie had finished medical school and Dr. Joseph L. Johnson took over as the dean. Dr. Johnson remembered how many improvements Eddie made in the operations of the bookstore and the expansion of the inventory.[22] Eddie remembered how he ran it so efficiently that the new dean came to realize it was a mistake that the university did not operate the bookstore itself:

> The bookstore was successful while I was there. Over the summer months, I ventured to take some of the instruments outside into the city and sell them to

various doctors in their respective locations throughout the entire medical community. I would receive goods on consignment, which meant that those I did not sell I was able to return and I would get a 10 to 20 percent commission. It proved to be very lucrative. In my senior year and my last year as the keeper of the bookstore, I was called in one day by the dean of the school, who requested I submit financial statements regarding the sales of the bookstore, and I complied. The custom was that I should designate some other student whom I felt was in need financially and this would be the individual to take over. My selection proved to be in vain when Dean Johnson looked at me and said, "Eddie, the day of the gravy train at the bookstore is over. Howard University is going to take over the bookstore." This they promptly did after I had brought it quite a long ways from where it was in the beginning.

Through the bookstore job, combined with waiting tables on weekends and during the summer as well as working in the post office during the holidays where I served as a mail clerk and a mail carrier, I managed to do pretty well. Occasionally, I would go as far as Annapolis to wait tables on New Year's Eve. I also served as a chauffeur for a salesman and worked in a filling station and pumped gas and greased automobiles in order to continue financing and funding.

It was not long before we could buy a Ford automobile for which we paid $125. It was running even though it was about a 1930 model. Soon I was carrying some of my fellow students out to other places where we would study medicine, like St. Elizabeth's, which, at the time, seemed like quite a distance away.

In 1941, Eddie graduated from Howard University with his medical degree. Opportunities for internships at that time were fairly limited. Generally, black graduates could continue their education only at Freedmen's Hospital in Washington, Meharry in Nashville, Homer G. Phillips Hospital in St. Louis, Harlem Hospital in New York, Provident Hospitals in Chicago and Baltimore and, in the 1930s, Cleveland City Hospital, which was the first white hospital to take blacks as interns.

There had long been a close relationship between Freedmen's Hospital and Howard University. The original "Freedman's" Hospital, as it was called then, had been situated at two different locations in the city since its founding in 1863. In 1869, when the influx of freed black men after the Civil War was reaching its height in the District, a new hospital was erected by the Freedmen's Bureau on grounds belonging to Howard University. This new facility was used by the Medical Department for instruction. In 1870, it was mandated that the hospital's residents should be appointed from the medical students graduating from Howard University. The administrations of the university and the hospital were also interlocked, including a professor and sometimes dean of the university who also served as surgeon-in-chief of the hospital. Starting with Secretary of Interior Harold Ickes's recommendation in 1937, Freedmen's Hospital was eventually transferred to Howard University. By 1939, all members of the hospital's professional staff were nominated by the university for appointment.[23]

With the inception of World War II in 1941, Eddie's internship at Freedmen's proved to be even more hectic and more of a challenge than is usually required by such a demanding position.

> In 1941, I graduated from medical school and received a commission as first lieutenant in the army. I was doing an internship at Freedmen's Hospital. There was no other choice. The places where blacks could practice were limited. None of the leading universities permitted blacks to participate in any residential programs or internships. However, Freedmen's was a fine place to do an internship, lots of work. Indeed, when the war broke out the medical staff at Howard University as well as Freedmen's Hospital had been exhausted to the point that we had to use "externs" who worked under the interns—they were senior medical students. By this time, there was such a grave shortage of physicians that the federal government decided to set up what was called an ASTP (Army Specialized Training Program) wherein funds were granted by the federal government to train medical students to become physicians since they were needed in the military.
>
> On one occasion, after working all day and having stayed up to work the entire night before, there was a

terrible automobile accident. One of the injuries sustained was a compound fracture of the leg involving the tibia as well as the fibula and it took us pretty much all night to wade through this one and get it done. Finally I was able to get off my feet at about five in the morning. Then, I had to come back for surgery again to do a radical mastectomy at eight. When I got to the operating room I was tired, sleepy, and exhausted but nonetheless I had to go right on through with the procedure, which involved continuous work. We were in surgery from eight in the morning until three o'clock when I suddenly experienced severe pain in my left leg and I began to develop chills and fever. When I came out of the operating room, I hastened to come home and the fever and chills and pain in the left leg persisted.

The next morning, I was carted from home to the hospital, where I was hospitalized and was under the care of Dr. Charles Drew and Dr. Clarence Green in neurology. When they examined me, it was found that I had a thrombophlebitis of the left leg and I was placed on bed rest for an indefinite period of time. Antibiotics were not known in those days but sulfur was. Finally, I got papers to come and be examined to head out for Tucson, Arizona, to carry on military work but when I was examined by the physicians of Walter Reed Hospital they found that physically I was unable to go because there was a residual of the thrombophlebitis in my leg. I was supposed to come back in ninety days for another examination. When I did go back, the hospital was so seriously depleted of help that they needed me there.

In the meantime, because of the shortage of doctors at Howard University and Freedmen's Hospital, I was appointed to several jobs. I was in charge of the health services at Howard University and had to take care of all the ASTP programs for the aspiring young physicians and that meant that I had to be on duty at four o'clock in the morning and again at four in the afternoon. In the interim, I worked filling in taking care of the internal medicine in the clinical area at Freedmen's Hospital plus teaching internal medicine to the medical students and

> the dental students as well. I carried out this work throughout the entire tenure of World War II. I proceeded to stay in the field of internal medicine and served a residency for a period of three more years. It was not until 1945 that I went into private practice.

Despite the hectic nature of his experiences and the toll that the phlebitis took on his health, Eddie remembered his time at Freedmen's with a great deal of fondness. The relationships he formed with the professional staff were closer than he had experienced since beginning his medical quest. A fellow Mississippian, Riley Thomas, urged Eddie to go into internal medicine and gave him constant encouragement. Later on, Eddie was to become his physician.

One of the most eccentric people Eddie was to meet during his residency was a patient at Freedmen's.

> I was the chief resident in internal medicine at the hospital. This fellow was from East India and he had dabbled in all the techniques of hypnosis and transcendental meditation. I discovered him as a patient through my work on the ward. He could put himself into a trance or a hypnotic state. I found him fascinating, so during my leisure time I would go there and we would talk. His name was Reverend Shadd.
>
> He kept on saying, "I want you to take a needle and stick it anywhere on my body and there will be no blood and no pain." He kept after me to do it. Finally, one day, I went to Mrs. Sterling, who was head of the ward, and asked her to give me a sterile needle for a puncture. I decided that I had to try this guy. I figured it couldn't hurt him. I went in there quietly and closed the door. He went through his routine of repeating that there is no blood and no pain. I took the needle and I stuck it in, then I tried another spot and another. There was nothing there, not even a hole.
>
> I talked to E. Y. Williams after that to see if he would like to use this man as a demonstration for his class. E. Y. was a psychiatrist and neurologist. This man made a good example of mind over matter. The first time I presented him before the senior class in medicine in the

autopsy room of old Freedmen's Hospital, he came into the room and stood up as if he were fixed. He picked up a long hat pin and ran it through his arm and then pulled it back. Each time before he did it, he always said, "No blood, no pain." Each time there was no blood and he said he didn't feel it. I took him to E. Y.'s classes for about three or four years. From that point on, the Reverend Shadd and I became lifelong friends and he was a patient on the outside when I started practicing medicine. Later, when I was going through some difficult times and started to see E. Y. as a counselor, the phrase "No blood, no pain" became a signal between us as to how I was feeling.

The Reverend Shadd introduced me to many unusual experiences. He began to hold séances and invited me to go. I had read about séances but can you imagine me going to one? Naturally, though, I was interested. We were in a room like this with about a half-dozen people sitting around, many of whom were psychiatrist friends of mine from over on Connecticut Avenue. While he was waiting to call up the dead, the visitors sitting there would be put into a state of hypnotic suggestion to get their minds ready. I decided I was going to do this thing scientifically. I carried my stethoscope and my blood pressure equipment. I would take the pressure before and after. By God, when they were supposedly communicating with the dead, their blood pressure would drop way down and then afterwards it would come back up. I don't know whether they saw things or not, or whether these were visions or hallucinations or things of fancy. But I do know that their blood pressure dropped. It is a fascinating thing.

Out of this, I developed an interest in hypnosis and took a course. Before I knew it, I was doing a hell of a job and I got a degree in hypnosis. They had at that time what was called the Washington Hypnotic Medical Society. It is a very valuable technique and it is utilized a lot.

The Reverend Shadd was very prominent among the followers of Father Divine. Upon one occasion, on

> Seventeenth Street, they had this luncheon. I had never met Father Divine although he was the students' friend because, in a lot of places, there were shops opened by Father Divine where you could go and get a whole meal for fifteen cents. He had a word you had to say—"Peace"—then he would let you have the meal for fifteen cents. Upon this occasion, I was invited to participate in one of the exclusive affairs with Father Divine present. It was a long table and every item on anybody's menu was served. You name it: every vegetable, every meat, every kind of salad, every kind of food. When he got up he waved his hand and said the blessing; everyone was immediately quiet. I was very impressed with that.
>
> There came a time when Father Divine decided to marry. He married what he called his angel. She was a beautiful girl, about twenty-three or -four years of age and white. Of course he was black. He picked her as an "angel," not to be touched. He said he never thought of her in terms of sexual contact. What he was trying to do was to bring forth or project an image of brotherhood regardless of race, religion, or stature in life. This was the concept that he was trying to stress—a love that would be all-encompassing rather than the base type of sexuality. I did go to that wedding.

Throughout Eddie's tenure in medical school he never had the opportunity to return home. Eddie's mother, Addie, remained healthy and living on China Grove, gardening and selling the vegetables with Eddie's older brother Alex assisting. As always, there was little surplus. Eddie's sister Maude had been married and was living in Natchez with her two children. Theodore had gone on to college to become a pharmacist and Douglas had completed medical school at Meharry, the same year Eddie graduated from Howard.

Soon after graduation, Eddie and Jewell purchased their first home on California Street, N.W. It was not long before it was filled with many boarding students who were attending Howard, a venture that Jewell handled with great expertise. After Maude divorced her husband, she and her two children, Dolores and Mildred, came to live with Eddie and Jewell for a while. Maude got a job at St. Elizabeth's Hospital and the children were enrolled in school and did well. To get to St. Elizabeth's, Maude

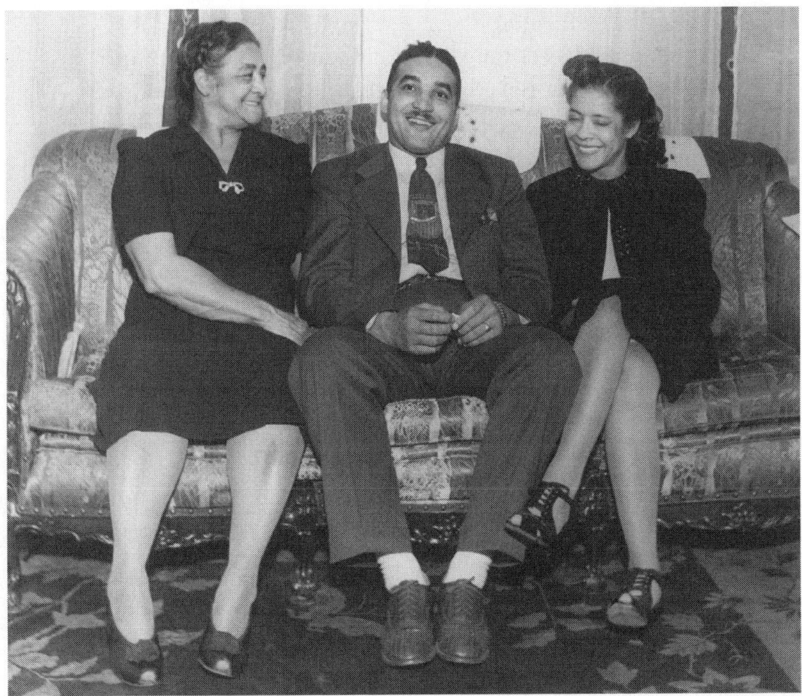

**Fig. 13:** Eddie, his mother, Addie Wilkerson Mazique, and Jewell. Photo courtesy of Maude Mazique and Dolores Pelham.

would take a bus. She could sit wherever she wanted until she reached the Maryland border, and then would have to move to the back of the bus. Maude stayed for two and a half years and then moved to Detroit.[24] Addie Mazique, Eddie's and her mother, became ill and was living with Theodore, and Maude went to care for her and to work with her brother in his pharmacy. In the meantime, the house continued to fill up with Jewell's relatives: two brothers, two sisters, and a maid and her small daughter who were brought from Georgia. Although there were inevitable complications, Eddie seemed to enjoy having family close once again.

> During this period of time, the warm family relationships continued to develop and I felt quite secure in spite of all the differences that do exist when you have family living together. Jewell's mother was flown up very sick from Georgia because she had a huge fibroid tumor in her uterus. We put her in Freedmen's Hospital and I

> personally assisted in the operation in which her hysterectomy was done. The relationship between me and Jewell's family developed very warmly and when her father got sick, he, too, came up and we were able to take care of him. Her uncle, who we called Uncle Lum, was living in Florida with one of his sons at the time and when he got sick, they called up and stated that he refused to go to any hospital unless I would take care of him. He was brought from Florida to Freedmen's Hospital, where he was under my care as well. It made me proud to know they all had such confidence in me.

There was something special about Eddie's manner with patients. No matter how hectic his schedule, he seemed to give them undivided attention when he was with them. His genuine caring came through when he dealt with his patients, and he seemed especially sensitive to those who had little or were older.[25] Emmie Perkins, a registered nurse who developed into one of Eddie's dearest friends, remembered their first meeting in complete detail. It was 6:45 one morning, when she heard this voice behind a curtain talking to an elderly lady and gentleman. There were no senior citizen's programs then and there was no Medicare or Medicaid. Yet this doctor behind the curtain was gentle and caring with the couple, treating them with a great deal of respect. Mrs. Perkins had waited outside the curtain, wanting to give the doctor and his patient and family some privacy. But she had never heard any doctor be this kind to a patient and so finally decided she had to see just who it was that showed such compassion. She pulled the curtain back and there stood a most handsome gentleman with the blackest hair and the reddest mustache that you could ever see on any human being. In her heart she felt such joy that she grabbed him and hugged him. Eddie was so shocked, he demanded to know who she was. Mrs. Perkins introduced herself as the head nurse on the ward and thus began their life-long friendship.[26]

In 1945, when Eddie finished his residency at Freedmen's, he was fortunate, as he explained, in being able to take over the practice of a well-known physician on Riggs Street, N.W.:

> When I was the chief resident at Freedmen's Hospital, one of my patients was a prominent surgeon, Dr. William ("Billy") Welch. Dr. Welch was a relatively young man, in his fifties, but in spite of everything that

> was done, he died. The family was very pleased with the care I had given to the doctor and developed a strong affinity for me. His mother, "Mother Welch" as I later learned to call her, said to me: "I want you to be my son now to take the place of my boy." Upon the doctor's death, "Mother Welch" and his widow, Sue, who was the secretary to the dean of the Medical College, came to me and said they would like it if I took over the doctor's practice. They said I could take the office just as it was when he had been stricken. It was in the basement of their home on Riggs Street. They knew I did not have much money—in those days you were paid ten dollars a month for an internship and twenty for a residency. They told me I could begin my payments after I began to build up a practice. When I walked into the office in August of 1945, it was just like he had left it. I enjoyed a very rich and good relationship with this family and we all thrived.

Eddie next moved to a facility on W Street, where he joined with another doctor in a venture to build a medical diagnostic and treatment center. It was one of the first of its kind. They had participants in surgery, pediatrics, obstetrics and gynecology, and dentistry, and a laboratory and a drugstore. Their undertaking was productive, and they all flourished. In 1948, with the money Eddie was starting to accumulate, he was able to buy a summer place at Highland Beach, the resort community founded by Frederick Douglass's son, Charles. It functioned as a township with its own elections and mayor. Before the founding of Highland Beach there was no place where professional blacks could go in the summertime to get away from the hectic Washington city life. A patient of Eddie's, a dentist named John Washington, who had built one of the first Highland Beach homes, offered to sell him a lot on his property. Eddie had a modest but well-constructed house built. Once the schools closed for the summer, the town would be bustling with activity until after Labor Day. Such notables as Paul Laurence Dunbar, Langston Hughes, and Booker T. Washington were all frequent visitors, and Mary Church Terrell had her summer home at Highland Beach. The beach bordered on a white beach, and not only was the land partitioned but there were stakes as you went out into the water to separate the white and black bathers while they were swimming.[27]

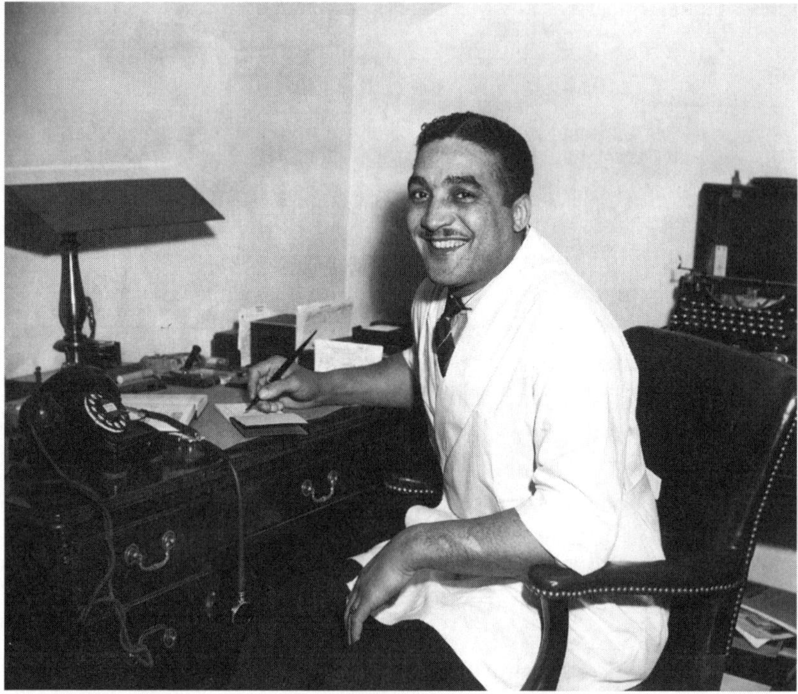

**Fig. 14:** The young Dr. Mazique in his office. Photo courtesy of Maude Mazique and Dolores Pelham.

Eventually Eddie left the group practice and started his own office on Ninth and S Streets, N.W. in the Shaw area ghetto, where he practiced for a number of years. Finally, in 1970, he moved to the site on Kennedy St., N.W. where he continued to practice until his death.

Eddie never had much trouble attracting patients. He instilled a great deal of confidence in those who came to him and they were willing to wait until he had time to see them.

> When I did go into private practice, I felt honored that the individuals with whom I had worked at Olney Inn, numbering about twenty-odd, the bakers, the waiters, the barmaids, easily 94 percent of them became my patients when I began to practice. It was also good to know that once I got out into practice, so many of the doctors themselves chose me as their private physician. This inspired me with a great deal of confidence.

Eddie's female patients were especially devoted to him. Dr. Herman Stamps was a dentist who was one of Eddie's students at Howard and later went into practice with him in 1947, shortly after Eddie had opened his group practice on W Street, N.W. When his grandmother was in need of a new physician, Dr. Stamps took her to see Eddie. When she first went to see Eddie, she was quite elderly and had suffered a stroke. Dr. Stamps brought her into Eddie's office, where she proceeded to look at him very carefully. Finally she said: "My, my, you are such a handsome young man; I don't think you had better treat me." Eddie wanted to know why. She said, "I have buried so many physicians and you are too good-looking to die."[28]

Eddie's early practice of medicine included a bit of everything. He recalled how a doctor at that time, specialist or not, had to know how to meet all the physical needs of his patients:

> Medicine has changed so tremendously since this period of time that it is difficult to relate to the things a doctor was required to do in order to survive. Even though you were specializing in one particular area, it was difficult to exist unless you would do other procedures such as taking care of a little bit of everything for everybody, like obstetrics and gynecology, internal medicine, pediatrics, and even surgery in the same office. Many minor surgeries, such as the removal of tonsils, cysts, abscesses, and the like, were performed in the office. I did all of these joyfully and started my journey into my profession with exuberance.

## CHAPTER FIVE 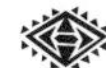

# Being a Doctor Is Not Enough

Basically, you can't separate medical problems from social, economic, and political ones, nor can you neglect the health of one racial segment or class without damage to the health of all.

— *Edward C. Mazique,*
*The Milwaukee Sentinel,*
*14 August 1958*

Eddie was now a doctor, a man respected by the black community. No longer living in the South, his relations with whites were clearly an improvement over what he had experienced in Natchez and Atlanta. Yet all of his professional achievements did not make him immune to the discrimination suffered by blacks in the nation's capital and the surrounding areas. Memories of some of these incidents would always remain in his mind.

For some reason, my car wasn't running one day and Dr. Jimmy Gray and I decided we would take the bus over to Arlington to this particular place to study. We were received very well until we were ready to get on the bus to come home again. It was pretty much empty so we sat in the front of the bus. This was in Virginia, right across the bridge from Washington. The bus driver came and told us, "I'm sorry you have to move to the back of the bus." I told him we were tired of sitting in the backs of buses and we were not going to move. He told me he was going to leave me in

> Virginia. Anyway, we had to leave the seats where we were, to go sit in the back of the bus to cross over the Potomac River into D.C. The man had a black curtain that he drew across so that we couldn't see where we were going. That was in the early 1940s. Imagine going through that as a doctor and being relegated to this type of thing. It just didn't make any sense.
>
> Things like that will do something to you. Life goes on, but when you keep on facing events like this you have to develop a way to get around it without having to stoop. I made a statement at that time that I would never cross the Potomac River to live over there in Virginia. I decided, because of that incident, I wasn't going south or southeast any more. I always moved towards Maryland and headed north or northeast in the city.

It was not just Virginia and the southern states, however, that were still segregated. The 1940s saw discrimination in Washington housing greater than that evidenced in the 1930s. Although restrictive covenants were struck down in a 1948 Supreme Court decision, voluntary adherence to covenants still limited the areas in the city in which blacks could live. Places of recreation including restaurants, movie houses, theaters, and District playgrounds were still segregated. Major organizations for the city's youth such as the Boy's Clubs and the YMCA fought any integration efforts. Public schools were still separate and given unequal funding. And equal opportunities in employment, even at the federal level, came only after battles that were to spread over the next several decades.[1]

No matter how dismal this view of the city seemed, there were good people working at all levels to change it. One of the most effective of those challenging the segregated world that was Washington, as well as injustices everywhere in the United States, was an active civil rights lawyer named Charles Hamilton Houston. By the time they met in 1948, "Charlie," as Eddie called him, had been vice-dean and a professor at Howard University's law school and had refused lucrative offers to serve as its dean. He had directed the NAACP'S legal campaign for equal rights from 1935 to 1938 and served as a special counsel until 1940. He had successfully pleaded some of the Supreme Court cases most crucial to eliminating segregation. In 1938 he argued before the Supreme Court in *Missouri ex rel. Gaines v. Canada* and won one of the first major court battles for equal educational opportunities. The decision denied the state's right to exclude blacks from state-supported educational programs that were offered to whites. They would no longer be allowed to meet their obligation to black students by paying their tuition and sending them to another state for their education. Now the states either had to admit blacks or create an equal facility for them.[2]

In 1948, in *Hurd v. Hodge,* the Supreme Court accepted his arguments, and restrictive covenants were ruled unenforceable by the courts. Mr. Houston did not limit himself to educational issues or housing. If it were a case of discrimination, Charlie could be found slashing his way through the legal roots that supported the injustice. It seemed he had a hand in most of the important cases, usually to the detriment of his own private practice.[3]

The year 1948 brought Charlie and Eddie together. Charles Houston became a patient and close friend, and it was his beliefs that were to prod and drive Eddie until his death. Although Eddie had achieved his goal of becoming a physician, Charlie Houston convinced him this success was not enough. He had to remove the stumbling blocks that blacks as a group faced. Charlie gave a focus to combating all the slights, injustices, and inequities with which Eddie had to deal. Eddie's upbringing and education in the South had taught him how to maintain his dignity while tolerating the system—how to get around prejudice. It was Charlie who taught him how to confront it and change it. Life was never to be the same.

> In 1948, a big thing happened to change my life. Until I met Charles Houston, I don't know that I had a conception of doing very much about others in their struggle for freedom and equality. I didn't have any great sense of civic or community involvement. I was just starting out. I didn't have much. I thought it was time for me to get about my work, finding a home, having children. I was thinking about family.
>
> But something happened in 1948. I had a patient by the name of Charles Hamilton Houston. Charlie Houston was a great constitutional lawyer—in some ways, the father of civil rights. In my opinion, he was the greatest black attorney who ever lived. He and I became very good friends and I admired him a great deal.
>
> During the time of our relationship, he began to talk to me about discrimination and segregation and how it could be fought. He began to tell me about curbs that

were present in my life, curbs as far as the medical field is concerned. The fact that blacks were not permitted to join the AMA and physicians were not permitted to go into most of the hospitals in the Washington area: Garfield, Providence, and Sibley. You name them and they had no black doctors, hardly any black patients—no one to admit black patients or care for them. He talked about this and he talked about it in the framework of medical professionalism. At the same time, he began to broaden my vision and increase my horizon about the total environment of black people and all minorities who were subjected to this kind of treatment and entrapment and the true meaning of segregation and discrimination in housing and all this type of thing. You couldn't buy a house, you couldn't go to a restaurant, anything like that.

Charlie Houston was an attorney who served for causes rather than money. He had a rich father but Charlie died very, very poor because his life was devoted entirely to causes. He turned out to be the greatest lawyer that the NAACP would have. He was also a professor of law at Howard University. Then he would take a few private cases in between, but not many. His time was devoted to teaching and going around fighting cases, sometimes for the NAACP and sometimes on his own, that had to do with injustices in housing or education or any other area.

The Charlie Houston story and the John Hope story are things you don't forget because they are turning points in your life.

It was not until I met Charlie that I began to focus on what was happening. A lot of turmoil had been brewing in the country. The people were starting to feel oppressed. It was not just Jews and blacks but also labor. There began to be an upsurge in the labor movement. The old separation of the AFL and CIO was finally bridged so that one stronger group could be formed.[4]

Henry A. Wallace was the secretary of agriculture and later became vice president under Franklin Delano Roosevelt. Wallace represented the first man I had heard who was white who had come out in the open on the radio and later when television came into play and said all people should be treated equal and they should be given an opportunity.[5]

Charlie nudged me into this stream of discontentment. He pointed out there were still a lot of things that needed to be done in order for me to improve myself. I was denied the possibility of going into other hospitals for residency. I was not allowed to join the American Medical Association. I was not allowed to practice in most hospitals in Washington or to send my patients there. It just wasn't right that people should be living this way. I thought, "What the hell can I do? I'm just one person." But anyway I listened to him.

Charlie had an uncle who was a doctor, named Ulysses Houston. Dr. Houston was fond of me because he knew I was taking good care of his nephew. He pulled me in one day. He said, "Eddie, we are going to start you out here with the medical society." It wasn't long before, through his efforts, I was made president of the Medico-Chirurgical Society in 1951. Then I began to fight. The society increased my awareness of what was happening as far as the hospitals and I decided I would tackle them. So I began to take on the matter of eradicating barriers in hospitals and medical organizations and to get blacks admitted to the hospitals.

Charlie was not specifically pushing for the integration of hospitals or the medical society. He was working on a national basis, dealing with things relating to lynchings and civil rights, personal and individual liberties. Charlie's goal, however, was to eradicate discrimination and segregation wherever it existed and so he focused me on areas within my own field that needed to change.

Just as with his community involvement, Eddie's family began with the assistance of Charlie Houston.

I told you about the affinity and closeness and friendship that had developed between me and Charlie Houston. He began to question why we didn't have any

> children. He said, "I have a friend in New York named Peter Marshall Murray, a well-known gynecologist and obstetrician."[6] He was the only black at that time who had been admitted to the County Medical Society of New York City. Eventually, he was in the House of Delegates of the AMA, which was unheard of at the time. He also became president of the New York State Medical Association, which was the constituent organization of the AMA. He was quite a man and he had the advantage of having been exposed to medicine that was more than black because they permitted him to come in to see other procedures that were going on. So he knew the latest surgical procedures and what was behind them and all this. So Charlie said, "I want Jewell to go see Dr. Peter Marshall Murray in New York City." She went there in 1950 and he found she had fibroids and did surgery.
>
> I went up to get Jewell and I told Dr. Murray I was grateful for what he had done and I wanted to pay him. He insisted I owed him nothing. You are a fellow colleague and I am grateful to be doing it for you and for Charlie Houston. I'll consider it paid when you call to tell me your wife is pregnant. He was very overjoyed when I called. Skipper was born in May of 1951 and Jeff followed in 1952.

When he first began his private practice, there was little else Eddie could afford to do other than concentrate on his work and his family. Cash flow was limited. Eddie's first nurse, receptionist, and jack-of-all-trades, Charlotte Walton, remembered those first days of working in the office when she was just a teenager. There were almost no patients and little money even for food. They would split a few Little Tavern hamburgers for lunch and pretend that they were busy when a patient would come in.[7] No doubt Eddie managed to convince himself those hamburgers tasted wonderful just as he had done at Morehouse when his diet was limited to peanut butter.

By the late 1940s, Eddie's reputation had been established and he could start taking an interest in public affairs. It helped that he had patients like Charlie Houston. This made other people believe in him. But mostly, it was his diagnostic skills and his love for and devotion to his patients that won him an enthusiastic and large following. Essential to his success, as his patients frequently stated, were his ability and willingness to really listen when they spoke:

> As a physician, he can tell you what is wrong with you without doing any tests. He doesn't even have to put a hand on me. Before he does anything, you feel better all the time because of the conversation he is having with you. At the same time he is learning more about what the problem might be.[8]

Dr. Mazique made house calls. He paid special attention to the elderly, caring about them instead of medicating them.[9] As one of his elderly patients said, "You know a lot of times, a word does as much good as the medicine."[10] Many of them just felt better when he kissed them and said, "Hello sugar, how are you today?"[11] As his friend the comedian and civil rights activist Dick Gregory put it: "He was just a force. Just going to his office to see him made you well."[12]

No matter how hectic his schedule, he always made a patient feel like he or she was the most important thing on his mind. They never felt he slighted them or rushed them. By the time he was ready to leave his Riggs Street office, the patients were lined up outside to wait for a chance to see him.[13]

In 1957, when Ricardo Hawkins, the stenographer and clinical attendant at Freedmen's Hospital, needed assistance with an ailing mother, Eddie was willing to go beyond what would be expected of a physician. He accompanied Ricardo on the long drive to Pennsylvania, necessitating a two-day absence from his practice, so that he could personally evaluate Ricardo's mother's condition. Mr. Hawkins attributes the extension of his mother's life to the care Eddie gave her when she was subsequently brought to Washington.[14]

Eddie's monetary position began to improve as his practice expanded. Eddie and Jewell were ready to buy a new home and Eddie wanted the best. At Charlie Houston's urging, it was to be in one of the least accessible neighborhoods. When Charlie knew Eddie was planning on buying a home, he suggested Eddie test the recent Supreme Court ruling in *Hurd v. Hodge* that restrictive covenants were unenforceable and look in areas that formerly had been limited to whites.

> My practice was growing and things were coming along great. I decided to move into a white neighborhood.

Charlie had a lot to do with this, too. Until 1948, they had restrictions on properties and things wherein they would not permit you if you were of African descent or Jewish to live in certain areas of the District of Columbia. He went to court and Charlie won this one. Shortly afterwards, he said to me, "You go out and get yourself a house in one of those places." So I went out and purchased this piece of ground to build a house west of Sixteenth Street. It was unheard of at the time. Negroes didn't go there unless they were working. I had made house calls over there to see some of my patients who were in those beautiful homes working as maids. I was astounded! I had never seen such luxury.

I saw a lot in Crestwood one day and I wanted it. When they knew I was trying to get it, they quoted me a tremendous price which I couldn't afford. One of my white patients, Johnny Garne, a good friend who now lives in Virginia, went and bought it for me. I took care of him and his whole family when they lived in the District. They sold it to him for a song. I got a white builder and a black contractor. I built the house but I had to keep it in Johnny's name until I got ready to move in. The day I moved in, Johnny and I went down to the Court of Deeds to transfer it from him to me. That's how I got the house on Upshur Street. I was the first black to move up there.

We moved in 1952 and the first weekend we were there, beer bottles and bricks were thrown at the windows. I got my shotgun and a rifle and I said, "If a sucker puts his foot on this damn lawn, I'm going to let him have it." My wife in the meantime was having fits. I said, "I'm going to protect my home."

The chief of police of our precinct said, "Oh, Doctor, it's nothing. Those fellows are coming in from Maryland and do it all over the city. On Saturday nights, my lawn is all messed up. Everyone's is." I said, "Come on, Chief, you know and I know that that is not true. It is my duty to let you know that this is my home and I have to protect it and I'll let you know that I have a couple of guns in there (in those days you didn't have to register guns)

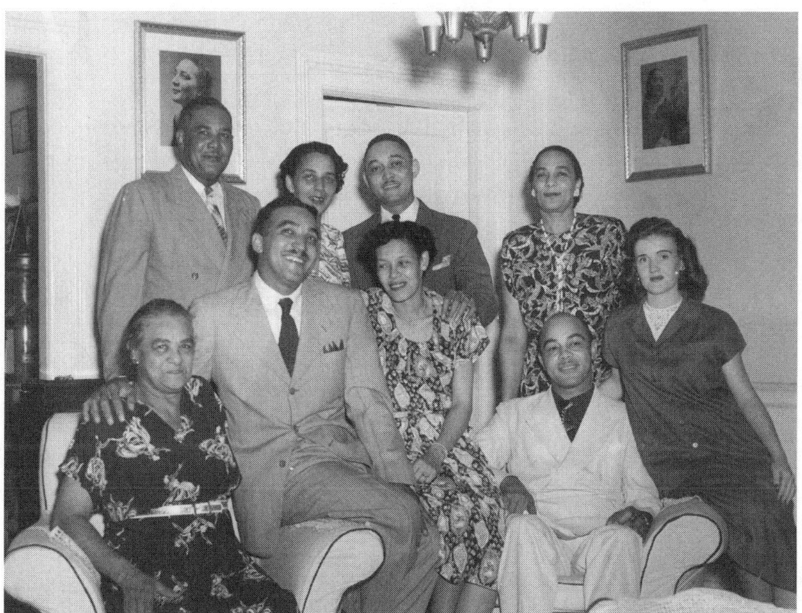

**Fig. 15:** Eddie with his mother and his siblings and their wives in 1949. Top, left to right: Alex II ("Buddie") and his wife, Eloise; brother, Theodore; sister, Maude. Middle row, from left to right: Eddie; Theodore's wife, Juanita; Doug's wife, Shirley. In chairs: mother, Addie, and brother Douglas. Photo courtesy of Maude Mazique and Dolores Pelham.

> and if anybody tries to break into my house there are going to be some problems." He said, "I believe you. I tell you what, don't worry. I'll put a cadre of protection around you for a while until things simmer down." He did. I would see cops coming around all during the day and all during the night—surveillance, you know. That was good. It quieted things down. It so happened that I was living next to a congressman named Anderson. We became good neighbors and everybody was fine.

Life seemed to be going well for the young Dr. Mazique. He had a beautiful and intelligent wife, two healthy sons, and his own practice, and he was beginning to develop a following of patients. The happy image that Eddie was projecting, however, was not reflective of the actual situation at home. Eddie and Jewell were just two very different personalities.

Eddie was gregarious. He loved dealing with people and being surrounded by friends. He liked to joke and kid and just have a good time. He enjoyed fishing, dancing, and going to movies. He was far from being a frivolous person, but he cherished his moments of fun as an escape from all the problems that he faced in society and work. The warm home life, full of socializing and people, that Eddie so desired was missing.

Jewell believed that life should be centered on causes. Given her perspective, she must have viewed Eddie's need of a social life as unimportant at best. That isn't to say that they did not do "social" things. During the 1950s, the magazines and newspapers were replete with articles about the latest party the Maziques hosted or affairs they attended.[15] Jewell explained this apparent contradiction in an interview she gave to a newspaper reporter in 1958:

> Ever since I was a student in college, I have looked upon the emphasis which many of our educated group place on social life and so-called society as a waste of time an [*sic*] energy. . . . The frills of social life hold no charms for me, I am more concerned for instance with what the political leaders of Paris decided to do about their colonial possessions than what the Paris designers decide about what women will wear.[16]

The diplomatic receptions she hosted were an outgrowth of her cultural study group and served to introduce ambassadors from African nations to Americans of African descent. Some of them were elaborate events that received mention in not only the black newspapers but also in *Hue* and *Jet* and even the *Washington Post.* Jewell worked in the Library of Congress and then as a medical technician and wrote newspaper articles to support her positions. She was honored for the contribution she made to the crusade for human rights and was a leader in the United Givers Fund Campaign. Yet instead of bringing them together, the leadership and the good works that Eddie and Jewell did drove them farther apart as they had less and less time for each other. Eventually friction ensued.

Perhaps Eddie would not have slipped so wholeheartedly into community service if his family and social life had been more fulfilling. It is also possible he would not have been at the forefront of so many civil rights causes. What he felt was missing at home was, at Charlie Houston's urging, soon to be replaced by constant devotion to any cause he considered just.

Most times, an individual you are married to has to do with your reactions to things. I can say this: Jewell was very strongly motivated, very brilliant, and very active. I guess maybe her activities made for an unusual home situation. That may have in part been due to the fact that I was so devoted to my medicine and to study.

I married her in 1937 and went to school the next week. So it started like that. She had a good job at the Library of Congress. She worked there for years. Initially, she had a job and enrolled at Howard University to take her master's degree in history. She accomplished that maybe the year after we were married. She made many acquaintances during her work at the library and got involved with a lot of organizations, mainly labor organizations. There were a couple of professors at the university who I am sure influenced her. What I am trying to say is it seems that she found her own way of doing things. But then there would be no one at the house when I would come home in the evening. She would be at this meeting or that one. So I would keep busy with my work. We made that kind of an adjustment over time.

By the time I graduated from medical school, there was not the close-knit type of family relationship that you usually see. One of the things that I never forgot was, whatever business she was doing, she did not come to my graduation from medical school. I felt that rather deeply. I had a sense that I had to be involved with other things.

When I got out and started practicing medicine the same thing prevailed. I found myself working hard, working late into the evening hours, making house calls and putting in two shifts. Coming home and having dinner and going back to the office. Getting home, twelve or one in the morning. That was no bother since Jewell would be away for the most part.

Jewell never cared much about socializing or dancing or playing. So there was no problem about social life—we simply didn't have any. Something had to fill that vacuum and I found it easy to slip into something that was positive. I got into community work in this

> way. I never got involved in her type of affiliations as far as organizations and people because their time was different from my time. This was during the time of the McCarthy era and there were questions regarding the groups with which she was affiliated. To what extent or even if she were involved with Communist groups, even to this day I don't know.
>
> I had nothing else prepared at home or someone to say "Hey you do this" or "You do that" or someone who could steer me into the social limelight or the arts or song or plays. This wasn't brought into it at all. During the time I was in med school, I would always make it a point, however, of going to the movies once a week on a Friday night. That was it. Usually on weekends, I would be very busy working as a waiter or something like that. I think these may have been the factors that motivated me because there was nothing else that had already been set up or planned around the family.

Washington in the late 1940s was the perfect arena for a young man who wanted to do battle with social injustices. It was a city deeply entrenched in segregation yet rich in black culture, with Howard University, the medical school, and numerous black professionals. In 1939, there were already 191 doctors, 72 dentists, 98 lawyers, and nearly 600 public-school and university teachers.[17] Perhaps this wealth of educated black men and women was one of the reasons why Washington began to feel the nudge toward equal rights five to ten years earlier than the remainder of the country. From 1946 to 1954, movements for desegregation were going on in all aspects of the society from recreation to employment, in housing and the school system, and in professional societies and organizations.

In 1948, a strong push came from the federal government in Truman's Civil Rights Message to Congress when he stated that "all men are created equal and that they have the right to equal justice under the law.... they are entitled to equal opportunities for jobs, for homes, for good health and for education.... that all men should have a voice in their government and that government should protect, not usurp the rights of the people."[18] Truman backed up his speech with an executive order instituting equality of training and opportunity within the armed services.[19] By 1950, the military had moved a long way toward implementing the order, as had the executive departments of the federal government. The governing body of Washington, the District Council of Commissioners, was much harder to sway. "Although the makeup of the board of commissioners changed several times between 1946 and 1953, only Commissioner Joseph Donohue openly expressed a personal wish to see segregation curbed in Washington."[20] An outspoken advocate of integration, Commissioner Donohue, before resigning, publicly prodded incoming president Dwight D. Eisenhower to end segregation in the District once and for all. On local radio and television shows, he said Eisenhower would have the support necessary to have Congress put an end to segregation. "'I think Gen. Eisenhower will keep his promise [to end segregation],' the commissioner replied. 'He not only will be able to do it, but he will do it.'"[21] On the December 8, 1952, program, Donohue also suggested that desegregating the District's schools would end up saving a great deal of money despite the school superintendent's stating otherwise.

Harry S Truman was a consistent and staunch supporter of civil rights. Yet in several instances he had failed his black supporters, as in 1945, when he did not back the Fair Employment Practices Committee in its dispute with the Capital City Transit Authority, allowing it to continue as an employer of "whites only" until 1956.[22] This failure prompted Charles Hamilton Houston, who served on the committee, to resign in protest. When Truman dismissed Henry Wallace as secretary of commerce in 1946, the sympathy of many blacks was to lie with Wallace. Wallace had always been an outspoken advocate of the common man. He was the first white man of note that Eddie and probably many other blacks could remember speaking out publicly against discrimination. Although Truman's record was sound on civil rights, it was Wallace to whom many minorities felt an allegiance. In 1948, when he left the Democratic Party to run as a presidential candidate on the Progressive ticket, it was a logical step to aid in Wallace's campaign. Eddie, along with other black idealists, including Paul Robeson, was to join in support of the Progressive Party.

The greatest differences between Wallace and Truman lay in their positions on international affairs. Wallace was a supporter of coexistence and felt Truman's military muscle-flexing was a betrayal of the Franklin Delano Roosevelt legacy. He was a strong supporter of the United Nations and believed we could peacefully coexist with the Communists.[23]

Wallace's position was to prove very unpopular at a time when the United States felt especially threatened by Communism. Russian domination of Eastern Europe after the end of World War II had led to tension with the West. The overthrow, a few years later, of Chiang Kai-shek by the

Communists in China and the friendship pact between Russia and China strengthened the justification for a cold war military buildup.

It was not just events on faraway shores that were upsetting Americans about communism. The House Un-American Activities Committee (HUAC) was established in 1938 and became a permanent committee in 1945. Threats from within the system were believed to exist because of the disloyalty of many government workers. Members of Nazi, Fascist, and Communist organizations were discharged from federal employment as early as 1940. In 1947, the investigation of Hollywood led to the blacklisting of actors and filmmakers. With Whittaker Chambers's confession in 1948 that he had been a member of the Communist Party during the 1930s and had passed on secret government documents provided by Alger Hiss, a former State Department officer, to his party superiors, the loyalty question became foremost in the minds of some politicians and the public. Charges of Communists in the State Department in 1950 were enough to drive a hitherto unknown senator named Joseph McCarthy and the HUAC to headline news for the next four years.[24] The atmosphere was such that the loyalty to the U.S. government of a Wallace supporter, especially a black one, was in question.

The Eighty-first Congress in its "Hearings Regarding the Communist Infiltration of Labor Unions" stated directly that an affiliation with the National Wallace for President Committee was proof that a man had Communist leanings. They called it "the outstanding Communist front movement at the present time."[25]

Those groups such as manual laborers and minorities that were believed to be the unhappiest with conditions in the United States were thought to be most susceptible to the propaganda of the Communists. Paul Robeson's speech to the Paris Peace Conference in April 1949 touched off a furor at home. He stated: "It is certainly unthinkable for myself and the Negro people to go to war in the interests of those who have oppressed us for generations."[26] Despite their recent performance in World War II, the loyalty of black citizens came into question and special hearings were held in the summer of 1949 "Regarding Communist Infiltration of Minority Groups." The purpose of the hearings was supposedly to attempt to combat Paul Robeson's statement and the propaganda boost it gave to the Communists.[27]

A letter was sent from General Dwight D. Eisenhower to the committee to attest to the loyalty and devotion of the "Negro" soldiers who served in the Second World War. He went further by stating that "I have seen or experienced nothing since the close of hostilities that leads me to believe that our Negro population is not fully as worthy of its American citizenship as it proved itself to be on the battlefields of Europe and Africa."[28]

The investigator for the committee, Alvin W. Stokes, found no serious inroads of the Communists among the black population but did claim that almost half the white population surveyed believed that "Negroes" were communistically inclined and would be disloyal given the opportunity.[29]

The famous Brooklyn Dodger baseball player Jackie Robinson was called in as the epitome of the "good" black man to dispute Robeson's statement. Although strongly denying the legitimacy of Robeson's statement, Robinson did not fail to take the United States to task for the treatment of black people. He stated, "Negroes were stirred up long before there was a Communist Party, and they'll stay stirred up long after the party has disappeared—unless Jim Crow has disappeared as well."[30]

Eddie found himself entangled in this fray. Being called before the House Un-American Activities Committee proved to be a frightening experience.

> I worked in 1948 with Henry Wallace on his ticket for the Progressive Party. They branded that as Communist. At the same time, they banished Paul Robeson because he began to come out with a lot of stuff about mistreatment of minorities and so on. They called Robeson before the House Un-American Activities Committee. Robeson said in essence, the black man will never fight Russians because they were people who believed in equality and would give equality to their citizens. Blacks had freedom there. I was caught up in the same type of whirl. These are the twists that make life what it is.
>
> They called me down before the House Un-American Activities Committee. Charlie was living then. This was in 1949, right on the heels of Jackie Robinson. I never shall forget when Charlie called me. He laughed and said, "Eddie, we are going to have some fun today." I wasn't in the same good mood. "Charlie, I've never been in anything like this." He said, "You don't have anything to worry about. You have done nothing wrong. What you have said and done is honorable. Not only is it honorable but it is democratic. Not only is it democratic but it is constitutional. You are fighting for what

> we should have had all the time and that is freedom. So we are going to have fun."[31]
>
> We went down and we sat in this hearing. I've never seen anything in my life like it—it was enough to scare the hell out of me. We listened for about an hour or two to others. Finally the chairman got up and banged down his gavel and called for lunch. Charlie got up. "Mr. Chairman, before you leave may I say a word? I have my client here who is Dr. Edward Mazique. He's a busy physician in this city and he wants to leave here and get back to his patients in his office who are waiting for him. For whatever reason you called him down, I'm his attorney and I am here to defend him. But if you need him, I wonder if you wouldn't mind letting us know. If you can't take care of it now, what time can you take care of it? We will be back at a given time. Or if you don't need him, I'll come back and defend him." The chairman said, "Just a minute," and he turned this over to his number one attorney, who got out the book and flipped it and looked and finally they said something to each other. Then he said, "I'll tell you, Houston, I see no reason for the doctor to come back." That closed it.
>
> When we were coming back near the Supreme Court, Charlie said, "Come let's walk through the Supreme Court, I want to show you something." We looked up and there was a sign which said "Equal Justice Under the Law." He said, "I want you to read that. That is what you have been doing, so don't you be ashamed of what you have done. Be proud, you hear?"

Charlie Houston had always been under enormous pressure with more cases and more causes than any one man could handle. He made no time for a social life to provide himself with a temporary outlet from the pressures of his crusade. In the fall of 1949, he suffered a heart attack. The added strain his illness placed on Charlie's wife, Henrietta, who was emotionally unstable, necessitated her hospitalization in November. Charlie wanted her to go to the best possible place for treatment but there was none available in Washington. Eddie agreed to take the train and accompany her to New York so she could receive proper medical care.[32] Their young son, Eddie's godson Charles, or "Bo" as Eddie called him, lived part of the time with his great-aunt and uncle, Dr. and Mrs. Ulysses Houston, and the remainder with Eddie and Jewell. Upon his release from the hospital in December 1949, Charlie came to stay with Eddie and Jewell. Eddie slept in the room with his patient, and each night Charlie would talk and talk and Eddie would listen.

> When I would come home at night we would talk at length, hours and hours about the problems that I've expressed. About the necessity to participate in this, about you not going to do anything to disturb the status quo unless you do this. And when you do this, you're going to get called a whole lot of things and they're not going to be good ones, because you are doing it. But do not be afraid. This was his advice.[33]

After Christmas, Charlie returned home and soon got up and went back to work. His chest pains grew more frequent and more severe over the next few months and eventually Eddie hospitalized Charlie again. They wouldn't let Charlie in Walter Reed, even though he had served in the military.[34] Eddie remembered his own frustration at not being able to treat Charlie in any hospital other than Freedmen's:

> Charlie wanted to go to one of the other hospitals. I'm his doctor; I have no privileges because I'm black. Well, this had to disturb me, and he saw to it that I was disturbed by keeping after me, "I want to go to that hospital!" And I said, "Charlie, you know you can't go to that hospital.[35]

Finally, a white friend pulled strings to get him into Bethesda Naval Hospital, where the hope was to keep him secluded and quiet. He suffered another heart attack and asked Eddie to have him moved to Freedmen's where Eddie could treat him and he could receive visitors. On a beautiful April day, while Eddie was visiting his room, Charlie died suddenly and Eddie was left without one of his dearest friends and his greatest inspiration.[36]

Instead of discouraging him from crusading for the causes that were of such importance to his friend, Charlie's death served to spur Eddie on to a stronger commitment. It was time to attack all those stumbling blocks, all those impediments to being a great doctor that

Charlie talked about. Charlie's uncle, Dr. Ulysses L. Houston, supported Eddie for offices within the Medico-Chirurgical Society, and he became chairman of the Committee on Programs in 1949, vice president in 1950, and was elected to the presidency in 1951, 1952, 1953, 1957, and 1958. From Eddie's standpoint, the fight was on.

Although it became of premier importance for Eddie in the late 1940s, the struggle to integrate the Medical Society of the District of Columbia and the Washington hospitals did not begin with his entrance on the scene. It was to be a long battle, beginning with Reconstruction and fought for almost an entire century.[37] In 1869, Drs. Alexander T. Augusta, Charles B. Purvis, and A. W. Tucker were proposed for membership in the Medical Society of the District of Columbia, the local affiliate of the American Medical Society. When their applications were rejected, Senator Charles Sumner of Massachusetts introduced a resolution attempting to repeal the charter of the District Medical Society and further argued for whatever legislation might "be necessary to secure for medical practitioners in the District of Columbia equal rights and opportunities without distinction of color."[38] The Senate refused to act on Sumner's bill and a new strategy was necessary.

A group composed of black and white physicians petitioned Congress for a charter, stating:

> It is a fact worthy of note that this is the only country and the only profession in which such a distinction is now made. Science knows no race, color or condition; and we protest against the Medical Society of the District of Columbia, maintaining such a relic of barbarism. We, for the reasons stated, and in accordance with the spirit of the times, ask Congress to grant a charter to a new Society, which will give all rights, privileges and immunities to all physicians, making only the presentation of a diploma from some college recognized by the American Medical Association, and good standing in the profession, the qualifications necessary for membership.[39]

After formation, the National Medical Society of the District of Columbia, a biracial group, then tried to seat its delegates at the annual convention of the American Medical Association in May 1870. They were unsuccessful, and the AMA ruled that the wishes of the Medical

Society of the District of Columbia regarding membership should be respected. It maintained this "hands-off" policy toward the local affiliates until 1950, when, at their annual convention in San Francisco, it was urged that the race question be studied "in the light of prevailing conditions with a view to taking such steps as they may elect to eliminate such restrictive provisions."[40]

In the meantime, black physicians in Washington were left without a society with which they could affiliate in an effort to improve themselves and their expertise in their chosen profession. In 1884, the Medico-Chirurgical Society of the District of Columbia was formed to fill the gap. It was open to doctors of all races. It was biracial in the beginning and throughout its history had white members at various times. However, it has been largely composed of black physicians so is regarded as the "first and oldest Negro medical organization."[41]

Black physicians were not only barred from associating with white physicians in their professional organizations, they were also excluded from practicing in local hospitals. Black patients were treated at most of the hospitals in the District but on a strictly segregated basis, and they were generally assigned to the older and less well equipped parts of the hospital. As mentioned, the only hospital open to black physicians in the District was Freedmen's. This meant that black patients could not be treated by their black doctor unless they were patients at Freedmen's or at one of the six privately owned hospitals operated at various times between 1894 and 1953 by some industrious black physicians.[42]

Beginning in 1945, under the presidency of Dr. Montague Cobb, the Medico-Chirurgical Society began an unrelenting attack on discrimination in health-related areas. One of the prime targets was Washington's chief health official from 1935 to 1949, George C. Ruhland, whose outlandish statements provided his critics with numerous openings. Speaking about the number of cases of tuberculosis in the city at a hearing on the D.C. appropriation bill, he stated: "Our record is not so good. But as I stated in the beginning, our record is largely caused by the colored population."[43] In the 1943 hearings, he continued on the same theme: "The racial composition will determine what will happen in the matter of public health."[44] Little change was reflected in his thinking by the 1945 hearings when he said: "The colored are really our health problem in the District."[45] By 1949, he was "almost ready to suggest screening of Negroes planning to move to Washington."[46] Although Dr. Ruhland made it clear that he was well aware of the connections between poor housing and overcrowding and disease, in his public statements he still treated race as a causative factor. Dr. Cobb, in an article in the *Bulletin of the Medico-Chirurgical Society of the District of Columbia,* was scathing when pointing out the absurdity of Ruhland's position.

Gallinger was the first of the hospitals the doctors challenged since it was tax-supported and the majority of the patients were black. The National Medical Association supported the protest against Gallinger at its Louisville meeting. With the assistance of Federal Security Administrator Oscar R. Ewing, Gallinger agreed to admit black physicians in 1948.[47]

Next on the agenda for the Medico-Chirurgical Society was the attempt to gain admittance for black physicians into the District Medical Society. Entrance into the District Medical Society was crucial for a physician, as Eddie noted, since without membership, a doctor could not be a member of the American Medical Association and could therefore be denied a staff position in the hospitals.

> We took on the District Medical Society first. Black physicians had been subscribing to the black organizations like the Medico-Chirurgical Society and the National Medical Association because we had no choice. They were established largely because of bias and prejudice.
>
> You had to be a member of the AMA before you could apply for hospital privileges in the District of Columbia. So the number one problem was becoming a member of the District Medical Society. This had been lily-white. There had been no way for me to get into it. Black doctors had been working under the aegis of the Medico-Chirurgical Society, which was a constituent medical society of the NMA, which is a black organization.
>
> The AMA was largely a white organization and most of its constituent organizations such as the District Medical Society were also limited to white members. In order to become a member of the AMA, you had to belong to the local medical society. When you would go and file your application to become a member of the hospital the first question that was asked is "Are you a member of the District Medical Society?" The answer would have to be "No, but I am a member of the Medico-Chirurgical Society." They may

> be synonymous in function, have all the ethics that go along with a good medical society, but it was not a satisfactory answer. You simply had to be a member of the District Medical Society. So that was where we started.

When the push for this acceptance began in 1949, Eddie was vice president of the Medico-Chirurgical Society and part of a special committee formed to integrate the District Medical Society. Dr. John Sinclair Perry, president; Dr. Ulysses L. Houston, past president; and Dr. Montague Cobb, past president and chairman, comprised the remainder of the committee.

The twists and turns of the negotiations are difficult to follow even with all the newspaper coverage the struggle received and the eyewitness accounts of the happenings provided by Eddie, medical historians, and another of the key participants, Dr. W. Montague Cobb.[48] Success seemed imminent several times when something else would arise to block progress. From both Cobb's and Eddie's accounts it is clear that the black physicians strove to gain membership in the District Medical Society in as amicable a way as possible. No demonstrations or threats of legal action were made, nor was any legal action taken. The white doctors of the District Medical Society were to become their colleagues and the black doctors were well aware that the animosity caused by threats would only hamper their working together in the future.

The committee first met with the president of the District Medical Society, Dr. John Minor, and its executive secretary, Mr. Theodore Wiprud, in June 1949 and explained that recent events indicated a liberalization of attitudes as evidenced by the entrance of black physicians into medical societies in other parts of the country. If these opinions were reflected in the District Medical Society, there seemed a possibility that the Medico-Chirurgical Society could achieve its goal without the rancor involved in a legal or lobbying effort. No response to the subject of this meeting had been received by November 1949. Dr. Cobb wrote a letter inquiring as to the status of the matter and was informed that while it had been "discussed at nearly every meeting of the board since that time, no satisfactory conclusion has been reached."[49]

Over the next year, some overtures were made from both organizations. In March 1950, the Medico-Chirurgical members were invited to attend the scientific sessions of the District Society. Dr. Freeman, the president of the District Medical Society, was invited to present the Charles Sumner lecture in May 1950, and his address was published in the *Journal of the National Medical Association* in July. A scientific manuscript by a Medico-Chirurgical member was published in the *Medical Annals of the District of Columbia.*

The American Medical Association was beginning to pressure local groups that still discriminated to rethink the race issue. In the meantime, just across the Potomac River, the Arlington County Medical Society dropped its racial ban of black physicians in February 1951.[50]

Finally a ballot was taken by mail of the membership of the District Medical Society on the admission of blacks. In May 1951, it was announced that 674 had voted for admission and 290 were against. Newspapers hailed the end of the "color bar," and it was assumed that applications from black physicians for membership would be accepted. Within twenty-four hours, Eddie had sought an application for membership to the District Medical Society. On May 7, Wiprud sent a letter and application to Eddie. Three other black physicians followed suit during the month. All four applicants were interviewed by the Board of Censors on December 12, 1951 and found qualified.[51]

Despite the vote and the interviews, victory was not to be gained without further struggle. Eddie was to learn that the ballot was not considered as a mandate and that a further vote would have to be taken. On April 2, 1952, members were asked to vote on the issue at an all-day ballot, in person, at the Society headquarters. Nonmembers were barred from attending a previously scheduled open panel discussion on malpractice held by the District Medical Society on April 16. A last-minute switch to a closed meeting left Eddie and some friends standing on the outside of the secured doors; a slight that was deeply felt.[52]

> In the interim, I went down with a friend of mine, a white lawyer named Dorsey Offutt. We attempted to enter the meeting to watch the proceedings but we were denied admission because neither of us was a member. We stood outside on the sidewalk and talked about inequities and discrimination and this type of thing. Dorsey was quite a fighter in his legal way.

It was announced on May 8 that the number voting on April 2 was fewer than half and that a new mail ballot would be taken and held valid if more than half of the members responded. Finally Dr. Frank D. Costenbader, the retiring president, announced, on the evening of June 30, that the 735 in favor to the 296 opposed was a mandate to add to the bylaws the phrase that "no qualifying physician applying for membership shall be denied membership because of race, creed or color." Only 57 more physicians had voted than over a year earlier. Costenbader also noted that the four applications for black physicians that were pending would be processed through regular channels.[53]

Finally, on September 22, 1952, at forty-one, in Eddie's second year as president of the Medico-Chirurgical Society, he and four other black physicians were accepted for membership in the Medical Society of the District of Columbia.[54] The October 1 form letter from Theodore Wiprud, with Eddie's name typed in the blank space after "Dear Dr.," was a rather anticlimactic end to the long struggle.

The news of the integration of the Medical Society was not universally hailed by all segments of District society. The Federation of Citizens Associations ousted them from membership after they admitted black physicians.[55] Eddie sent a letter of protest but to no avail, as the bylaws of the federation specified only white membership. Such maneuvers made it clear to all observers that there were still many changes to be made if equality were ever to become a reality in Washington.

Now Eddie and the Medico-Chirurgical Society were ready to turn their attention toward the integration of the hospitals. Although hospital integration was of paramount importance in Eddie's life, other involvements were also demanding attention in 1952.

# CHAPTER SIX 

# The Battle Continues

Let us be reminded that segregation, whether racial or religious, voluntary, or enforced inevitably leads to boundless conflicts—conflicts which restrict and deny opportunities, penalize a nation and create universal dissension and final destruction.
— *Edward C. Mazique, 1957*

After the District's collapse as a territory in 1854, agreement was difficult to attain on how it should be managed. Everyone seemed to want control. The stormy debate was finally settled by an act of Congress in June 1878, which detailed a plan that was to hold sway for the next ninety years.[1]

Under the new arrangement residents of the District were to be denied control over taxes and local problems. In exchange for their giving up these rights, the federal government was to share expenses equally with the District taxpayers. Three presidentially appointed commissioners and Congress would govern. Two of the commissioners were to be civilians with at least three years of local residence and the third was to be an officer of the Army Corps of Engineers. The public works functions were assigned to the engineer commissioner, public safety to one of the civilian commissioners, and social programs to the other. Administration and appeals were handled jointly, and some functions were assigned to other federal agencies and autonomous boards and committees. In the final analysis this new system gave extensive power to three people who were not in any way responsible to the local residents.

Throughout the years, those who were interested in social change were interested in some kind of "home rule" for the District.[2] In 1961, the

Twenty-third Amendment to the Constitution finally granted the citizens of the District the right to vote in presidential elections. It was not until 1967 that the District government was to have an executive branch with a mayor and deputy mayor who were presidential appointees and a separate legislative council. Since 1970, Washingtonians were allotted a nonvoting delegate to the House of Representatives. Congress approved partial home rule in 1974 when they allowed residents to elect a mayor and a city council.

As part of this continuing struggle toward enfranchisement, in July 1952 the commissioners created the Citizens Advisory Council.[3] It was an attempt to simplify and strengthen the city government while giving the citizens a larger voice in their own affairs. Since the council was appointed, not elected, the actual increase in control was minimal. Eddie was one of the first nine people appointed, with one other member being black. His work with the Medico-Chirurgical Society and the integration of the District Medical Society had made Eddie a well-known figure in the community. Woolsey W. Hall, the other black appointee, was the former president of the Federation of Civic Associations and had served in a similar advisory capacity to the commissioners in 1931.

On July 2, 1952, Eddie and the other eight council members took the oath of office at the District building. Robert V. Fleming, the president of the board of the Riggs National Bank, was elected to serve as chairman of the council. That night a reception was held at the Washington Hotel and the two black councilmen were in attendance at a hotel that had not seen a black guest over the many years of segregation in Washington. It was a heady experience for Eddie to view Washington from the balcony of the hotel, but he was promptly brought back to the reality when Robert Fleming, in a gesture of kindness, made it clear how little he understood about black men and black achievement.

> That first night after I was sworn in I was permitted to attend a reception at the Washington Hotel. From that terrace you could see all of Washington. I had never seen such beauty. I just stepped out on the terrace alone because I didn't know too many of the guys.
>
> He walked out. Robert Fleming. He was a powerful man. To be chairman of the board of Riggs Bank was quite a thing. He said to me, "Dr. Mazique we are mighty glad to have you on the board. I want to let you know as chairman of this board that I have no prejudices. I like

> you people. I like the colored people. I'll tell you what I did for Jamie. Jamie was our maid, just like a member of our family. When Jamie was living with us we just loved and adored her. Jamie would always say she wanted a big funeral and she wanted a white coffin and she wanted lots of flowers. And Dr. Mazique, I want to let you know that when Jamie died we gave her the most beautiful white coffin you ever saw and we had flowers all over the place."

Eddie had some positive experiences and made some lifelong friends in what was to be a very short term. A fellow council member who frequently sided with Eddie on issues, J. C. Turner, then the president of the Central Labor Union, remembered Fleming as a good chief executive. Despite being conservative on some issues, Fleming would listen and he could be persuaded. He would look at things, think about them, and sometimes go along.[4]

One of the recommendations the council accepted was Dr. Mazique's argument in support of fluoridation.[5] There was a public outcry when the District introduced fluoride into the water supply in June 1952. It was not an issue particularly well known at the time, and it became Eddie's responsibility to make a presentation to the board about the benefits and disadvantages of fluoridation. Eddie did a lot of research and presented the council with a whole history on what had been done in other states and cities and convinced them to go to the commissioners with a strong recommendation in favor of continuing to fluoridate the water. The commissioners concurred and fluoridation was maintained in the District.

An experience Eddie remembered with particular pleasure was his lunch with Joe Kaufmann at the exclusive Occidental Restaurant.

> When we finished our work one day a member of the council, Joe Kaufmann, said to me, "Ed, lets go across the street and have lunch." Casually we walked across the street and there stood the Willard Hotel, which, of course, was in those days segregated. Then he headed for the big sign that said Occidental Restaurant, which was a first-class place where all the big fellows, like the senators, congressmen, and all the high government officials, would go.

> He was headed in that direction. It just never occurred to me where he was going to take me for lunch. I figured since I was a member of the Advisory Council, maybe I was accepted in the inner circles.
>
> We got there and almost got to the door. Joe went to open it and suddenly he stopped dead and turned around and faced me and said: "Damn." I said, "What's wrong?" He said, "We can't go in there. I'm not going to walk in there and get you embarrassed." He said, "Nobody will give us a seat; nobody will wait on us. It would be hard for you." I paused a while and I looked at him and smiled and I said, "Joe, how do you feel about it?" He said, "I feel just like I told you." I said, "I'll tell you something. If it doesn't hurt you, it's not going to hurt me. You see, I'm accustomed to this stuff and I've developed a type of immunity to it. So let's go and see what happens." He looked at me and said, "If that's the way you feel about it."
>
> We went in. They had Negro waiters there. The guy who came to greet us, his eyes got big. After he had regained his composure, without any hesitation, he led us to a table and we sat down. We were served at that table without any problems. You could see the black employees huddling together making note of the fact that something was happening there. But they were gracious even though they were surprised. You could see their eyes were gladdened by the incident. After that, we walked on out. Joe said, "That is a new one on me."

Although the federal government led the way in the desegregation of restaurants, including the one at National Airport that came under the jurisdiction of the Civil Aeronautics Administration, this did nothing to open up privately owned restaurants. In an attempt to end segregation in public places, a biracial Coordinating Committee for the Enforcement of the District Antidiscrimination Laws was formed in 1949 to try to get the 1872 and 1873 laws, which had never been repealed, enforced. As a test case, the John R. Thompson Restaurant Company was sued. It was not until the case reached the Supreme Court, in 1953, where the justices unanimously affirmed the validity of the eighty-year-old Equal

Service Acts, that restaurants were officially opened to all races. The District Commissioners refused to act on any ruling until all appeals had been settled.[6]

From 1950 until the Supreme Court decision in 1953, much had been accomplished to desegregate restaurants by peaceful sit-ins in which Eddie and numerous other concerned blacks participated. One of the larger department stores, the Hecht Company, opened its lunchroom in November 1951 and other department and drugstores along lower Seventh Street followed in a few months.

The importance of the opening of restaurants to black customers was more than a matter of ethics and justice. It was also a very practical issue that had a great impact on the ability of black people to enjoy what downtown Washington had to offer.

> What whites failed to take into account were the bodily discomforts to which racial barriers had subjected colored citizens. For fifty years, any Negro who worked downtown, out of reach of a government cafeteria, had to travel several miles to get a bite of lunch. And as long as eating places excluded Negroes, restrooms which colored people could use were few and far between. For that reason, colored parents had rarely taken their children to shop in the big well-supplied downtown stores.[7]

Many other parts of the country were even slower to desegregate than the District, which made travel to them difficult. Eddie's friend, a priest named Father Patrick Nagle, who accompanied Eddie and his two sons on trips to visit historic sites remembered how, in going to see Gettysburg, they had to bring their own lunch since there was no place that would serve blacks. Then when the two young boys needed to go to the bathroom, there was absolutely no place to take them. He remembered little Jeff crying and finally Eddie's having to just stop the car by the side of the road. It turned out to be a much harsher history lesson than Eddie had intended for his sons.[8]

Eddie had a manner and style that helped him win people to his position. J. C. Turner remembered how there would be a tense moment in the Advisory Council meeting and Eddie would josh someone or tell one of his funny stories. There was a warmth that Eddie projected and a grace that made his accomplishments possible. But in 1952, even all his charm was not enough to make up for the waves Eddie was creating. There were just too many things Eddie wanted to alter, and it clearly worried those not anxious to make changes.

> When I got on the board, I knew I was locked in by hierarchy and bureaucracy in terms of what I could accomplish. How are you going to fight discrimination if you don't start somewhere and make the public aware of the affronts of segregation? I felt the best place to start was in the government, in the political arena.
>
> There was a labor leader who worked well with me. His name was J. C. Turner. He is still a very dear friend of mine. He is white. He turned out to be the best friend I had on the council. He would ride along with me on things. I was in charge of health issues and I did manage to push for fluoridation in the District of Columbia.
>
> I wanted the council meetings to be open. I wanted the newspapers to be there and all the media, whoever could be there. I wanted exposure. I wanted them to hear what everyone would say on any given issue that would come up. In order to let the public know about segregation and discrimination, I was for open hearings of the council each time we would meet. They didn't want that.[9]
>
> They had another black on the board named Woolsey Hall who was pretty much a figurehead. He was an older fellow, a nice guy, but he "ain't going to ripple no water." Anyway, I started rippling a little bit too much so they got dissatisfied and decided they would try to do something to get me off the council.

As head of the committee to study fluoridation, Eddie admitted the press to two of its sessions. The newspaper articles about the council meetings reflected the importance to the public of the issue of open meetings, but not the bitterness of the debate within the council.

> Without going through a lot of stuff, it was really rugged. I began to become uneasy. Soon after I was sworn in, it was clear a feeling was developing that I was too liberal-minded. They felt they could do without me.

The main thing that happened was they concocted a lot of stuff about me and dug up the old thing with the House Un-American Activities Committee, that I was Communist and all that junk. Nonetheless, I weathered it out.

They became restless on the board. The members, mainly Mr. Fleming, the chairman of the board, went to the head commissioner, whose name was Joseph Donohue—we called him "Jiggs"—and told him to see if he could get me in line. "Jiggs" was the most liberal white commissioner that we ever had in the District.

Nothing happened right away. But soon after, my wife got a telegram stating that she was being subpoenaed. At this time, she was in her third trimester of pregnancy with Jeffrey. She was going to have to appear before the House Un-American Activities Committee to face charges of being a Communist. I really didn't want my wife to be exposed to this type of thing, especially given the pregnant state she was in. I thought it was unjust. At that time, there was no Charlie Houston around whom I could go to. I had a lawyer but he was not that kind of fighter. I sought legal advice on it and I didn't know what to do. I mulled it over and developed ulcers over it. Another telegram followed. I didn't know what steps to take.

Finally, "Jiggs" called me in. He told me he knew what was happening to my wife because they had sent him a letter to this effect. I said, "Well that does not affect me. You know damn well that I have never been a member of the Communist Party. I don't know anything about it. So I don't see where I am involved." He said, "They aren't after your wife, they are after you to get you off the council. I know you are concerned about it and I can stop her from being called." I told him I was grateful. He said, "The only way I can stop it is if we have a deal. You resign because they are really after you. They are not after her. You are too open-minded and too outspoken about discrimination and segregation. I feel the same way about it as you do, but you got a choice to make between your family and the life of your child and

> whether you want to stand and fight this type of hypocrisy that exists. I want to let you know that if you come off the council, I can get all the charges dropped."
>
> Well, you know, it took a whole lot of time to make that decision. I tried every way I could to figure out what steps to take. Whether to fight it and then know they would come up with some other damn manner in which to do the same thing. After long thinking and consultation with others, my decision was to leave the board. I left it because of my family. I issued a statement that I was leaving. I never shall forget when I went in to see "Jiggs" to tell him I had arrived at a decision. I said, "People are going to want to know why." He said, "Give no answer, and make it short." He was a lawyer. He said, "Simply use one sentence. Say you resign because of personal reasons." That was my statement.
>
> I don't know who it was on the council who had the connection with McCarthy to get me off. But this is the way the system works. How are you as an individual to work courageously and manfully within a system like that and still achieve in spite of it, knowing that these innuendos are developing to swallow you up?
>
> That's how and why I left the council. After experiencing that kind of a pressure, I know now and understand why politicians are faced sometimes with charges that are unjust. I can understand the undercurrents of things. It is bigger than just that—there is the plum they are after and the way they are going to get the plum is to chop the tree down.

At the November meeting of the Citizens Advisory Council, the paper reported that Eddie, J. C. Turner, and Joseph A. Kaufmann, the three liberals, had sided together in an effort to recommend keeping the public assistance rolls closed to public view.[10] On December 9, five months after Eddie took his oath as a councilman, Brigadier General Benjamin O. Davis, a retired, seventy-five-year-old, black army general, was named to replace Eddie on the council. The article stated simply that "Dr. Mazique, a colored physician, said he was leaving the post for 'personal reasons'."[11] In February 1953, when Eddie was named to the *Washington Afro-American*'s Honor Roll for 1952, the article noted that he had resigned the honorary post on the Citizen's Advisory Council when "he found that he would have to swallow his racial pride to maintain the job."[12]

In 1952 there were plenty of vehicles other than the Citizen's Advisory Council through which Eddie could work toward integration. As president of the Medico-Chirurgical Society in 1951, 1952, and 1953, ending the segregation in the District hospitals was one of his top priorities.

A 1945 study conducted by the American Hospital Association found that the segregated system of hospitalization in the United States was denying black physicians the opportunity to develop professionally and relegating black patients to inferior health care.[13] Yet despite the breakthrough with Gallinger Hospital in 1948 and the admission of Eddie and four other black physicians to the District Medical Society in 1952, the voluntary hospitals in Washington still denied privileges to black physicians.

Dr. Montague Cobb, the authoritative scholar on the medical history of the District, described the integration of Hadley Hospital that occurred in 1952 as a very genial affair. Several years before the hospital was built, Dr. Hadley made the unprecedented move of seeking approval from the Medico-Chirurgical Society for the policies under which the new hospital would operate. Dr. Cobb reported that the society cooperated with Dr. Hadley and almost immediately a black surgeon was appointed to the staff. Several other black physicians were given consultation and courtesy privileges and patients were not segregated. The nursing staff and technical personnel were given assignments according to their qualifications.[14]

Eddie remembered the integration of Hadley a bit differently. His account makes it clear why Dr. Hadley would choose to approach the Medico-Chirurgical Society instead of the District Medical Society for approval.

> Hadley was a small, private hospital in southeast Washington. They were just getting established. In order for them to become recipients of Blue Cross–Blue Shield they had to be approved by a recognized medical organization. Dr. Hadley went to the Medical Society of the District of Columbia for this approval. For whatever reasons, they turned him down. He came over to see me and we had a talk. The upshot of it was that I carried the matter before our board of governors and we decided what to do. The strategy was, we'll give you approval so you can get your insurance money but the price tag

> is you must give us black physicians on the staff of Hadley Hospital. We gave him the names of four men to serve on the staff. We got a letter back from Hadley saying yes we will accept them to serve on our staff. One of the men initially on it was P. Wilkins Davis in radiology, and he is still serving on the staff over there as chief radiologist. That was the first one that we got down. And of course I went on the staff over there.

The National Association for the Advancement of Colored People (NAACP) and the Medico-Chirurgical Society in 1953 launched a public offensive against the segregation still existent in the District hospitals. Letters were sent to eighteen directors of voluntary and federal hospitals from the chairman of the Health Committee of the local branch of the NAACP, Dr. Montague Cobb, as well as from the president of the local NAACP, Eugene Davidson, and from Edward C. Mazique, the president of the Medico-Chirurgical Society.[15]

Despite numerous applications to District hospitals, no black physicians were admitted to the staffs in 1953. The summer of 1954 saw a similar assault by the NAACP, this time with Eddie as Health Committee chairman. The NAACP claimed it was illegal for the District hospitals to discriminate since they were recipients of federal and District tax monies. They threatened the hospitals with a proposed petition to Congress to add an antidiscrimination clause to all hospital appropriations.[16] A local black newspaper urged support from all civic groups, claiming that the barring of "Negro" physicians from the staffs of hospitals and "Negro" patients from admittance or segregating them once they are admitted are "incredible" given the "tremendous progress made in other areas."[17]

Finally, it was announced on September 23, 1954 that Dr. Edward Mazique and Dr. Frank Jones were to be admitted to the staff at Georgetown University Hospital.[18] Providence Hospital also announced that it would remove restrictions against "Negro" physicians on the staff, but it would be later in the year before they would appoint any. It was clear that changes were going to be made throughout the District health care system and all the newspapers carried articles on the breakthrough. One newspaper entitled its article "A Quiet Transition."[19] It may have seemed quiet to the casual observer, but to Eddie and the other physicians who were slowly entering the bastions of white medicine it was a time of tension, uncertainty, challenge, and exhilaration.

They had actually won! Now it was up to those who went first to prove themselves and their race capable.

There were different problems associated with getting on the staff of each hospital. One thing clear from Eddie's experience was that since the system was so dominated by white physicians, initially entrance was possible only through the kindness and open-mindedness of a few white doctors. Nowhere was this reality more evident than at George Washington University Hospital, where Dr. Walter Bloedorn was willing to take the risk necessary to support the appointment of its first black physician.

> I went to see about gaining admission to George Washington and got the forms. I filled out the part about academic training and the next thing required were references from two doctors currently serving on the staff. This was a real stumbling block for black doctors. How in the world are you going to know white doctors if you have had no opportunities to interact with them? I did know one fairly well, Walter Bloedorn, who at that time was dean of the Medical School of George Washington University. He was quite well known and respected throughout the city. Walter had taught at Howard University and served as the chief of staff at Freedmen's Hospital so he knew about the institution and the caliber of people there. I had called Walter in on some of my cases for consultation and he would come and make house visits. We had a good, wholesome relationship.
>
> One day, I called him up and told him what my problem was and explained that I would like to have his endorsement. He said all right, Mazique, come on up. His office was on I Street in downtown Washington. He gave me a time to be there. I was there on time. I was greeted by the secretary and told her my mission. She said, "The doctor is expecting you." I gave her the paper for him to sign. I thought all he would do is sign this and send it back instantly. Instead I waited for fifteen minutes, thirty minutes, an hour, and started getting very restless.
>
> Finally after about two hours, he came out and said, "I will see Dr. Mazique, send him in." I went in. He told me, "Mazique, you probably wondered why I kept

> you so long. Usually we don't keep our colleagues that long but I am going to be perfectly frank with you. This is the very first time that this has been done here. It is historic and I wanted to make damn sure of what I was doing. I don't mind telling you that I called up and searched all of your academic records and checked on your standing in the community. I have even searched your police records and they are all clear. I know I am taking an individual stance here, but I am going to sign this and endorse you." I smiled and thanked him. He said, "You have got to have someone else's signature." I said, "Doctor, I don't believe I know another white doctor in the city except you." At that time he had a youngster working with him whom I have come to know well. His name was Dr. Kirchner. He specialized in diabetes. He called his associate in and asked him to sign under his name endorsing me. He didn't even question it, he just signed. He gave me the papers, shook my hand, and said, "I wish you luck" and that was it.
>
> I submitted the application and the board passed on it favorably and I was admitted as the first black physician at George Washington University Hospital. I took several of my patients there and was the object of a great deal of curiosity.

Getting into a few hospitals did not mean that the barriers in all the hospitals would automatically be lowered. Eddie was optimistic and was quoted in one of the newspapers as saying "the rest is just a question of time."[20] In 1954, although significant inroads had been made, there still existed various types of segregation in many of the District hospitals. Black doctors were still barred from the staffs of many of the private hospitals. In hospitals where they were admitted, black patients were often put on separate and inferior wards. Two hospitals, Sibley Memorial and Homeopathic, were still refusing to even admit black patients. The name Sibley had become synonymous with the injustice of segregation. It did not seem likely that Sibley would change policy of its own accord. Eddie recalled how the pressure was brought to bear on Sibley.

> There were other hospitals still around which were not even touched yet. The next one on the list was

Sibley Memorial. It had its facility on Second Street, North East, down by the post office.

The records will show that Sibley was so segregated they would not only not admit Negro physicians but they would not treat black patients. There came a time on a cold snowy night in January that a colored female went into labor. She went to the emergency room of Sibley, which was close to her home, for delivery. They told her they would not accept a colored patient. She had to leave in pain and agony and go out on the street. Before she could get somewhere else, her baby was delivered in the snow in front of the hospital.[21]

Sibley needed funds. I knew that. It was a Methodist hospital so I contacted a friend of mine who had done a lot of infighting with me with labor and the YMCA, Reverend Charles Webber. He was an active, Christian gentleman. He and I marched together on the picket lines for the YMCA. Knowing that he was Methodist and held in high esteem in the Methodist hierarchy and also a friend of the bishop, I went to him and we had a long talk.

Reverend Webber was working with the labor movement. He was a counselor and pastor for the AFL-CIO and had an office in D.C. He knew all about labor and was a friend of Meany's.[22] I explained to him what the problem was. He says, "I got it. The AFL-CIO is in the process of making a contribution to Sibley Hospital. We'll stop that contribution unless they admit Negro physicians on the staff." Right away, he sent a telegram to Meany and the bishop. It wasn't more than two days when a reply came through. "We are for it. We will cut off all funds unless they have Negro physicians on the staff. Labor will not donate this money for the construction of a new hospital."

I went right over to Sibley and got my application and filled it out and sent it in. Almost the next day, I got a call stating that I was admitted. The man in question who was heading the hospital was Dr. Owen. He was in orthopedics. He turned out to be a wonderful man once I got in there. Every year when it was time to renew, he

> would call up and remind me to pay my dues. He would say, "Look, we don't want to lose you as a member of the staff, you know." He turned out to be a great friend.

Staff positions became easier to obtain once the black physicians started to have some interaction with their white colleagues.

> Providence was an interesting story. By the time I applied to be on the staff at Providence my contacts with white doctors were increasing. I had quite a few friends, among them Doctor James Kane. He was a Catholic and a good man in obstetrics and gynecology. I was dabbling in hypnosis and Jim was also interested in hypnosis. We worked in a group and received certificates in hypnosis together. I had referred some of my patients to him. We had a good understanding. He would talk to me about what a beautiful hospital Providence was.
>
> When I needed an endorsement to get on the staff at Providence, I called on Jim. I said: "Jim, how about an endorsement? I need two people. I have the application." "Well," he said, "Ed, I'll tell you what I'll do. Let me pick you up and I'll see if I can get another friend of mine who is active on the staff of Providence, Dr. Leo Gaffney." Dr. Gaffney was a team physician for all the Catholic schools, particularly Dematha, which had a good basketball team.
>
> Jim said, "I'll come by and pick you up and we'll go to the basketball game, watch the game, and then at the half we'll go see Leo and see if I can get him to sign with me to endorse you." I said, "I could meet you there, you don't have to come by." He said, "No, go on home and enjoy yourself. I know where you live."
>
> At the time I was on 1824 Upshur Street. I was the only black up there. He came by at the allotted time, in the afternoon on a Saturday. I was ready to cut out when he arrived but he asked me for a drink of water. I went down the four steps in my split-level house into the kitchen and he followed me. He took the water and took his time about drinking it. I noticed that he was looking around. He looked out the window at the backyard, he

> looked up the stairs. I thought nothing of it. The kids were hanging around. He met them and my wife and the maid. Finally we left to go to the game.
>
> At the half we went over to Leo and he introduced me to him. At that point he asked Leo if he would sign. Leo listened to him and looked at me and asked me a few questions. He said to me: "Mazique, don't let me down." I said, "I will try not to, Doctor, and I appreciate it very much." So he signed. I carried it over to Providence and I was in.

Years later Jim Kane spoke to Eddie about that incident:

> "Hey, Ed, did I ever tell you why I didn't want to pick you up at the office? . . . I wanted to see what kind of home you were living in. I never knew any colored folks other than the maid and the janitor. I didn't know if you all lived the same way. I looked around and saw you were living better than I was."[23]

Once on the staff, Eddie derived a great deal of satisfaction in seeing how much it meant to blacks to have a black physician on the premises.

> You will never understand how much pride it gave other blacks and coloreds to see someone make a dent in this thing. One day I was going through the parking lot at George Washington and I saw a family come along. It was a woman whom I had known at the hospital. She pointed me out to her children, saying there goes the only black doctor on the staff.

It was not only doctors, medical societies, or antisegregation organizations who played a part in making it possible for Eddie and other doctors to succeed in getting on hospital staffs. There were countless other people whose influence will never be fully known. A nurse in a hospital with only white doctors related how in talking with black patients who were not very seriously ill, it would be suggested they request a black doctor. The patients would ask for a black physician, saying they had never been treated by a white doctor. They would explain how they would feel more comfortable with a doctor of their own race. Eddie attributed a lot of the success of his and others' admission to staff privileges to this kind of pressure brought by patients upon the administration of a particular hospital.[24]

Receiving staff positions in the hospitals did not automatically guarantee equal treatment of the doctors or their patients. Some of the most obdurate problems arose after Eddie was accepted on the staff of Providence, a hospital where, ironically, he would one day serve as president of the medical-dental staff.

> Of course most of the hospitals were highly segregated when it came to patients. You worked within the climate of things as best you could.
>
> One of the most traumatic experiences I had in Providence was with a patient whom a friend of mine, Dr. Spellman, admitted. Dr. Spellman came in after I did and was doing chiefly surgery. Before then, I had to use the white surgeon.
>
> One night a patient of mine needed to be admitted for surgery. When Dr. Spellman called, he identified himself and said he wanted to admit a patient named so and so whose diagnosis was appendicitis. The admission clerk said, "Yes doctor, colored or white?" Dr. Spellman said, "He's sick." Oh boy, that did it. Next thing Mike Spellman was on the way out.

This was not the only incident with Dr. Mitchell Wright Spellman, who apparently became known at Providence as a bit of a troublemaker.[25] A dean of Harvard University Medical School when he was interviewed, he recalled how on another occasion a black physician asked him to admit a patient of his who was a legislative assistant to Eugene McCarthy, then the congressman from Minnesota. The aide was white. The question of race never arose during the conversation with Dr. Spellman. The hospital staff simply assumed the patient was black.

The patient was placed in a two- or four-bed unit with black patients until they realized he was white. He was then quickly transferred. In the past, when Dr. Spellman had questioned the placement of patients he had been told it was simply fortuitous that the black patients all ended up together. This case seemed to be clear-cut discrimination based on race.

Dr. Spellman arranged a meeting with the administrator, Sister Eleanor. She listened to his story and his protest and responded by explaining that as a manager, it was her responsibility to see that the hospital was run efficiently and remained on a sound financial basis. The attitude of white patients had to be considered.

A few months later, when Dr. Spellman called in to have another patient admitted, he was informed he was no longer a member of the staff. Apparently when his renewal came up, they chose not to renew his courtesy privileges and did not even inform him. At the time, he was a full-time member of the staff at Howard and was not dependent on the use of Providence so it did not seem the time for him to fight it as a major battle. Nor did Dr. Spellman remember any great rallying by the other physicians around his cause. The newly admitted black doctors were choosing their battles carefully and holding onto their hard-fought positions to work inside the system.[26]

Eddie tried to lobby some behind the scenes for Dr. Spellman but to no avail.

> I had developed a pretty good rapport with Dr. Philip Caulfield, who was white and proved to be a very good man, a Christian and a Catholic. I went in and we began to talk about intolerances and injustices springing up in a Christian institution. We were both Catholic. The answer was, we are sorry but the decision of the committee is that we will have to suspend Dr. Spellman from staff privileges. So Mike was out. I got a warning and stayed on and kept up the fight. But that was how it was.

Eddie and Dr. Spellman were deeply hurt by this experience because they were Catholics. It was difficult to reconcile their faith in and commitment to the Catholic Church with the way in which this Catholic hospital was managed. They felt such treatment relegated them and their race to beings of lower worth and made a mockery of the Church's teachings about brotherhood. The height of irony, as Dr. Spellman noted, was that when Sister Eleanor left Providence she was elevated to the highest position in her order.

Racism within the Catholic institution was not something new to Eddie. For many years, he had stopped attending the Catholic church because of the experiences he had when he first came to the District.

> On Main Street in Natchez there was a Catholic church. The whites would take the front seats and the

> blacks would have to sit in the back. There was another church which was named Family Church which was called the Negro Catholic church. When you went there for Mass in the morning, the colored or Negroes would all go up front but if whites came in they would have to sit in the back.
>
> I could understand that—that was in Mississippi. You learned somehow that you are going to have to accept and live with the situation there because you can't do anything about it. It's not vulnerable. Timing is a great thing. There is a time to do everything. There is a time for striking, a time when you don't strike. There is a time when you move forward; there is a time when you retreat and think and refurbish your forces and make new plans to go out again. There is a right time to do these things. There was no timing then to challenge this type of seating arrangement. You had to know that.
>
> When I came up to Washington and walked into a Catholic church I went up front to sit. They told me to go to the back. The timing was then to make my statement. I just kept walking and walked out of the church and didn't go back in the 1940s.

Attitudes did begin to change slowly at Providence, as Eddie's later encounter with Dr. Caulfield showed.

> It was not until I was there about a year and a half, when I was walking out to the parking lot alone, that Dr. Caulfield approached me. For the first time, he put his arm around me as we walked out to the parking lot. He said, "Eddie, do you mind if I call you Eddie? I'd like for you to call me Phil. I don't mind telling you that when you first came here you were under a lot of surveillance. We didn't know whether you had the capability to practice here. It was the first time a colored doctor had been out here. We watched everything you were doing. Everybody looked at you as a colored doctor. Now, I want you to know, they look upon you now as another physician and I would like to be your friend." I thought

> that was a victory well won. He's living today, he's retired, and we are still good friends.

The hospital eventually came full circle when, in the 1960s, Sister Eleanor's replacement at Providence called Dr. Spellman to offer him privileges once again. At this time he was getting ready to leave for California and turned the offer down.

Eddie's Catholicism or the lack of it became an important issue when he decided he wanted his children to go to a Catholic school. The District public schools in the late 1950s and early 1960s were still not fully integrated. In 1953, the Medico-Chirurgical Society presented the Consolidated Parents Group a one-thousand-dollar donation to aid in their Supreme Court suit against the Jim Crow practices of the District public schools.[27] Jewell was one of the leaders among the doctor's wives who raised the funds. May 1954 saw the Supreme Court hand down a decision in *Brown v. Board of Education* declaring that segregation in the public schools was unconstitutional. Integration began with the fall enrollment for 1954. Yet six years after integration began, whites were still asking and receiving transfers for "psychological reasons" from predominately black schools to predominately white schools. However, the problems involved in the physical placement of students were much less difficult than the disparity between the education whites and blacks had received in previous years in their respective schools. It was impossible to rapidly compensate for differences in funding that had left the black schools understaffed, overcrowded, and in poorer-quality facilities.

With the public schools in a turmoil, Eddie's oldest son, Edward, or "Skip" as he was called, was enrolled in kindergarten at the Sidwell Friends School in 1956 as its first "Negro" student. Skip's admission caused Senator James O. Eastland, a staunch anti-integrationist from Mississippi, to withdraw his son from enrollment.[28] The irony was that Skip had been recommended to the Sidwell School by other white southerners from Texas and the Delta.

As his sons grew older, Eddie felt they needed a bit more discipline and looked for a school that would instill in them strong values. He decided he wanted them enrolled in a Catholic school and found he had to reconsider his own relationship with the Church if he wished them to be students.

> I thought the boys needed more discipline, someone to help rear them. There was no one in the house

> most of the time. There was no one to pick up the business of right and wrong and ethics and Christianity and discipline, all things I believed they needed. Me, I was out most of the time. I hired help, I always did. We always had a man and wife in the house, continually. As they began to grow up, they needed more than that. I had to get someone so I went back to the Catholic Church.
>
> I was told if I came back they would take my boys into the school. I told the monsignor I had left the church earlier because of the segregation and he said, "We are not the same way anymore." So I went back to rejoin the church. One of the newspapers carried an article saying I was converted. I don't know if I was converted or not but I came back. The next Monday, my kids went to Catholic school. Then I began to take them to church every Sunday at Sacred Heart.
>
> I was trying to be a role model, the kind of father who always makes some kind of a positive presentation. I had to be twice as strong because I had no one to lean on. In order to get that strength I probably went overboard in religion into Catholicism, into prayer and into the Bible. I think all that helped.
>
> I married Jewell twice. When we agreed I would come back to the Catholic Church, the priest said to me, "We are not done with you yet. You have got to marry because you are not really married since you were not married in the Catholic Church." So we went inside the church. There was someone kneeling down. The priest went and touched him on the shoulder and asked if he would stand up and witness a marriage ceremony. He stood up and we got another marriage certificate.
>
> And sure enough, the church had changed. It wasn't long after that that I was invited to speak before the Catholic club that was meeting once a week. There must have been a thousand members of the club that I spoke to, down at the Presidential Arms Hotel. I even have that speech.[29]

As time went by, getting on the staff of other hospitals was not a problem for Eddie. By 1957 he knew enough white physicians to secure endorsements, and this was true for more and more of his black colleagues. Once on the staff, it was unlikely the hospitals would ever ask Eddie to leave. His practices always ended up being larger than anyone else's. As Dr. Spellman commented, "The hospitals' response was commensurate with their economic interest."[30] Therefore Eddie not only remained on staff but had a great deal of clout once his practice was established at the hospital.

This degree of integration, however, had not been achieved uniformly in all areas of the country. Dr. Montague Cobb was still working on a national level to try to have the health care system improved for blacks. In 1956, when he was editor-in-chief of the *Journal of the National Medical Association,* Dr. Cobb suggested the establishment of an organization whose goal would be the end of discrimination in the country's hospitals. It was called Imhotep ("He who cometh in peace") after the early Egyptian physician.[31] During Dr. Cobb's chairmanship in 1957 and 1958, conferences were held under the sponsorship of the National Medical Association, the National Association for the Advancement of Colored People, the National Urban League, and the Medico-Chirurgical Society of the District of Columbia. They were continued later under the chairmanship of other prominent black physicians for another five years. Despite the "golden opportunity to broaden understanding of the problem and unify action in respect to the elimination of one of the present major barriers to making the best in medical facilities available to all of the people of the nation,"[32] the effectiveness of the conferences in changing practices was limited because of lack of full support and participation of the most powerful health-related organizations: the American Medical Association, the American Hospital Association, and the Protestant and Catholic hospital bodies. In 1964 President Lyndon Johnson forced participation by convening a conference with the leaders of the power structure of the hospitals to stimulate voluntary compliance with the 1964 Civil Rights Act. Dr. Cobb labeled this the "Eighth Imhotep Conference."

Although integration was continuously moving forward in the 1950s, there were still many individuals in the District opposed to the changes. A 1956 newspaper article reported the founding of a "White Citizens Council" whose goals were halting the integration process in Washington, reestablishing segregation, putting the NAACP on the attorney general's subversive list, and eradicating "Rock and Roll" music.[33] Although some organizations were less obvious in their stated goals, many of them were no less determined to preserve segregation. One of them was the local Young Men's Christian Association (YMCA).

Chauncey Longdon was the first corresponding secretary and a member of the Board of Managers for the YMCA, which was established in Washington in 1852. One of his coworkers, Anthony Bowen, a free black man who had become the first "Negro" clerk in the U.S. Patent Office, was attracted by the aspirations of the YMCA. With Longdon's assistance, Bowen founded the Young Men's Christian Association for Colored Men and Boys in 1853. It was the first YMCA for blacks. In 1908 the building of what was to become known as the 12th Street YMCA was begun. This was where Eddie and Mr. Sampson stayed when they first arrived in Washington. In 1972 the name of the building was changed to Anthony Bowen Branch of the YMCA, but in the 1950s it was still known as the 12th Street Branch and was the only YMCA in the metropolitan Washington area where blacks were allowed admittance.[34]

Because of his very high visibility with the Medico-Chirurgical Society and the integration of hospitals, Eddie was becoming more and more sought after by boards of organizations in the city, especially those who wanted a strong leader to push for integration. The YMCA was to be one of the toughest groups Eddie ever lobbied. As head of the Interracial Practices Committee, Eddie annually challenged the membership of the YMCA of metropolitan Washington at their December meetings to display "Christian acceptance and brotherhood."[35] His challenges and the appeals of numerous others were ignored throughout the fifties.[36]

Eddie remembered his YMCA battle as "rough" but had a special fondness for those who fought with him to make it possible:

> Meantime, the community began to pick up and say, "Hey what goes with this fellow Mazique?" I began to get calls and demands to participate in various organizations. So I went to the Y. Naturally, it was segregated. No swimming pools. I began to appear every year at their annual meeting. I couldn't vote but I would talk. I would just let them know there is no place in America for this. That was a rough fight.
>
> We had several conferences with the board of what they called at that time the Central Y, which is located on Eighteenth and H Street, North West. We were down at Twelfth Street North West. We also had occasional meetings with the general secretary. The only entree we had to the proceedings was through this general secretary

who in this instance was a fellow named Randolph Myers. Randy was a stalwart segregationist. Not only was he the general secretary of the Central Branch but also of the Metropolitan Y. The Metropolitan Y included all the YMCAs in the surrounding areas of Virginia and Maryland as well as Washington proper. We always had one representative who would be asked to sit in on the hearings, but the representative was only there to sit and nothing more.

Randy would come when we would have our meetings at the Twelfth Street Branch and see what we were doing and indicate whether he approved of this or that. In order to get some of the funding to have things done in our branch, we had to get approval from the Metropolitan Y.

The YMCA had a school called Southeastern University and also another one called Woodward School for Boys. These schools were segregated. We tried to break through by request and peaceful negotiations but to no avail. We finally decided there would be nothing wrong with going and filing an application to become a board member when they would have their annual elections and meeting. I would do that knowing full well that they would not accept me. There was nothing to prevent someone from getting up on the floor and nominating a person to become a member of the board. We tried that on several occasions. I would sit down and that would be it.

Each year I filed and they would permit me to make a statement. So time after time I would get up and make a statement about the injustices and the fact that it was a shame that an institution that was called a Christian association was practicing such un-Christian-like activities. They were promoting inequities, prejudices, and discriminatory practices by keeping people away from education and not permitting them to fully develop themselves. They would all listen and that would be the end of it.

That procedure kept up and every December, I would go down to do this.

Finally, one cold day in November, Reverend Charles Webber, the man who had helped me with integrating Sibley Hospital, and I decided we would picket the YMCA before the election. We made signs and the two of us went down and started picketing in front of the Y, calling them to task for not permitting colored to come into their schools. For several days we marched up and down and talked to each other. One day, from way up top at the Y where someone was living (people lived there and down below there were swimming pools and other places for activities), urine came out the window and we were doused with it. We smiled at each other and went into the bathroom and washed up and kept on picketing. That was in November. In December I once again appeared before the board and I told them that I was not going to appear before them again. This was my last time. I made what amounted to a farewell speech there.

About the next year, they sent down this fellow from New York. I don't remember why Randy Myers left, whether he retired or was sick or what. Anyway, they replaced him with James Bunting. I was then chairman of the board at the Twelfth Street Branch. Anyway Jim Bunting and I developed a very good and warm relationship. His attitude was totally different from Randy's and we began to work positively to remove barriers and to get this thing going. We had several closed sessions with members of the board and we decided, okay, we'll try one more time.

Finally the agreement of the board was to permit blacks to be integrated into the other Y facilities. Jim Bunting came to my office on Ninth Street; this would have been in 1961 or '62. He said to me: "Dr. Mazique, I want you to be the first to become a member of the Central Branch of the YMCA. I brought you a membership card."

This was all right for me but I asked, "What about my people? I want the kids to know they can come to the swimming pool, the kids in the street to know that they can make application for Southeastern University and Woodward School for Boys." He said, "I don't want you to do it that way. We've worked together this long. I'd appreciate it if we don't have any publicity about it because it will incite some of the members of the board to take away some of the privileges that we have already decided to go along with. Just pick out some individuals whom you know and let them file an application for the school and let them do it in a quiet way and it will be done without fanfare and it will be accomplished that way." That was fine with me as long as the job was done. The hell with the fanfare! So we did it that way and it was quietly integrated.

That was the story of the Y except to say that Belford Lawson, one of the foremost attorneys in the District, was chosen as the first black member to serve on the board of the Metropolitan Y and subsequently became president. Shortly after the integration began, I was nominated for and did serve on the board of the Metropolitan YMCA and have until the present time. After that many other blacks became board members. The barrier was torn down.

# CHAPTER SEVEN 

# A Year at the Helm

Doctors, for many reasons such as complacency, economic security, busy schedules, and fear of public sentiment have failed miserably in their exercise of suffrage and developed a political inertia that America can no longer afford. Physicians are challenged to take their rightful place as citizens and share in the problems and aspirations of society. Medicine is in politics for better or for worse. It cannot be considered separate from socio-economic problems or cultural and physical developments.

— *Edward C. Mazique, 1960*

The fight for equal treatment was far from over in the District, but 1959–1960 afforded Eddie the opportunity to reach a national audience with his ideas. At the relatively young age of forty-seven, he had succeeded in his chosen profession and was rewarded with the highest honor for a black doctor among his peers, to serve as the president of the National Medical Association (NMA).

The opportunities Eddie's position afforded him to act as a spokesperson made the late fifties and 1960 an exhilarating time. Eddie first won a seat in the House of Delegates of the National Medical Association in 1957 and moved on to serve two years as a member of the Board of Trustees. Then the opportunity arose to actually lead the organization. Eddie remembered the day in 1958, at the Schroeder Hotel, when he received the telephone call asking him to run.

I'm lying in bed in Milwaukee, Wisconsin, when, eight o'clock in the morning, my phone rings and

> someone said, "Ed, we decided we want you for president of the organization." No one had said anything about it to me before. I'm young—I'm forty-six years of age now and have a lot of energy. To make a long story short they ran me and I was elected president of the NMA in 1958. Then I began to really get out and do a lot of organizing and visiting a lot, going to a lot of states and lecturing.

The election was far from a sure thing. Eddie's opponent was the outgoing chairman of the board for the National Medical Association, Dr. James T. Aldrich, an older, well-established physician. The victory was only by a two-point margin. One of Eddie's key supporters summed up why he had been chosen by saying, "We wanted someone to head the national who had something else on his mind besides making money. Dr. Mazique is one of those too-few physicians with a genuine interest in civic affairs."[1]

Eddie certainly lived up to his supporters' expectations. He was no sooner elected than he began making his views known. In press interviews he hit hard at the discrimination that still existed in the Washington, D.C., medical system, claiming that some of the hospitals only had one "Negro" on the staff as "window dressing." "Negro" patients were still assigned to certain rooms or areas of the hospital and might even be refused admittance if the quota of "colored" beds was full.

As with most things with which Eddie was involved, even the meeting in Detroit at which he was officially inaugurated was surrounded by controversy.[2] Detroit's mayor, Louis C. Miriani, was scheduled to address the convention at its public meeting held in the Detroit Civic Center on Tuesday, August 11, 1959. The mayor sent his regrets and, in his stead, sent a deputy to present the key of the city to the outgoing president, R. Stillmon Smith, and to welcome the record registration crowd of 1,563 doctors, 1,127 spouses, and their 411 children.[3] Thurgood Marshall, at that time the fiery counsel for the NAACP, was scheduled to speak at the same public session. He delivered a scathing address leveling charges of "Jim Crow" treatment at Detroit's Mayor Miriani. Marshall told the doctors, "[Y]ou haven't escaped discrimination in Detroit, Illinois and New York. . . . The fact that the mayor was not even here to greet you is proof that Jim Crow is not limited to the South."[4]

Eddie and Dr. R. Stillmon Smith, the retiring president of the NMA, called Mr. Miriani and invited him to attend the President's Luncheon on Thursday. Realizing the monetary clout of the doctors and his political error, the mayor was quick to accept the invitation and spent almost four hours with the medical men, not only re-giving the key to the city to Dr. Smith and inviting the NMA to return to Detroit for another conference, but also handing out small souvenir keys to almost everyone present.[5]

Eddie came into the office of president of the NMA with an agenda. His speech, delivered in Detroit on August 13, 1959, was not a bland inaugural address in which he thanked everyone and said what a great organization it was. His prepared copy of the address, entitled "Integration Enters Medicine," was twenty-six pages long.[6] When it was printed in the *Journal of the National Medical Association* it covered a full seven pages, almost two pages of which were very specific recommendations. The speech reflected Eddie's concern that doctors and medicine could not and should not remain aloof from the political processes that affect the social and material well-being of their patients. The housing conditions, the income level, the ability to buy food, the types of literature to which an individual was exposed, all play a part in his or her mental and physical health. The year ahead was spent trying to convince other doctors of the necessity of becoming involved in the political process to pressure for changes that would enhance the lives of citizens and especially the elderly.

Eddie listed specific recommendations that not only stated his goals while he was president of the NMA but pretty much summarized what had been important to him in previous years and for which he would continue to strive during the remainder of his life. One recommendation was about recruitment of membership for the NMA, but the others were issues that reached far beyond the narrow confines of the NMA to the broader issues facing blacks and other disadvantaged groups in the United States and throughout the world.

There was a recommendation for a committee that would redefine the NMA's basic aims and objectives. Eddie saw this committee as having four functions, the most important of which would be making recommendations on national legislation before Congress. Included under his list of legislation that should be of concern to NMA members was support for an increase in appropriations for Indian Health Services, the Johnson Newberger Bill "establishing a voluntary medical hospital insurance for government employees and their dependents under 21," the Keogh Bill allowing for "tax exempt reserves from physicians' income to establish a retirement plan," and the bill of supreme importance to Eddie, the Forand Bill, "designed to provide medical-hospital benefits to the elderly through the Social Security System."[7]

Various aspects of Eddie's speech were reported in the press. Several articles concentrated on his call for more black physicians and an end to segregation in medicine.[8] Other reporters focused on his overall perspective as reflected in the challenge to the physicians to look beyond their own narrow world into the interrelationships of medicine with environmental elements that affect health. The vast majority, however, caught the importance of Eddie's plea that black physicians take a more active role in the political process. As one Detroit paper stated: "A vigorous program of medical and social action was charted for the National Medical Association by Dr. Edward C. Mazique in his presidential inaugural address Thursday at the association's convention held at the Sheraton-Cadillac Hotel."[9]

The way in which this speech was reported by the more conservative American Medical Association is of particular interest since they fought so hard against the Forand Bill and any other legislation that would institute nonvoluntary health insurance. The *American Medical Association News* had two pieces relating to Eddie's recommendations. The article that appeared in August 1959 focused on Eddie's support of a compulsory national health insurance program. Interestingly enough it quoted as its source not Eddie's speech or an interview conducted with him but a report in the *Michigan AFL-CIO News.* Clearly they were monitoring the labor publications, since the AFL-CIO was one of their major opponents in the AMA's attempt to defeat the Forand Bill. They quoted Eddie as saying the voluntary health insurance proposals of the Eisenhower administration would fail to meet "the medical and health problems of our nation's 17 million Negroes, nor is it an answer for other underprivileged groups."[10] One can imagine the raised eyebrows after learning of Eddie's position at a time when the American Medical Association was mustering all its resources to fight compulsory health insurance for the elderly, but no opinion was expressed in the article.

A second article appeared in September noting Eddie's request for the "Formation of special committees to establish a unified policy for the National Medical Association on congressional bills in the health and medicine fields . . ." and his plans for an "accelerated campaign against segregation in medicine."[11] Again no position was stated in the AMA publication.

Another publication designed "as a service to the medical profession" and published by CIBA Pharmaceutical Products, Inc., entitled *Medical News* carried an article headlining the proposed support of the NMA for "Forand-Type Coverage." CIBA Pharmaceutical Products, a prominent advertiser in the *Journal of the National Medical Association* in 1959 and

1960, took the trouble to interview Eddie as well as to familiarize themselves with the inaugural address. The article was fairly detailed and without bias, claiming that "[f]or probably the first time, the leader of a national physician's organization has advocated compulsory health insurance and opposed voluntary plans."[12] The article explained Eddie's reasons for support of a compulsory plan as stemming from a belief that voluntary plans fail to meet problems presented by "our exploding population, the greatly increasing numbers of our aged, the tremendous rise in medical care costs and the obvious economic inability of the lower and middle thirds of our population to meet these soaring costs."[13]

Even though the press coverage was much more limited than it would have been if Eddie were heading a white organization, some of the general public and the major groups of physicians were made aware of his stand on health care and the direction Eddie would try to push the NMA in his year as president. Although there were other issues of importance to Eddie, much of his effort during the late fifties and early sixties was on passing a bill that would make it possible for the elderly to have sufficient medical care. Many of Eddie's patients were elderly and poor. He was quoted as saying that "[t]he time has come for doctors to put desire for personal profit second to the need for their services by the public."[14] Until his death, Eddie still made house calls to see his poor patients in Washington, D.C. He would leave their apartments with a pocket full of candy, his "pay" for the visit. It was widely known that he only charged those who could afford his services, yet he did not believe the medical care of the elderly could be trusted to charity. After all, there were hospital bills, surgery, prescriptions, and nursing home care, not to mention that all doctors might not be as humanistically inclined.

A concern about health care for the elderly was not new in the 1960s. Originally it was part of the Social Security Act sponsored by President Franklin Delano Roosevelt. It was considered so controversial that it was dropped for fear that the bill would not pass. Over the ensuing years various health insurance bills, many covering all citizens, were placed before Congress, but they received little support despite having presidential backing when Harry Truman was in office.[15]

In 1957, a small group of health insurance advocates decided to try again with a new bill. They wanted to expand the Social Security system to include health insurance under the same "contributory payment system administered by the Federal government."[16] They sought sponsorship from the ranking Democrats on the House Ways and Means Committee. It was not until they reached the fourth in rank, Aime Forand from Rhode Island, that they located a Democrat who would even take a look at the bill. To everyone's surprise, Congressman Forand put the bill in for consideration and requested a hearing just before the end of the Eighty-fifth Congress in 1957.

Forand decided he wanted to ease the burden on the elderly but was not aware of what a vital and controversial issue health care was in the public's mind. The reaction from Rhode Island workers was overwhelmingly favorable and that from the American Medical Association (AMA) was vehemently negative. Forand had little backing even from fellow Democrats, only four of whom on the House Ways and Means Committee offered support. The powerful chairman of the committee, Wilbur Mills, was so opposed that he refused to schedule hearings until Forand threatened to make it public that it was Mills holding up the process. When the hearings were finally held in 1959, Mills refused to show up and Forand had to chair them.

The hearings made it clear that labor and those involved with the Social Security system favored health insurance for the elderly. As a rule, doctors, Republicans, and conservative Democrats argued that federal health insurance for the elderly was just a step toward compulsory health insurance for everyone. Some opponents went so far as to call it "un-American" and a step toward "socialized medicine."[17] At the hearings, the president of the American Society of Internal Medicine asked, "Does it not seem inconsistent that we should be fighting Communism in Geneva while introducing legislation supporting it in Washington?"[18]

From 1957 until the passage of a Medicare bill in 1965, the American Medical Association hired a public relations firm and spent millions of dollars lobbying against Medicare. In 1961, fearing their lobbying efforts might not be strong enough, they founded a new organization called the American Medical Political Action Committee (AMPAC) whose sole purpose was to fight Medicare.[19]

Eddie was not only going against the preponderance of white physicians. The National Medical Association had a mixed history of support and rejection of compulsory health insurance. As early as 1946 the NMA went on record as being in favor of national health insurance when its president testified before a Senate committee hearing on a National Health Program. Yet their support was anything but consistent.[20]

The Medico-Chirurgical Society of the District of Columbia became the first regular medical society to endorse national health legislation. C. Austin Whittier, president of the NMA for the 1948–1949 term, took a firm stand in favor of President Truman's national health legislation in the speech he delivered as outgoing president.[21] After overtures from the American Medical Association indicating they might finally be willing to make a stand for the integration of the local societies, the NMA adjourned its 1949 meeting without taking a position on the plan, prompting a warning by their new president: "If you support the stand against Truman, you will receive a pat on the back from the AMA, but condemnation from ten million Negroes and the NAACP."[22]

Dr. Herbert Marshall, while president of the NMA, in 1951 had tried to get the organization to support the Truman Health Insurance Bill. He was also among several of Washington, D.C.'s prominent black physicians who came out strongly in 1954 against President Eisenhower's proposal to have a national pre-pay health insurance plan. Drs. Marshall, Paul Cornely, and Montague Cobb all denied that such a plan would help the vast number of poor people who could not afford the payments. Yet there was little doubt that some black physicians were as conservative as their white brethren about allowing the federal government to interfere in any way with their profession. At the meeting at which Eddie was inaugurated president in 1959, the NMA once again postponed a decision on the issue of their support for voluntary versus compulsory health insurance.[23]

Eddie knew he was up against a tough audience when he pushed for support for the Forand Bill. In one interview after his inauguration, he even acknowledged he did not believe the NMA would go along with his position.[24] A Detroit newspaper reported that "Despite his personal opinion, Dr. Mazique predicted that the NMA would go along with the administration and the AMA." In what was an uncharacteristically cynical statement, Eddie verbalized his doubts.

> The question is will the members of our House of Delegates vote as doctors or as Negroes? If I were a betting man I would bet that they will vote as doctors, rather than as champions of the underprivileged people in our country of all races, colors and creeds.[25]

Eddie also presented resolutions to do with integration, a top priority and a necessary condition if other gains were ever to be made. He pushed for the study of problems that arose from the inferiority due to segregation of the primary and secondary schooling of minority medical students, for continued support and an increased budget for the Imhotep Conference on Hospital Integration, and for urging the U.S. Department of Health, Education and Welfare to appoint Negro physicians to the Health Advisory Council study sections and committees.

There was a resolution for the formation of a Special Committee on Problems of Gerontology and Geriatrics to study the special problems of those persons over sixty-five, problems Eddie believed were beyond the powers of the individual or of private philanthropy to resolve. He pushed for the support of the Sparkman Bill, which would provide federal aid to homes for the aged.

He advocated the establishment of a Foreign and International Health Program. The purpose would be to "study environmental factors affecting diseases; to promote goodwill between the U.S. and other countries; and, to exchange ideas toward the development of better health programs for all the world."[26] This program would necessitate visiting other countries. The trips he would later make to study how socialized medicine worked in other countries and his extensive work to build a hospital in Ojike, Nigeria, were some of the ways he sought to bring this resolution to fruition over the years.

Eddie also wanted a Special Committee on Socio-Economic and Environmental Factors affecting health. He strongly believed that doctors could not succeed in securing the health of patients without attending to factors in their surroundings that affect their mental and physical well-being. The theme of the Detroit convention had been "environmental hazards and the rising incidence of disease and accidents traceable to consumer and industrial factors."[27] Eddie went further and also attempted to focus attention on the socioeconomic factors affecting patients with which many doctors made no attempt to deal. If people do not have "good food, clothing and good shelter," their health is bound to be affected negatively.[28]

Although most of Eddie's s views would be considered liberal, he also advocated the formation of a special committee appointed by the president of the United States that would "make a comprehensive study and review of pornographic materials and the effect of alcohol and narcotics on present day society."[29] He was convinced that "the operation of pornographic materials sets off a chain reaction of anxieties, prostitution, sadism, sex violations leading naturally and ultimately to widespread mental illness, serious crimes and social deterioration."[30] Eddie was not unaware of the threat that any restrictions might place on freedom of speech and freedom of the press. He pointed out in his inaugural address that it was of the utmost importance that these rights be protected. However, he strongly believed that no matter how hard physicians worked

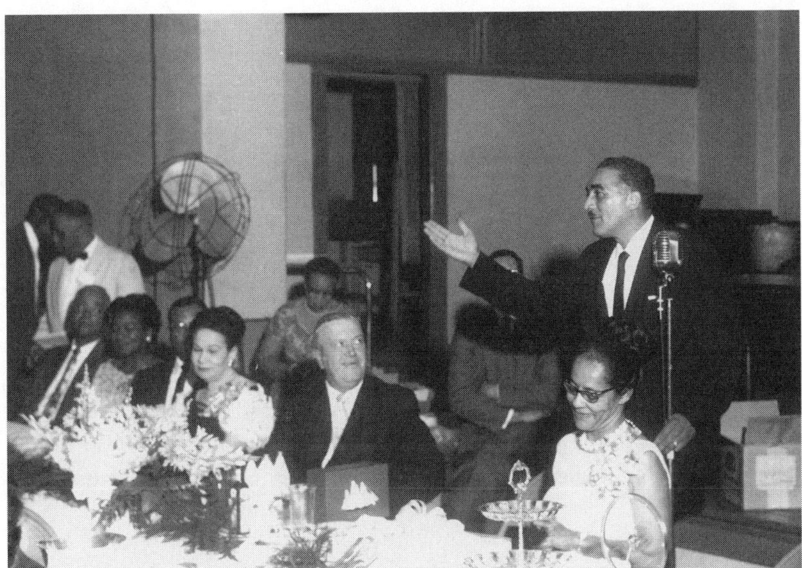

**Fig. 16:** Dr. Mazique addresses Arkansas Medical Association in June 1960 when he was president of the National Medical Association. His wife, Jewell Mazique, is seated at far right. Photo from Edward C. Mazique files.

to cure physical diseases, they would be undermined if social factors such as drugs, alcohol, and pornography, which initially posed the greatest threat to the lower classes, many of whom were black, were not curtailed.[31]

These proposals to the National Medical Association were a crucial part of the general philosophy that guided Eddie's life. More socially aware than most physicians, he spent much of his time trying to convince his colleagues to get involved in political issues. It was also part and parcel of what one of Eddie's teachers at Howard had recognized in him earlier: that he was one of the few students who were interested in public health and preventative medicine.[32] Even at that young age, he understood the connections.

His term as president provided Eddie with the opportunity to widely promote his political beliefs. The travelogue for his 1959–1960 term shows he made over twenty trips to conferences and meetings, where he frequently delivered the main address. Texas, Arkansas, Louisiana, Maryland, Florida, New Jersey, and Mississippi were among the many places Eddie visited. He was invited to the United Nations Headquarters in New York City in December to confer with officials and delegates. He traveled to Michigan at the invitation of its governor, G. Mennen Williams, for the Governors Health Conference. Williams was a giant of a man who always sported a bow tie and was known for his liberalism. He impressed Eddie so much with his concern for the health needs of the poor that Eddie invited him to be one of the featured speakers at the sixty-fifth convention of the National Medical Association in August 1960.[33]

Eddie also made numerous speeches to groups in Washington, D.C., such as the Capital Press Club and the District Health Department. Although his speeches varied, the common themes of civil rights, aid to the elderly, worldwide cooperation on health issues, and the necessity of political involvement of physicians were ever present. The black physician, Eddie believed, was or should be especially attuned to the problems facing society.

> Collectively the Negro physician, out of his experience of personal suffering and struggle for a share in the fruits of this Nation, can well become the dominant figure in constructive health planning. It is easier for his activities to encompass the physical, the mental, the moral, the social and economic and for him to support a program which embodies the whole field of human endeavor. [F]or recent racial segregation taught him well the inter-relationship of all social forces that affect man. He has [not] forgotten that only recently and still in some parts of this Country, [it] mattered not how well-trained a Negro physician nor how dedicated he might have been, social customs and political law excluded him, nevertheless, from participation in the larger community. The historic tradition of common concern of the National Medical Association together with the collective experience of its membership presents new currents of medical power and a sense of responsibility essentially unique for medicine in this period of transition. And until peace and good will and dignity are restored to all humanity and equal access to good health is enjoyed by all without fear of nuclear radiation and atomic annihilation, the NMA will remain vibrant, potent and powerful and progressive.[34]

Eddie used his position as president of the NMA to give him credibility to push for legislation that he believed was important. Even before his inauguration, as president, Eddie testified twice in 1959 before Congress in support of the Keogh and Dowdy bills.[35]

At the Annual Interim Meeting of the Executive Committee of the Board of Trustees of the National Medical Association in February 1960, two resolutions that Eddie presented to the Board were approved.[36] One was to endorse the administration's Civil Rights Bill "providing that the Federal Courts be authorized to appoint referees to register qualified Negroes and to watch over the balloting and vote counting."[37] The second resolution was in support of the Delaney Amendment and other legislation proposing more rigid control of food additives. The NMA questioned what the ultimate impact of chemicals added to foods and pesticides used on crops would be for the individual consumer. The NMA came out in support of Secretary of Health, Education and Welfare Arthur S. Fleming, who had been attacked by those with economic interests for his attempting to act as a "watch dog" over the health of the nation. The resolution unanimously endorsed Secretary Fleming and informed "him and the public what he has done in the Nation's interest is not to his discredit."[38] The NMA resolution was transmitted to "responsible legislators" and, according to Eddie, played a role in Surgeon General Burney's receiving over twenty-five million dollars for Public Health expansion.[39]

A Pittsburgh newspaper, discussing the interim meeting, reported that the Executive Committee of the Board of Trustees voted to establish an office of legislation and community action, something that Eddie had requested in his inaugural address. "This new office would work for the passage of desired health bills, sponsored by the NMA and would serve as liaison for the Negro physicians with the President of the United States, the United Nations, the Congress and the Department of Health, Education and Welfare."[40] A proposal to establish such a committee again shows up in the "Recommendations of the President to the Board of Trustees of the National Medical Association at its 65th Annual Convention" in August 1960 when Eddie attempted to get the entire Board to accept such a committee.[41]

It was also noted by the Pittsburgh paper that Dr. Mazique called for support of the Forand Bill "because it could be used effectively to eliminate discrimination in hospitals receiving federal allocation of funds."[42] Racial discrimination in hospitals was still a very serious problem for many physicians and therefore an argument Eddie frequently used when talking in favor of a Social Security–based health care system. As Eddie described it,

> [b]lack patients were admitted to some of the hospitals but no black doctors were allowed to attend them. At some hospitals, blacks were not even admitted. One of the reasons that we pushed hard for Medicare was we found out that any time a program is supported by the federal government they have to constitutionally uphold a citizen's right to utilize any facility in which federal funding was instrumental in getting it established. This is what happened in the case of Medicare. The AMA was strongly opposed to Medicare and one of the reasons was it would serve as a tool for black patients and physicians to gain admission to the hospitals. All you have to do is file a case against the hospital and that would be it.

During his term as president, complaints of such discrimination were still pouring into the NMA. In a speech to the Cook County Medical Society in Chicago in January, he discussed a few examples of the accusations brought to his attention since becoming president. They were more frequently from the South, but by no means limited to that geographic area. If black physicians could see their own self-interest in the Forand Bill (that they might be allowed to practice in hospitals where they were presently barred), he was hopeful they would be more likely to favor it.[43]

Eddie also asked for support of the proposed tour to Socialist countries to study how their health care systems worked.

In April 1960, Eddie got his chance to appear before the McNamara Sub-Committee on Problems of the Aging and Aged, where he spoke as an individual physician, never using the word *we*. However, with his title as president of the National Medical Association and his discussion of its history and purpose, it seems likely that some of the committee members believed Eddie was speaking for the NMA when he endorsed a program to provide medical care for the aged and aging with the cost covered by an expanded Social Security system. Yet at this point there was no NMA endorsement of such a program.

Eddie launched an all-out attack on those who claimed such a program would mean "socialism" and a "loss of freedom" to choose their doctors and hospitals.

> Over half of the 16 million aged today or 9 million are without insurance policies, have no major savings and are on their "medical" own, enjoying no freedom but the choice between sudden death or withering away in suffering and neglect. Millions of former war workers, farm and factory employees, domestic servants are outside the protective walls of any private, fraternal or religious institutions. Of the fortunate few among the aged finding places in nursing homes, the majority receives little more than custodial care from untrained personnel and, consigned for the balance of their lives to pitiable vegetation, they gradually fade away. Is this the freedom for which in our youth we have aspired and offered our lives and fortunes in war?[44]

Since he saw the use of the word *freedom* by opponents as but a propaganda technique, Eddie suggested to the committee that they abandon the words *volunteer* and *compulsion* in their discussion. He went on to support "a division or department under Health, Education and Welfare for supervising the whole range of problems affecting the aged and aging, such as exists in the Children's Bureau."[45] Finally, he expressed support for plans for building hospitals and training personnel under government sponsorship.

Eddie's personal scrapbook for the term of his National Medical Association presidency is full of letters from congressmen and government officials. From William P. Rogers, the attorney general, and from Barbara Rathe of the president's staff, there are notes about the NMA resolution pertaining to civil rights; from Adam Clayton Powell about the resolution regarding chemicals employed in food production; from Wayne Morse to thank Eddie for campaign help; from Stuart Symington on health care; from Hubert Humphrey containing warm wishes for the success of the medical delegation to Europe; a Christmas card from Senator John F. Kennedy and his family. It is clear from the correspondence that Eddie was a politically active president and that he lent his support to those who favored health insurance for the elderly funded through the Social Security system.

Although one would never know it from the smiling family picture of Eddie, Jewell, and their two sons in the *National Medical Association, Inc. Bulletin* of June 1960, as Eddie's professional career was thriving, his home situation was worsening. By this time, Eddie and Jewell had very little time together. Jewell was pursuing her interests and Eddie his. Yet it was clear that despite their differences, Jewell was using her talents to assist Eddie in his political efforts. Eddie's scrapbook also contained letters addressed to Mrs. Mazique thanking her for sending copies of NMA resolutions and answering requests for information on bills.

Eddie's year was not totally devoted to standard political issues. A lengthy medical and moral battle was brought on by a paper presented at the twelfth annual meeting of the American Association of Blood Banks (AABB) in Chicago, Illinois, on November 6 by Dr. John Scudder of the College of Physicians and Surgeons of Columbia University and his associates. The ensuing furor was one of the highlights of Eddie's tenure as president of the National Medical Association. An Associated Press story of November 7, 1959, which received worldwide publicity, stated: "A noted medical researcher and blood specialist says transfusions are safer for patients when blood of their own race is used."[46]

Given the implications of this statement and the years of fighting to have blood banks remove regulations requiring the separation of Negro blood from white, the tone taken by Dr. Montague Cobb, the editor of the *Journal of the National Medical Association,* and by most of the black physicians was amazingly moderate. They made every effort to allow Dr. Scudder to explain his motives and the scientific rationale for such an outrageous statement. Scudder, after all, had been a mentor of and dissertation advisor to the late and very famous black physician Charles R. Drew, who had done his doctoral work at Columbia.

Dr. Cobb maintained that "[b]ecause of the far reaching socio-political implications which Dr. Scudder's thesis or 'new philosophy' would have if it were found to have scientific validity, it was necessary to examine his premises and evidence with the greatest of care."[47]

Although the *Journal*'s response was slow and methodical, Eddie's response was swift and emotional. Known for his humor and his ability to diffuse situations, Eddie did not shrink back when he felt the circumstances required strong words. On November 12, 1959, Eddie issued a press release on the National Medical Association letterhead entitled "Dr. Mazique Denounces Physicians' Recommendation to Separate Blood."

> Such a fantastic claim ranks with that of a distinguished scientist during the slave era, who, in discussing diseases peculiar to Negroes reported at length on dreptomania, 'a malady that gave Negroes a compulsion to

run away,' which condition forced them to run away from even happy plantation life, as reported by John Hope Franklin recently.

... It is ironic that at this precise moment when the Red Cross is collecting blood dramatically even in the South and distributing it regardless of race or previous condition of servitude that there should arise out of the 'liberal' North 'dreptomaniac' physicians with an up-to-date finding of the existence of a grave and sometimes fatal difference between the blood of Negroes and whites, and [*sic*] argument so convincing that it is expected leaders in other walks of life of this most advanced Nation may give these fantastic claims authenticity and publicity.

First, I would like to challenge Dr. Scudder's contention that the American Negro is a distinct racial group, rather than a social concept or entity. Is it possible that Dr. Scudder and associates are unfamiliar with the blood mixing that has followed cross-breeding between Negro and whites since 1619? Certainly, Dr. Scudder cannot believe that Anglo-Saxons who left Southampton centuries ago have a blood monopoly or certain component elements that may be more successfully matched with that of recent arrivals from Slavic countries than with his natural kith and kin—the American Negro, a difference dictated and identified by skin coloring exclusively. It is my belief that if there actually exist some common minor factors in the blood composition, granting Dr. Scudder's minor factor theory, Negroes and whites in close historic proximity would have more common blood elements than recently arrived white elements of the North. Scientifically, Dr. Scudder must identify his pure race before he can even begin the application of his new blood theory.

We suspect the anti-bodies Dr. Scudder and his associates have recently identified and are popularizing, are far more of a social origin for exploitative purposes than of a physically scientific nature, intended rather to combat the current campaign to eradicate

> differences of opportunity rather than blood substances. There is nothing new in the application of the scientific approach for segregation purposes and such findings can have no effect but to continue our people in an inferior role. Chattel slavery was conceived of and supported in its time by religious leaders on moral grounds, by scientists for physical reasons; statistically documented by the social scientists and politically activated by the politicians. . . .
>
> It is ironic that Dr. Scudder, who did so much to develop the technique of blood plasma extraction with the able assistance and cooperation of the late Doctor Charles R. Drew on the eve of the great war against Hitler to rout forever theories of racial supremacy, should himself participate in propaganda at this stage of world-wide rejection of racial-based theories, to restore the Aryan concept of racial differences. It is hard to believe that the school of thought which supplied scientific proof to the folly of the American Red Cross blood policy of segregation should now itself disclaim its former findings in favor of separation on the basis of a contrived 'pure race' theory. . . .
>
> Our major blow must be directed against those who would corrupt the natural sciences and resurrect the outmoded theory that Negro blood is somehow different and the Negro's brain capacity is limited; this latter is all there is left of the old slavery theory to be resurrected.[48]

Others were also quick to respond and disassociate themselves from Scudder's statement, although generally their words were more measured than Eddie's.

Realizing Dr. Scudder's comments might lend credence to those who supported racism, some of his colleagues at Columbia felt the need to publicly denounce what he had said:

> No new evidence was reported, and the so-called 'new philosophy' serves no purpose except to reinforce the old 'philosophy' of race prejudice, which has been shown repeatedly to rest on ignorance rather than biological or medical knowledge.[49]

The press, especially the black press, gave wide coverage to the debate, frequently quoting Eddie's press release at length. It was soon clear that this was more than an academic debate. By January 1960, Arkansas had reversed its former position of not separating blood according to race and passed legislation at the behest of the Capital Citizens Council requiring that blood once again be separated according to race.[50]

In the meantime the *Journal of the National Medical Association* offered Dr. Scudder the chance to clarify his position in a paper he would write specifically for them. The resultant article was printed in their March issue. Dr. Scudder repeated the categories he had mentioned at the AABB conference in Chicago. The best blood transfusion results from, in descending order of preference: (1) the patient's own blood, (2) an identical twin, (3) a family donor. If a donor is not available in the first three categories, one should next turn to (4) a member of the patient's own ethnic or national group, and finally, if that is not possible, (5) blood donors from one's own race.[51]

On April 13, Dr. Scudder spoke before the Manhattan Central Medical Society and, at their behest, Eddie attended to debate with Dr. Scudder.[52] An article in the *Washington Afro-American* reported that Dr. Scudder had partially recanted some of his earlier claims.

> In his statements, recently Dr. Scudder concluded his references to race were unfortunate, that references to possible blood differences had been grossly exaggerated by the popular press, and expressed concern over the unfortunate publicity and the possible reflection of bias on his part, or willful slander, which some interpreted into his findings.[53]

The photograph in Eddie's scrapbook of him with Dr. Scudder, taken at the meeting, shows Eddie smiling and friendly.

The Charles R. Drew Memorial Lecture was delivered by Dr. Scudder at the Forty-eighth Annual Meeting of the John A. Andrew Clinical Society at Tuskegee Institute, April 23–29, 1960. After praising Dr. Drew, he went on to justify the Hindu custom of marriage within the same caste, claiming that "marrying within the caste they are able to bring more intelligence to the nuptial bed than by random selection based on emotions as is the custom here in the United States."[54] It was a statement that must have raised more than a few eyebrows at the conference! And despite the earlier press report about his rethinking his views, he still claimed hemolytic reactions were linked to race and therefore that transfusions from one's own ethnic and national group were preferable.

Only after waiting out all these chances to allow Dr. Scudder to explain his views did the *Journal* finally conclude:

> Dr. Scudder is a distinguished scion of distinguished lineage. His own reputations rest upon scientific studies and good works in hematology. Perhaps it would be best if the nebulous statement and implications of his 'new philosophy' were forgot.[55]

And so they have been.

The skirmish with Dr. Scudder was behind him as the sixty-fifth convention of the National Medical Association was gearing up in August 1960. NMA support for the sweeping agenda that he proposed when he had taken office, however, was still an unrealized goal. The battle lines were already being drawn at a press conference that preceded the official opening session. Eddie, with the support of the chairman of the NMA board of trustees, Dr. Murray B. Davis, came out strongly in support of Forand-type legislation and recommended that the five-thousand-member NMA should come out in favor of the bill.[56]

On the morning of August 9, 1960, Eddie delivered his presidential address, "Medical Dimensions in the Nuclear Age," at the formal opening meeting at the end of his term. He challenged the audience of doctors with the same themes he had hammered on from his incoming address through his entire year as president. Doctors needed, he argued, to be involved in political and social issues.

> Thinking of oneself as an individual set apart from the rank and file of humanity, set apart by knowledge, skills, privileges, money and power—as an elite class, can expose us to a tragic condition diagnosed as "occupational hazards." These can serve as ill omens not to us as individual physicians, but to the profession as a whole and society at large and can do irrefutable damage to the new world now a'borning.[57]

Medical education and physician shortage, population control, environmental hazards, mental diseases, and social pollution were all covered. Eddie pushed strongly for the formation of an organization in Washington,

D.C., whose purpose was the "assimilation, action, promotion and dissemination of legislative health measures in the best interest of the health care of the American people."[58] Eventually this was to become the National Medical Political Action Committee, or NMPAC as it is called, the present lobbying group for the members of the National Medical Association. Since there was as yet no formal lobbying unit, Eddie prepared a handout that outlined seven bills pending in Congress that he believed the NMA should support because they represented "measures for the advancement of medicine and the general welfare."[59]

Eddie once again emphasized the importance of international cooperation relating to health issues with a special stress on the needs of the emerging African nations. He went so far as to recommend immediate help be rendered to the Congo in the form of a medical mission or financial assistance.

The way in which Eddie linked health with human rights in his speech strengthened his claim that federal legislation was justified in order to provide medical care for the aged and aging. Once again this issue headed his list of what the NMA should support. It was also the most controversial issue at the conference. Disputing the rationale of the critics of federal health insurance legislation, Eddie met the challenge of their arguments head on—the very arguments that would that evening be presented at the public meeting by their host for the conference, Dr. John S. Donaldson, president of the Allegheny County Medical Society. Eddie attacked directly by saying that

> [m]any have branded this as indicative of compulsory health insurance and socialized medicine. The only compulsion would be that of paying slightly increased Social Security taxes. Beneficiaries would have free and wide choice of physicians in hospitals. The bogus labels of "socialized medicine" and "take away freedom" from physicians is but propaganda, and a large segment of our population has been tranquillized by such statements. Today, the nine million aged outside of private insurance coverage, of which the majority are Negroes have no freedom anyway except to suffer and die in neglect.[60]

The address following Eddie's was given by Dr. Leroy E. Burney, Surgeon General, United States Public Health Service.[61] Dr. Burney told his audience that doctors must go beyond their strictly medical duties—nicely paralleling one of Eddie's main themes. While admitting to an increase in the proportion of the very old and the growing demand for physicians that could not be met by the current numbers of medical school graduates, Burney did not talk about any additional health care legislation. Instead of legislative solutions, he argued for use of the available assets to better advantage: "By concentrating the aim of the physician at the point where he can do the most good—detecting the chronic condition in its initial phase, where it is the most amenable to treatment—we can achieve much more with our limited resources."[62] Since he was an appointee of the Eisenhower administration, perhaps nothing else could be expected of his speech, although in the waning days of the Eisenhower administration, Arthur Fleming, the secretary of Health, Education and Welfare (HEW), finally broke ranks and announced he was actually in favor of health insurance for the aged.[63]

That evening the head of the local medical society, Dr. John Donaldson, greeted the capacity crowd at the public meeting. Knowing the main speaker who was to follow had very liberal leanings, Donaldson attempted to answer in advance any plea for support of a Forand-type bill by calling it "socialized medicine."[64]

Governor G. Mennen Williams of Michigan in the main address that evening delivered a hard-hitting presentation that did not let Eddie down.[65] Governor Williams linked civil rights and health, calling health, as Eddie had, a basic human right. He likened the opponents of health care to reactionaries who argue that "Negroes are happy with things as they are, why rock the boat."[66] The enemies of progress in civil rights, health care for the aged, and aid to education all used the same three arguments, the governor claimed: the legislation isn't needed, the government can't legislate social problems, and if government does anything about it there will be no stopping it. In fact the third argument was that presented by Donaldson and the first and the third arguments were those that would be proposed by Dr. James T. Aldrich, the president-elect of the NMA, in his inaugural address. By linking rationales against civil rights to those against health care, Williams made it exceptionally difficult for the detractors of health care legislation to argue their case, for who among them would challenge civil rights? It really was an ingenious presentation.

A pitched battle had been waging throughout the convention when Dr. Aldrich delivered his address in the closing session. His presentation was short, taking only two pages when it was printed in the *Journal.* The beginning was composed of the usual compliments to everyone, including the outgoing president and the editor of the *Journal* and the NMA Board and for that matter just about everyone associated with the NMA. A plea was made for more black physicians and the initiation of a student loan fund toward this end. Then, in the several paragraphs near the end of his speech, Aldrich got to the burning issue of the day.

> The clamor at the present moment has reached a dangerous pitch and 1960 and 1961 may well be the years for decision as to whether the physicians of this nation are to continue to be members of a free profession, responsible directly to their patients, or whether they are to be singled out and made agents of a Federal bureaucracy that will in effect pay the physician for his services and determine for whom and under what circumstances these services are to be provided. We must continue to fight all legislation that would bring 16,000,000 aged citizens into a compulsory tax paid system of Federal medical service without any regard for the individual's economic status or need. It would be nothing else than socialized medicine for all persons over the age of 65, eligible to receive social security benefits. We realize, as physicians, we must tackle the problem of the basis of a constructive program that will preserve intact the direct relationship between patient and doctor. The National Medical Association believes in the free choice of a physician and that a patient should be privileged to exercise that right of choice. . . .
>
> Now a word about the Forand Bill. This bill would not benefit 4,000,000 aged citizens, men and women, who are not eligible for social security. No provisions have been made for payment to mental patients or tubercular patients hospitalized. No benefits to retired teachers on pensions. The government would select the doctor, the hospital and pay for these services and the patient would not have a free choice of physicians. The Forand Bill HR-4700 would do nothing for those who need medical assistance most. No aged person today in the U.S.A. lacks adequate hospital and medical care if he seeks it. Our welfare programs, community chest agencies are taking care of the indigent. They are being

> taken care of on the community, state or city level. I am convinced that voluntary health insurance coverage represents the best means of helping most people that need medical care in this aged group. . . . Therefore, I shall recommend to the House of Delegates, the policy making body of the Association that the Forand Bill HR-4700, be defeated in its present form.[67]

One can only wonder how intelligent human beings such as Dr. Aldrich and Dr. Mazique could interpret the same bill in such a different manner. There was nothing in the Forand Bill to indicate that the government would select the hospital for a patient or take away his free choice of physicians. Only the strongly propagandistic material of the lobbying arm of the American Medical Association tended to go this far.[68] One even has to wonder if the two doctors were living in the same country. While Eddie stated there were "millions [old and young] who at this very moment, need medical attention, who neither can afford a doctor nor pay for treatments,"[69] Dr. Aldrich claimed "no aged person today in the U.S.A. lacks adequate hospital and medical care."[70] Eddie saw examples of this need every day in his own practice. Dr. Aldrich's practice must have been with a very limited segment of the population to not have recognized any such need.

The debate between the outgoing and incoming presidents was not limited to their speeches at the convention. In a county medical society debate that was televised on the local educational channel, Eddie and an ophthalmologist from the Pittsburgh area spoke in favor of Forand-type legislation while Dr. Aldrich and the president-elect of the Allegheny County Medical Society represented the opposition. The reporter for the *Physician's Forum News Letter*[71] noted that in his "unbiased" opinion "Dr. Mazique was the most impressive of the four participants."[72]

Eddie was very persuasive in the floor fight for his program. Just how successful he was depends on which publication you read. The House of Delegates did vote to oppose national birth control laws, favor federal subsidies for deserving medical students, send a Negro medical mission to the Congo, and support stronger legal controls on pornography. One headline even proclaimed "NMA supports Forand-Type Care for Aged."[73] Another article claimed the NMA "came out strongly and formally for 'Federal legislation for the medical care of the aged and aging,'" which put it in opposition to incoming president James Aldrich and the American Medical Association.[74] The position taken by the NMA was actually much less than Eddie had requested. He had strong backing from the Council of Trustees but could not win enough support from the House of Delegates to pass a resolution. The divided sentiment led to tabling the resolution for further study. A committee was appointed to study the pending federal laws in aged medical care and present its findings at the NMA Council meeting in February 1961.[75]

Thus Eddie left the office of President of the National Medical Association in August 1961 with a lot done and much more left to be accomplished. The battles he fought in the NMA were continued without a pause as he left Pittsburgh and headed on a trip through Eastern Europe.

# CHAPTER EIGHT 

# Health Care for All

We say we have the best medical facilities in the world. Yet they aren't made available to all citizens. Colored people, the aged, and poor whites are sadly neglected groups.
— *Edward C. Mazique, 1960*

In health as in liberty, the world cannot stand half sick and half well.
— *Edward C. Mazique, 1959*

His year as president of the NMA ended but the struggle for Medicare, aid to the emerging African nations, and the other causes Eddie believed in so strongly continued. While president, Eddie organized a trip to Eastern Europe that was to begin only three days after the convention ended.

Eddie stated four reasons "which prompted [him] to undertake a trip for studying advancements and medical care in Poland, Hungary, Czechoslovakia and the Union of Soviet Socialist Republics along with France and England."[1] The first was as a partial implementation of the NMA's international program, which endorsed exchange of medical personnel with other nations. Second, it was seen as an attempt to advance understanding and dissemination of knowledge with world neighbors who, because of transportation and communication advances, have become closer. The third rationale, and clearly the most important for Eddie, was to participate in programs of technical and medical exchange that would help in combating the ravages of disease. It was an amplification of this broad purpose that justified taking a close look at the nationalized medical programs of the Socialist countries so that their achievements, techniques, and services could be evaluated. This was the main reason for the trip, a chance to get more publicity for the cause of "nationalized" medicine. It was also a chance to dispel some of the myths promulgated by the AMA about the flaws of socialized medicine. The final reason given for the delegation was "a realization of the urgency for promoting goodwill and peace in this imperiled world between the American people and the peoples of the socialist countries."[2]

In that fall of 1960, when the black doctors who had signed up to take this educational trip were getting ready to make their journey, there was little doubt that goodwill was needed. In the initial stages of planning, relations with the Socialist countries were improving. Nikita S. Khrushchev, chairman of the Ministers of the USSR, had made a trip to the United States in 1959; President Dwight D. Eisenhower was to meet at a summit meeting in Paris with Khrushchev and other leaders in May 1960; and Eisenhower was scheduled for a visit to the USSR in the same year.

On May 1 the Soviet Union shot down an American Lockheed U-2 plane that was flying over one thousand miles inside of the Soviet Union border, and relations between the two powers slipped to a new low.[3] The United States initially denied that the plane was spying until the Soviets produced the American pilot, Gary Powers, and a confession. President Eisenhower took responsibility for the incident, and Khrushchev labeled it as an act of aggression and refused to participate with Eisenhower in the summit meeting scheduled for May 16 in Paris. To make his point even more strongly, Khrushchev went farther and postponed the Eisenhower trip to the USSR scheduled for June by stating: "At the present we cannot display such cordiality toward the President of the United States since the provocative flights of the American military reconnaissance planes have created conditions obviously unfavorable for this visit."[4] The Soviets brought their complaints to the United Nations Security Council but no actions were taken. A trip that would have aroused controversy even if relations between the nations were at their best now became a potential threat to the careers of the doctors signed on for the journey. To their credit, everyone who was scheduled did participate.

In April 1960, Lewis Giles Jr., a public relations consultant hired to organize the trip, called Larry Still, a *Jet* reporter, to see if he would accompany the doctors. Mr. Still had a great deal of difficulty selling his participation to his superiors because of the extensiveness of the tour and the controversy surrounding socialized medicine. After the U-2 incident made his editors even more leery, Still had to agree to use his vacation time and even pay much of his own way. Many of the details of the trip

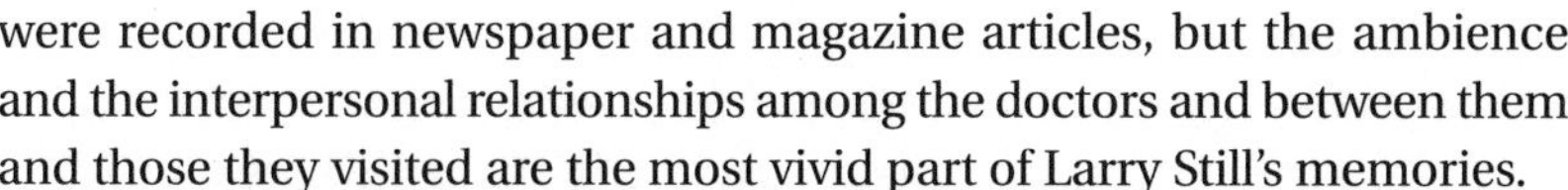

were recorded in newspaper and magazine articles, but the ambience and the interpersonal relationships among the doctors and between them and those they visited are the most vivid part of Larry Still's memories.

The learning began even before they enplaned. On August 14 the group assembled in New York City for orientation and briefing at the United Nations. A summary of the meetings was reported by one of the doctors on the tour, Dr. Leroy R. Swift, in his article "Medical Mission to Moscow," which was published in the *Journal of the National Medical Association* in July 1961.[5] One of the meetings not reported by Dr. Swift is the one that Larry Still remembered the best and the one that best reflects the tenor of the times. As Larry recalled,

> [b]efore we left we were being briefed by Public Affairs, I forget the exact title, they are the type of agency that briefs Americans when they are going into various countries. This Agency briefed us before we went abroad. They told us: "When you get to the Soviet Union the people will be friendly to you. You will see signs everywhere, Welcome Americans," and we did. But during the briefing they told us not to respond to them. "Be cold and curt." They were telling us as Americans not to respond to the friendship of the Russian people. Giles and Mazique emphasized that we were to accept the friendliness of the people. We didn't want to be ugly Americans. We wanted to be responsive to the people. We tried to do that. To the everlasting pride of the group they walked out on this briefing. I couldn't believe it and I wrote a story about it.[6]

Eddie and Lewis Giles made it clear to the doctors from the beginning that this was not going to be a typical junket. They viewed it as a history-making tour. Larry Still, and for that matter most of the doctors, did not understand the full import of the trip until it was underway. As Larry remembered it,

> [t]he trip sort of developed. When I left, I didn't know that it was going to be that kind of a trip. I didn't have any idea that it was going to be as significant as it was and as involved. I knew we had some key doctors who were all members of the NMA and were prominent.

A fellow named Swift who later became one of the first blacks to be assistant secretary of HEW. He was a prominent doctor from North Carolina. Dr. Logan who was Duke Ellington's doctor. Dr. Margaret Grigsby, she was at Howard, a specialist in African medicine and internal medicine. Dr. Ethelene Crockett, whose husband was a lawyer who became a congressman. These were top practitioners and prominent people. I was just excited to be in their company.

Frankly, from what I had written and observed about the NMA, I was questioning whether these guys really understood what they were after. I didn't know they were as committed as they were to what was then a revolutionary concept and really trying to make it work. I wasn't sure whether the focus was completely on the nationalized medicine aspect of it or on the so-called scientific aspects of it. This focus developed as I went along.

I don't think we realized the impact of the socialized medicine issue until we reached Czechoslovakia. Then it began to hit us that what we are doing here is trying to sell socialized medicine to America. Then some of the doctors began to hedge their answers and try to give me direction on what the story should be. I was beginning to have problems with that. I was glad that I had paid my way at that point because I began to get certain strong suggestions about you are along with us and we want you to do a certain type of story. Not from Giles and not from Mazique. I want to emphasize that! They were really top flight all the way.

Mazique was always ahead of his time even back in Washington. I knew that. Mazique spent time with Giles and me prepping us all along the way. The thing that stood out was here we were talking about nationalized medicine, medical care for all, at a time when the AMA was completely opposed to it. So I recognized here was something far-ranging.[7]

Getting press coverage had been a primary objective for Eddie from the beginning. If the trip was to have any impact on the battle between those supporting and those opposed to national health care for the elderly, then the people back home had to read about it. Larry was fully cognizant of the reason he had been asked to accompany the doctors.

> From the time we landed we knew we had to get the media interested in this because that was the reason Giles was asked to put this together. The reason why I was even asked to go along was not only to do the story for Johnson but to help get media attention back home. In other words, Mazique was always astute enough to know that you had to focus media attention on it to get people interested in it. After I got on the plane I found out that some of the group wanted media attention and some of them didn't. It was too controversial for some of them. It was all right as long as we were in England. There is no question about that. Everyone was pleased about what we were doing. They recognized the positive aspects. They thought these were good stories and something to focus on back home.[8]

The doctors learned from their trip. They learned about how the medical field was structured, the ongoing research, developments in medical instruments, and how maternity cases were handled, as discussed by Dr. Swift in his article. They visited hospitals and clinics, witnessed surgery, and met with the trade unions for medical workers. Eddie delivered speeches in Prague and Warsaw.[9] Eddie's article, which followed Dr. Swift's in the *Journal,* described the way that public health was structured in the USSR, new instruments, drugs, the provision for the aged, and some interesting medical statistics.

However, it was the nonmedical aspects of the trip that were having the greatest impact on the doctors. Larry recounted the events:

> We were beginning to get more and more involved in the socialist system. We were trying hard not to be ugly Americans, to be receptive, to be mindful of the fact that we wanted to bring back a true picture of what was happening in these countries. We wanted to focus on what was good for all of the people in medicine. As we became progressively involved in the trip, we were beginning to feel signs of indoctrination and there were concerns. Not so much in Bulgaria and in Hungary but

> as we arrived in Moscow we were beginning to really do the scientific part of the tour and we had tour guides. As we were trying to not show our Americanism we were subconsciously doing it. We began to have conflicts with the tour guides. We were beginning to become defensive about our system.
>
> It was hard not to react to criticism of your country even when they were critical of it because of the race problem. I tried to be dispassionate and keep my objectivity as a newsman but I found myself doing it. I found that it became a challenge for blacks, because in part, we were more American than we were black.
>
> Also we were having problems filing stories as we moved progressively through Soviet countries. It wasn't as much censorship as the mechanics of it. Before we got to the iron curtain countries we could file—we were writing our own stories, and I could file directly back to my office—to Johnson Publishing. We could put stories that we wanted on the wires. Not that they would go out but we could put the stories on the wire. After we left Poland, we couldn't file them, we couldn't go into the offices. They said, you have to give them to us and we will send them out. So we didn't know what got out and what did not. We couldn't tell what got out until we got back. I wouldn't say it was censorship though because in most instances the stories I wrote from there did appear.
>
> The embassy and the Western press were helpful to us but they weren't as cooperative as we thought they should have been. They were a little suspicious of the story I was after and what the group was after. They did arrange things logistically and it couldn't have been any better but they didn't seem to want to transmit the message we wanted to give. At one point there was some tenseness among the group about the message we saw and whether we should transmit it or not.[10]

As the trip progressed some of the doctors became more nervous about what was being reported to the folks back home. Larry remembered that by the time they arrived in the Soviet Union

> [s]ome of the members of our own group were getting squeamish about what to write about and all. Mazique made every effort to keep me informed. It was not a secret to anybody, anything we were doing. Whereas other members, I had problems getting all the information that would be helpful to me to do a complete story about the medical aspects.[11]

Their fear of publicity became so strong that some of the doctors put pressure on Johnson to kill the final story. As Larry recalled,

> [t]here was only one story which didn't appear and I'll tell you about that. That was my one overall story. But that wasn't censorship from the Soviets. I wrote the story when I came back. Certain members on the tour called Johnson and said they didn't want the story to appear.[12]

Although there were tense situations with some of the doctors, the overall tone of the tour was cheerful and adventuresome, thanks in large part to Eddie's leadership. There were new cultures, sights, and food to which the doctors tried to become accustomed.

> All this controversy wasn't that much. I'm taking it out of context by speaking about it as if it were a major issue. It was really one of the side issues because there were hardships: adjusting to the beds, the water and food. Dr. Mazique never became involved in that. He never let it bother him. It was like water off the duck's back. I remember we went on tours, boat tours, and it rained and we got caught in it and he was always cheering us up.[13]

It also took some adjusting on the parts of the people of the nations they visited. They did not realize that Afro-Americans came in such varying shades of color.

> Most of all, people didn't know what we were. They couldn't imagine that we were black Americans from what they had read and seen because we were so many

> different colors. They expected black Americans to be black or darker. They didn't call us black in those days, it was Negroes or colored. The range of complexions threw them off. We met people in the Soviet Union who were darker than us. The people in those countries were darker than us but they weren't Africans. They were dark-skinned Asians, I guess. That was amazing to us.[14]

Some of the incidents, though maddening, at the same time had humorous undertones, especially when viewed more impartially after time had elapsed. Larry Still recalled a visit to share an evening with a typical Soviet family:

> One Soviet family invited us over. I knew that they had prepared a special meal for us that day. We wanted to look at a typical family. There were rows and rows of high-rise apartments. I would later see similar ones built in Chicago and St. Louis. I had not seen the massive high-rise apartments like that before. This family was living in these kinds of dwellings. They served us fried chicken and watermelon. We didn't know whether to be angry or what. We figured the embassy must have told them that was what we liked.[15]

Always on the lookout for a chance to publicize national health care, Eddie wanted to call a press conference when they arrived back in England. As Larry Still remembers it, not everyone was as enthusiastic about the publicity as Eddie.

> I know when we came back to England, we agreed that Mazique would call a press conference which he was very emphatic about, making statements and calling for nationalized medicine. Even I was a little squeamish about that. Some of the group did not want to be associated with that but he did it. I must admit, I really thought he had guts and yet he was so affable and kept the group together.[16]

The press conference was held on September 16 and did receive some publicity even among the "white press." Both the *Washington Post* and the

*Star* carried articles the following day. The articles included quotations from Eddie that were sure to precipitate debate. "The free government health services are efficient and excellent and available to every citizen without annoying formalities," Eddie stated in his interview. "Their equipment is as good if not better than what we offer and the morale of the doctors is high."[17] If these statements were not enough to raise the hackles of the anti-nationalized-medicine people, he went on to state: "Patients admittedly don't have a free choice of which doctor to go to, but this is a small freedom to give up in return for complete and free medical treatment."[18] Eddie concluded that he would push the NMA for endorsement of "more comprehensive national health services in America."[19]

A few weeks later a semi-rebuttal of Eddie's views appeared in the *Star* under the title "Doctors Differ in Views on Soviet Medicine Gains."[20] The premise of the article was that two doctors who had not gone on the trip, one a Washington psychiatrist and the other the associate director of the National Cancer Institute, disagreed with Eddie's "rosy diagnosis" of the situation in the Soviet Union.

The doctors argued that the medical equipment was only good in several of the top institutions but that the majority of the medical facilities lagged way behind the United States. The morale among doctors, they argued, is only high among the few who are well paid, but the majority of doctors are poorly paid and their "social prestige is about the same as a school teacher's here."[21] This was perhaps as strong a statement about American values and priorities as those of the Soviets.

On the whole, the article was actually a surprisingly mild attack on Eddie's statements. The doctors joined him in praising the free tuition for Soviet medical students. They agreed the Soviets were ahead in preventive medicine, although they argued that lead followed from their centralist beliefs; immunization was not something a Soviet citizen would be likely to refuse. They questioned whether comparisons could be made since the systems were so different. Overall, they believed the medical care in the United States was superior but they did not defend the lack of equal distribution of medical care in America.

In the long run, Eddie's career did not suffer for his taking an unpopular stand. Larry Still was writing for a middle-class audience in *Ebony* and *Jet* and found the stories were reasonably well received.

> These stories were in *Jet*. Remember the readership. I was writing mostly for the middle class. They just thought it was unique and odd and recognized it was

> far-reaching. I think they thought it would never come to pass. I never realized in those days that what Mazique was talking about would eventually become Medicare or those kinds of programs.
>
> Eddie really moved the NMA. He made a statement. I didn't realize until after the trip was over how significant it was. I knew that he was in the vanguard but I didn't know that the NMA was opposed to socialized medicine.[22]

It is hard to gauge the impact of the trip on the NMA or the Medicare debate. In the overall picture of Medicare, the trip is but a small footnote, yet it had a decisive impact on Larry Still. If he is any indication of the impact of Eddie's thinking on others, we can be certain that he managed to change some minds about the importance of national health care for the elderly and the poor.

> I covered medicine and conventions after that and as a result of the trip I had a lot of insight. It was the first time I started thinking about the need for a more socialized approach. It radicalized me. It helped me get some insights into the changes that we needed.
>
> Since then I really became attached to Dr. Mazique. He became my personal physician. People like Eddie Mazique demonstrate that you can be black and excellent. He doesn't lower his standards. He makes people feel that we all want to aspire to his standards.
>
> I began to do stories at every opportunity. I don't think he really suffered any from the leadership of that trip. I think most people recognized that he was ahead of his time even though what he was saying may never come to pass. But I think most black people realized that what he said made sense and that the group made sense. I think it helped to focus the total community. The black press was really positive about it. I think that not only *Ebony* and *Jet* but other papers carried stories about it. I think it helped focus on the contrast in the way that the NMA and the AMA were addressing the issues at that time. I know it helped us to focus, as a country, on nationalized medicine.[23]

Overall, the newspaper articles tended to be neutral in their reporting, stating just the details of the trip without any editorial comment or slant.[24] The Soviets used it for propaganda for their purposes but, at least in their western publications, not to the fullest extent possible. In the Soviet Embassy's publication *USSR*, there were two pages of photographs with captions of the doctors on their visit and several articles touting Soviet medical advances but there was no mention of the problems the black physicians were having attaining equality with their white counterparts in the States. A short Associated Press release from Moscow quoted Eddie as stating the delegation he headed "had learned many valuable and useful things during a two-week stay in the Soviet Union."[25] Similarly, reports of the trip that appeared in *New World Review* were mainly informative and emphasized Eddie's point about human relations not keeping pace with scientific advancements. As Eddie reiterated in many different ways, "The physician must become convinced that if science is divorced from people it ceases to be a creative force in life and that his medicine will not in the long run extend longevity. It will only prepare man for destruction."[26]

The clamor for some kind of health care bill continued to grow as Pat McNamara chaired hearings in the Senate in 1959 and 1960. The Morse and the Kennedy-Hart bills became the first in the Senate to propose a payroll-tax-deduction approach to financing health care for the aged. In 1960, with the election coming up, the pressure mounted for President Eisenhower to present some kind of positive alternative to the Democratic bills. Finally, in June, he allowed Secretary of Health, Education and Welfare Arthur S. Fleming to endorse a bill that proposed federal and state partnership in a program to assist low-income seniors. If passed, it would amount to an expansion of the public assistance program. The Finance Committee of the Senate passed what was to become known as the Kerr-Mills Bill. It created a new category called Medical Aged Assistance (MAA), which provided for those who were over sixty-five and could be classified as medically indigent. On the floor the Democrats ended up supporting it after being convinced by Wilbur Cohen,[27] the most influential of the health insurance advocates, that it would be a step toward getting Medicare passed at a later date. President Eisenhower signed the bill on September 13, 1960.[28]

The reaction to Kerr-Mills was mixed. Even though there were grave inequities from one state to another depending on the state laws or lack thereof, the Democrats, although initially opposed, saw it as a means to pave the way for further legislation. At first the American Medical

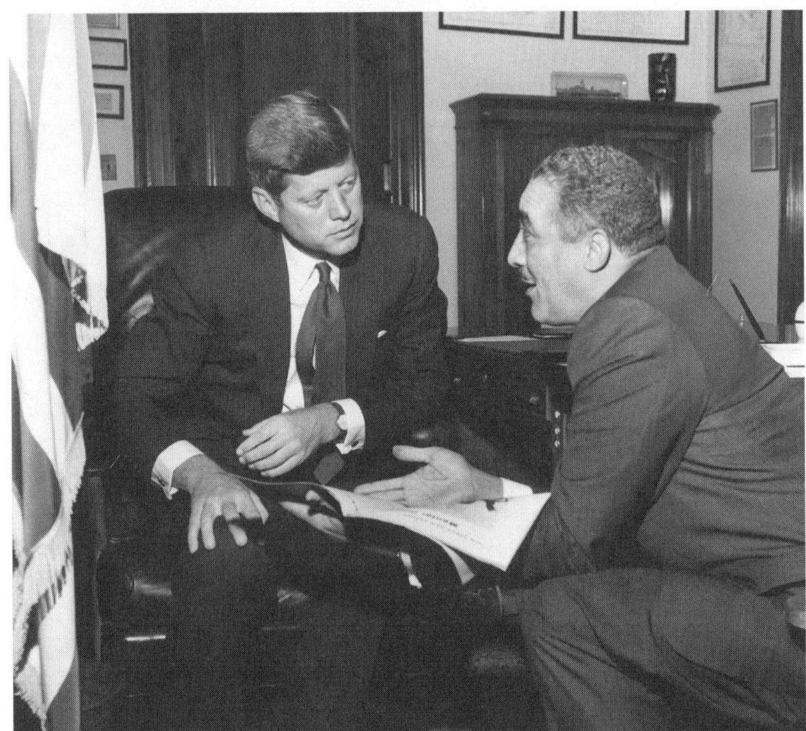

**Fig. 17:** Dr. Mazique consulting with President John F. Kennedy. Photo courtesy of Maude Mazique and Dolores Pelham.

Association opposed it on the grounds of resisting further expansion of the government into the health field. They eventually changed their minds and supported it in the belief it would forestall any further discussion of health insurance in the unlikely event that John Kennedy would win the election. The AMA argued that Kerr-Mills was the answer to the very small minority of seniors who needed some assistance with their medical bills, whereas the broader Kennedy-Anderson Bill "would be just the beginning of compulsory, government-run medical care for every man, woman and child in the U.S."[29] It ended up that most states just switched those who were on other public assistance programs to Kerr-Mills so that the federal government would pay a larger percentage of the cost. Very few new people actually benefited from Kerr-Mills.

During this time Eddie was giving political backing to those most favorable to Medicare. He was one of the twenty-five doctors who composed the National Committee of Doctors for Kennedy. He was pictured in the press with the then Senator Kennedy,[30] with a caption stating that, as the retiring president of the NMA, he urged support for the passage of the Democratic-sponsored medical care for the aged bill.[31]

With the beginning of the Kennedy administration, health care became a priority. The Speaker of the House, Sam Rayburn, and the vice president, Lyndon Johnson, both favored Medicare. With the barrage of new legislation on other issues such as education and tax revision, however, health care did not come to the forefront.

Throughout the remainder of 1960, Eddie used his recent trip to Russia as a means to engage the media in discussing a health care bill and an end to discrimination in the medical profession. The *Washington Afro-American* ran a two-part series on Eddie's views. Eddie stated:

> We say we have the best medical facilities in the world. Yet they aren't made available to all citizens. Colored people, the aged, and poor whites are sadly neglected groups.[32]

He claimed medical education and health care bear the scars of racial discrimination with lack of quality health care and a grossly insufficient number of "colored" physicians. Instead of increasing the opportunities for physicians, especially minorities, in our own country, we import them from other countries. Eddie said:

> We should be conscience-stricken. We are members of the most advanced nation in the world and known for our technical aid to other countries, yet we import their limited supply of physicians and interns to staff our understaffed hospitals.[33]

In 1961, fearing their present media campaign was insufficient to fight against Medicare, the AMA created an independent organization known as American Medical Political Action Committee, or AMPAC. Its advertised goal was for "educational purposes," although in reality they spent their funds attempting to elect conservatives who were opposed to Medicare.

AMPAC was to continue on after the passage of Medicare and in 1981 added another "A" to its title and became known as the American Medical Association Political Action Committee; AMAPAC was recognized as the legitimate lobbying unit for the AMA. This group, which Eddie fought so strenuously in the 1960s and whose very inception was rooted in fighting Medicare, would, ironically, in the 1980s solicit his membership.[34]

> You can understand the AMA being against Medicare. The AMA was and still is a very conservative and at that time a very racist organization. To show you how things take an ironic turn, in the office yesterday, one of the white doctors called who is a good friend of mine, wonderful man. He said, "I want to talk to you about something personal. You know we have submitted your name to become a member of the board of AMAPAC. I want to let you know that I am running for a member of the board of trustees of the District Medical Society and I want your support." What a change from then to now. Somebody has gotten religion! So the changes come but they don't come without a fight and without constant plugging.

The year 1961 was certainly a year for perseverance. Not much progress seemed to be made on the passage of a health care bill. In the middle of July, a San Francisco physician, Dr. Robert Mishell, met with Eddie and Dr. Lorin E. Kerr to try to assist in organizing a group in the District of Columbia similar to the Bay Area Committee, which was led by Bay Area physicians who favored President Kennedy's plan to finance health care for the aged through Social Security. The Bay Area Committee had been formed when area doctors had become angered by the AMA commercials claiming President Kennedy's plan would lead to socialized medicine.[35] One of the main purposes of the committee was to make public the "facts" about Social Security financing of health care and to testify on behalf of such legislation.

Hearings were finally begun on July 24 but no minds were changed and Medicare was put off for another year, with a promise from Kennedy to McNamara that Medicare would receive the highest priority in the next year's congressional session. Eddie again testified at the hearings, this time representing the American Association for Social Psychiatry as its president. His arguments were much the same, although framed differently, when Eddie mentioned the possibility of such a health care program forcing the opening up of hospitals to all races. "Could it be that one of the principal objections to the social security program for the aged is that this would permit the Negro doctors to put their 'foot in the door' of all hospitals that for so many years have excluded them from their staff because of race?"[36]

August 1961 again found Eddie leading the battle for support at the NMA convention. This year the battle was even more heated than in 1960. NMA President James T. Aldrich invited Dr. Leonard Larson, the president of the American Medical Association, to speak, the first time an AMA president addressed the group.

By all newspaper accounts Eddie made a "valiant fight on the floor of the convention with a well-documented speech, pleading with his brother physicians not to forsake the desperate elderly who are without means to pay for adequate medical treatment."[37] Apparently Eddie's presentation and that of supporters Drs. J. Herbert Marshall and W. Montague Cobb were enthusiastically received:

> Thus, they warmly applauded Dr. Edward Mazique of Washington, D.C., a past NMA president when he denounced the "means test" provisions of the present law and urged them to "let medicine remain a profession. Don't let it become merely a business."
>
> "Don't be fooled by these words 'socialized medicine,'" he urged; "the NMA exists to wipe out discrimination in the medical profession. We could use the King-Anderson Bill to open hospital doors from which we have long been barred, both in the North as well as the South."[38]

Although the delegates were more sympathetic and overtly appreciative of Eddie and his position than of the supporters of the AMA and the Kerr-Mills Bill, "the clincher," as one newspaper reporter called it, apparently was when Dr. Peter Marshall Murray, the only colored member of the House of Delegates of the AMA, took the stand to warn the NMA: "Don't take your eye off socialized medicine. We all remember the proverb that when a camel gets his nose under the flap of the tent, the whole camel may be in there very soon."[39]

Dr. Larson had no answer when questioned by Dr. Vaughn Mason, the incoming NMA president, about the implementation of Kerr-Mill by the states: "What faith can we have that states that do not even believe in the dignity of some of their citizens will treat sick, needy, aged, colored persons any better?"[40] He also had no answer for Eddie when he pointed out to the physicians that the King-Anderson Bill could be a way to get "the whole camel into the tent" of hospitals from which black physicians are barred.[41]

The major black newspapers in their editorials were supportive of health care legislation. They urged the doctors to support the Kennedy administration–backed bill and pointed out the hypocrisy of the policies of the AMA.[42]

> If Dr. Larson is sincerely interested in the problems and welfare of members of the NMA, as president of the AMA he would lash out at local medical societies which cruelly refuse to admit colored doctors, or humiliatingly allow them to join on a second-class basis only. Until he does, what he says about anything else has a hollow sound indeed.[43]

However, the show of newfound brotherhood from the AMA and the prestige of Dr. Murray seemed to sway the vote. The final vote by state was 171–44 to endorse the Kerr-Mills formula. Only Arkansas, the District of Columbia, Mississippi, and North Carolina favored Medicare under Social Security. The press coverage was less than sympathetic to the delegates,[44] especially since they had approved, without dissent, a resolution that not only called for the "inclusion of self-employed physicians under social security coverage but also determined 'to implement this resolution by appropriate lobbying locally and nationally.'"[45] One headline read "NMA Seen 'Duped' in Health Plan Vote." The article claimed that

> [w]hat happened was that the smart public relations experts of the AMA dazzled their colored colleagues with an unusual display of togetherness that succeeded in diverting their attention. . . .
>
> However, when the roll call was taken on social security for doctors, there was not one dissenting vote.
>
> Not even the siren song of the AMA could keep the doctors from looking out for their own old age and retirement.
>
> The big question is how will they be able to explain this to the elderly sick patients who need their help?[46]

Some publications even saw it as a case of "Uncle Tomism" within the NMA.

> Whereas at the previous convention in Pittsburgh last year the National Medical Association approved of medical care for the aged under Social Security, the incoming President, James T. Aldrich of St. Louis, Missouri, consistently opposed government aid to the aged, called similar members of his kind together during his presidency and quietly stole off to consult with officials of the powerful American Medical Association in Chicago. Following these consultations, the National Medical Association resolution on aid to the aged was withdrawn and local NMA organizations notified that the National Medical Association was no longer supporting health care for the aged, thereby violating traditional organizational procedure and the interests of elderly blacks. But Uncle Tom, in whatever walk of life he operates, has never understood nor recognized procedure.[47]

Apparently, as part of their strategy against Medicare, the AMA made an effort to influence black leaders, especially black physicians and ministers. It was reported that "the American Nurses' Association testified it had been subjected to similar pressures."[48] After the 1960 vote to study the federal laws regarding health care and report on them, "individual physicians reported a changed attitude on the part of former unfriendly white physicians, as well as novel invitations to join formerly segregated locals."[49]

It was clear from the press reports that the sentiment of many of the delegates was not represented by the vote in 1961.[50] Eddie stated he would join forces with other physicians across the country who were championing the King-Anderson Bill and look toward the next convention, which promised to provide a more receptive audience.

In June 1962, Larry Still wrote an article in *Jet* entitled "What President's Medicare Means to Negroes." The article was lengthy by *Jet* standards and was highlighted on the cover, indicating that the management of the publication "had come around" to supporting King-Anderson. Lawrence Oxley, the secretary-treasurer of the National Council of Senior Citizens, a group formed in 1961 to oppose the onslaught of propaganda of the AMA, told *Jet:* "This bill [King-Anderson Medicare Bill] is second only to civil rights in importance to us."[51]

At the Imhotep Conference of 1962, Roy Wilkins, the executive secretary of the NAACP, pressed the over one hundred physicians attending to

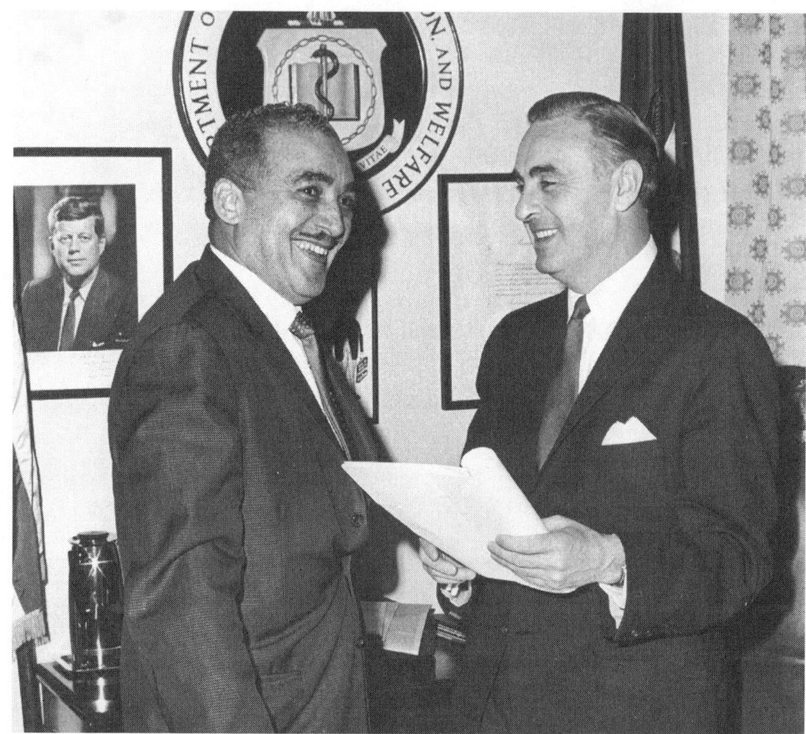


**Fig. 18:** Eddie in discussion with Abraham Ribicoff, Director of Health, Education and Welfare (1961–1962). Photo courtesy of Maude Mazique and Dolores Pelham.

support the bill.[52] Urban League Executive Director Whitney Young also spoke and also urged the doctors to support medical care through the Social Security system, arguing that it would "benefit millions of minority citizens."[53]

In January 1962, Eddie testified as an NMA Representative on Federal Health Legislation before the Interstate and Foreign Commerce Committee of the U.S. House of Representatives in regard to the problem of the shortage of doctors and the passage of H.R. 4999, which was designed to increase the opportunities for the training of physicians.[54] On February 10 he reported to the interim meeting of the Board of Trustees of the NMA regarding federal public health and welfare legislation that was likely to come before the Eighty-seventh Congress. No mention was made of King-Anderson since there was no sign of it coming up for a vote in 1962, but the *Bulletin* did carry a picture of Eddie conferring with HEW Secretary Abraham Ribicoff on "health legislation" after President Kennedy's State of the Union message.[55]

At the sixty-seventh annual convention in Chicago, pickets appeared outside the Sherman House urging the NMA to support President Kennedy's health care plan.[56] In a 106 to 71 vote, the doctors, going against their current leadership, voted to support a medical care bill for the aged financed through Social Security deductions, and the battle within the NMA was won. The Congress of the United States moved more slowly than the NMA, and in 1962 the health care bill could not be gotten out of committee in the House or Senate.

The National Medical Association at its Los Angeles Convention in 1963 reaffirmed its commitment to President John Kennedy's plan. The 1963 congressional sessions were used as a time for regrouping and planning. Meanwhile, the media were describing Medicare as the "forgotten issue" of the year.[57]

During the November hearings, Mills had apparently reached an agreement on how to fund Medicare and the bill would be brought out of committee. However, with the assassination of President Kennedy, the hearings were cancelled and all decisions put on hold.

Most of Kennedy's unfinished legislation was incorporated into Lyndon Johnson's Great Society. Civil rights was his first priority but Medicare, fair housing, and full employment followed closely behind. In a statement early in his administration, Johnson made his commitment to Medicare clear. In January 1964 he affirmed: "It does not seem fair to ask older people to stoop and bend and plead for funds to be shoveled out of the state and Federal treasuries by means of a means's test."[58] At a February news conference he reiterated his support for Medicare when he told reporters: "I can think of no single piece of legislation that I would be happier to approve."[59]

In the meantime the AMA continued its lobbying with one-minute spots on local radio and television stations. The Democrats won overwhelmingly in the November 1964 election, including replacement of three Republicans on the Ways and Means Committee, enough to force a Medicare bill out of committee. On November 11, 1964, Mills conceded in a statement to the press that he was ready to bring the stalled bill out of committee when the Congress convened in January. The 1964 president of the NMA, Dr. Kenneth W. Clement, testified before the Committee on Ways and Means of the U.S. House of Representatives on January 22, 1964, in support of a government prepayment plan for medical insurance.[60]

It was clear with the public support, the increase in Democrats, the change in Mills, and the presidential support that there would be some sort of Medicare bill in 1965. Dr. W. Montague Cobb, president of the NMA in 1965, testified in April before the Committee on Finance of the U.S. Senate on the continued NMA support for financing medical care for the elderly through the Social Security system. Dr. Cobb stated:

> The National Medical Association firmly believes that more than 20 years of study, observation and experience are enough, and that the time has come for broad definitive action.
>
> We are of the opinion that from the long period of attention given the problem has emerged the recognition that our senior citizens, those aged 65 years and over, are in the most need of financial assistance for medical care, and that the most effective and logical way to provide this assistance would be through the social security system.[61]

The form of the bill was partially determined by the AMA in a way they could have never imagined. Their final scare tactic was to criticize the administration's bill for not doing enough. The AMA argued that the bill would not mean any actual benefits for the majority of senior citizens. They pushed their form of coverage, called "Eldercare," which was little more than an extension of Kerr-Mills. John F. Byrnes, a Republican from Wisconsin on the House Ways and Means Committee, sponsored his own bill dubbed "Bettercare" that went beyond the other two in advertised services. It included drugs and doctor's fees that the others left out and was a voluntary program. It was clear that everyone was attempting to show they were looking out for the interests of the elderly.

Mills surprised everyone by suggesting all the bills be put together in a three-tiered approach that would best meet the needs of all the elderly. It passed committee and became known as the Social Security Amendment of 1965; the expansion of Kerr-Mills became known as Medicaid. It passed the House on April 8, 1965. Finally, with 513 amendments, the bill passed on July 30, 1965. Eddie received the following telegram to attend the signing, which would be the culmination of his and numerous others' long effort on behalf of health insurance for the elderly.

At the Cincinnati Convention of the NMA in August 1965, U.S. Surgeon General Luther Terry was one of the featured speakers. He praised the

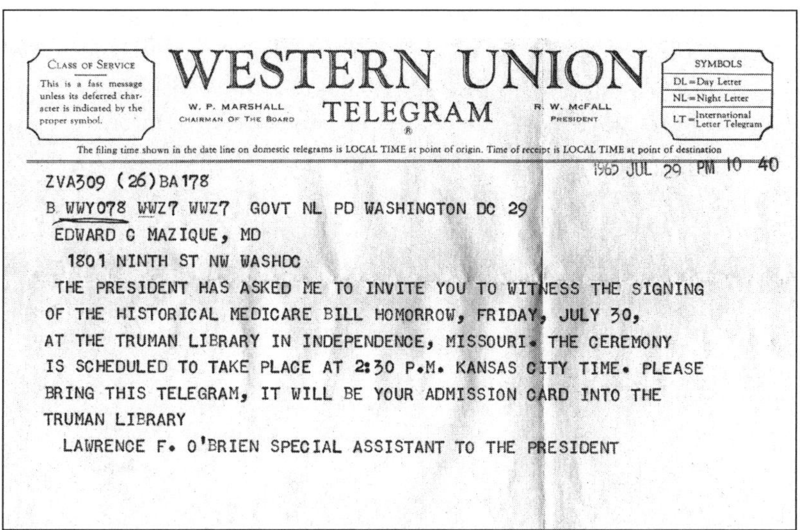

CLASS OF SERVICE
This is a fast message unless its deferred character is indicated by the proper symbol.

WESTERN UNION
W. P. MARSHALL CHAIRMAN OF THE BOARD
TELEGRAM
R. W. McFALL PRESIDENT

SYMBOLS
DL=Day Letter
NL=Night Letter
LT=International Letter Telegram

The filing time shown in the date line on domestic telegrams is LOCAL TIME at point of origin. Time of receipt is LOCAL TIME at point of destination

1965 JUL 29 PM 10 40

ZVA309 (26)BA178
B WWY078 WWZ7 WWZ7 GOVT NL PD WASHINGTON DC 29
EDWARD C MAZIQUE, MD
1801 NINTH ST NW WASHDC
THE PRESIDENT HAS ASKED ME TO INVITE YOU TO WITNESS THE SIGNING OF THE HISTORICAL MEDICARE BILL HOMORROW, FRIDAY, JULY 30, AT THE TRUMAN LIBRARY IN INDEPENDENCE, MISSOURI. THE CEREMONY IS SCHEDULED TO TAKE PLACE AT 2:30 P.M. KANSAS CITY TIME. PLEASE BRING THIS TELEGRAM, IT WILL BE YOUR ADMISSION CARD INTO THE TRUMAN LIBRARY
LAWRENCE F. O'BRIEN SPECIAL ASSISTANT TO THE PRESIDENT

**Fig. 19:** A copy of the Western Union telegram inviting Eddie, on behalf of President Lyndon Johnson, to attend the signing into law of the Medicare Bill on Friday, July 30, 1965.
Photo from Edward C. Mazique files.

NMA delegates for their organization's support of Medicare, telling them that it will stand with the Social Security Act itself "as a landmark in the nation's social history."[62]

Eddie's solicitude for the poor and the elderly was not limited to those within the boundaries of the United States. A strong concern for the emerging nations of Africa was clear from Eddie's inaugural speech, where he argued for the formation of the Foreign and International Health Program. He told his audience, "In health as in liberty, the world cannot stand half sick and half well."[63] As Eddie continued to champion Medicare after his presidency, he also persevered with his attempt to assist with the medical needs of those in the poorer African nations. He saw this as a natural extension of his humanitarian concerns as a doctor and of his African heritage.

The language of his final address as president showed a deepening concern for the extensive health needs of the African nations that had or would soon achieve their independence.

> Today, we are standing at the crossroads of our relationship with the people of Africa. The 230,000,000

> natives of the huge African continent are on the victory march to freedom and independence. The cauldron boils in the Congo. During 1960 alone, a minimum of 14 new African Nations will be admitted to the United Nations making a grand total of 22 Nations. The mills of the Gods are grinding out the sounds of freedom with an unprecedented and determined pace.
>
> Today, Africa is in great need of physicians and good health practices. . . .
>
> The Negro physician because of his African heritage, his traditionally rich culture and values as an American Negro, his technological and scientific knowledge of the Western hemisphere and his academic training, stands today in the unique position of being more capable and acceptable for ministering to the needs of Africa and more strategically designed to diplomatically cement Afro-American relations than any other group in North America.
>
> Your President has therefore recommended to the Board of Trustees that the National Medical Association render immediate assistance to the Congo in the form of a medical mission, or of finances or any such immediate action program that is deemed feasible by the Board of Trustees in collaboration with and approval by the House of Delegates.[64]

There was extensive press coverage of the proposal, and in several cases it even received the headline over his recommendation for NMA support of health care legislation for the elderly.[65] With the need for assistance apparent (as Eddie had noted in his speech, there was not one native physician in the Belgian Congo), there was wide support among the physicians of the NMA. The delegates decided to not only send a medical mission to the Congo but also to explore the medical needs of Africa as a whole. A study commission on the African project was formed that was to report to the board of directors of the NMA in February 1961.[66]

The Committee on African Affairs, as this commission became known, met with representatives from the African nations in an attempt to identify the major health problems and to better understand how the National Medical Association and the National Dental Association could be of the most assistance. A tour of Senegal, Ghana, Liberia, and Nigeria was arranged for eighteen physicians and dentists for August 1961.[67]

Of special interest to Eddie was the proposed Ojike Memorial Hospital in Nigeria. While on an official visit to the United States, at the invitation of President Kennedy, Prime Minister Abubakar Tafawa Balewa and his Federal Cabinet Minister, Dr. K. Ozuomba Mbadiwe, discussed Mbadiwe's idea to build a hospital in Imo State with a "few American friends."[68] The hospital was to honor Mazi Mbonu Ojike, a politician, teacher, and nationalist who championed independence for Nigeria and cultural pride and awareness for its people.[69] Unfortunately, he died in his early forties before he could see the fruition of his work. A university education in the United States led Ojike to consider the United States his "second country," making the project of heightened interest to those Americans who wished to offer financial and medical support. It also tied in nicely with President Kennedy's "People to People" movement, which emphasized improving international relations through private initiative.[70]

The building of the hospital was a slow and at times frustrating project. Eddie was made the U.S. general chairman of the foundation and attended the inaugural luncheon in Lagos, Nigeria, on August 11, 1962. In the speech he delivered that day Eddie noted the great need for the hospital: "The grim facts are that there are less than 1,000 doctors for all of Nigeria and less than 20 dentists. This means a rate of only one doctor for each 50,000 people and one dentist for each 2,000,000."[71] In his article for the NMA, Eddie gave more details about the deplorable medical conditions. "It may be noted that of all infants born, one-half die in infancy; of those who survive infancy one-half die before they reach the age of 17 years. The average life span for the inhabitants of Nigeria is 40 years of age."[72]

By 1963 Eddie had put together an impressive board, including such notable black leaders as Thomas Kilgore Jr., Martin Luther King Jr., Benjamin Mays, and Bishop James Pike.[73] Mrs. Eleanor Roosevelt, although in failing health, had initially agreed to be honorary chairwoman of the foundation. MEDICO (Medical International Cooperation), an organization founded by the late Dr. Thomas Dooley,[74] was committed to staffing the hospital once it was completed. After an impassioned plea for assistance from Dr. Mbadiwe at its August 1963 convention in Los Angeles, the House of Delegates of the NMA passed a resolution that "each constituent unit would voluntarily raise $5,000 for the Ojike Hospital project so that an amount totaling about $250,000 would eventually be presented."[75]

Despite these positive developments, Mr. Robert I. Fleming of the Rockefeller Brothers Fund in Nigeria, who served as national chairman of the Finance Committee, upon returning to New York, complained about the embarrassing lack of activity "at the American end" and the need for some coordination.[76] In 1963 Mr. Juan Trippe, president of Pan American World Airways, accepted the presidency of the United States–Nigerian Foundation For Ojike Medical Center Incorporated and provided the much-needed centralizing force.

Although moral support was evident in the NMA, the promised funding was not forthcoming. A committee had been appointed to help carry out the aims of the Ojike Memorial Medical Center but apparently did not function. Eddie again attempted to elicit support by writing an article about the Ojike Nigerian Hospital Project for the NMA *Journal,* detailing the project and outlining the extensive support from organizations and prestigious individuals. Yet by the August 1965 convention, the NMA had still failed to make a substantial contribution. A goodwill message from the prime minister was read before the NMA delegates by an embassy consul and an appeal made for the NMA to make good its commitment, but the final result was far from the anticipated goal of $250,000. Dr. Montague Cobb, then president of the NMA, recommended that the NMA donate $2,000 to the Ojike Memorial Hospital Foundation, urge its constituent and component societies to make separate contributions as they saw fit, and urge its individual members to make contributions. He supported his position by claiming that the initial action by the House was totally "unrealistic" and had "followed a stirring appeal by Dr. Mbadiwe of Nigeria and the action was taken at the height of an emotional tide which swept over the delegates."[77]

The political scene in Nigeria was anything but stable. In January 1966, Prime Minister Balewa, along with many of his supporters, was assassinated. A second coup occurred in July and new military leaders were installed. A split among the leaders in 1967 resulted in an attempt by the new state of Biafra to secede. The ensuing war lasted three years and resulted in hundreds of thousands of casualties, both military and civilian. After the war, with rebuilding underway, a bloodless coup was staged in July 1975. The new military government wanted to eventually return the government to civilian control. Although the leader was assassinated in 1976, the coup failed and the reforms were eventually instituted; elections were held in 1976, with the final constitution being completed by May 1978. The end of 1983 heralded another round of military rule. Turmoil of this magnitude was bound to create havoc with fundraising and slow down the building of any hospital.

By the fall of 1974, Dr. P. W. Ford from Oregon was recruited as the first doctor in charge of the Medical Center, construction work was in progress on the hospital grounds, and the out-patient department of the Medical Center was opened on November 30. Completion of the major sections of the hospital with a total of 120 beds was scheduled for opening in 1975. After having transferred the $150,000 they had raised to Nigeria, Juan Trippe and the Executive Committee decided to dissolve the United States–Nigerian Foundation For Ojike Medical Center Incorporated. Eddie and Dr. Mbadiwe argued for the continuance of the foundation in the letter they sent to all the board members, but no further official foundation correspondence is in Eddie's files.[78] The last letter of interest, dated July 1982, is from Mbadiwe, who wrote after many years to send Eddie a gift and let him know that the "Medical Centre project is going on progressively, except for the usual financial problems."[79] Eddie had at one time been advised not to make a trip he had planned to Nigeria because of his ties with the former Prime Minister Balewa. Yet at the time he was writing Dr. Mbadiwe was Special Adviser on National Assembly Affairs in the Office of the President. Not only had he survived all the coups and changes in government, but he still managed to be one of the national leaders.

# CHAPTER NINE 

# Battles on the Home Front

No blood, no pain.
— *Edward C. Mazique to his psychiatrist and friend E. Y. Williams*

There may have been no blood, but in 1961 Eddie experienced more emotional pain than at any time in his life. Eddie had learned to endure the insults to his dignity that were part of being a black man in the South. He had built a barrier of protection to keep himself from being hurt too deeply by the inconsistency and, at times, brutality of the white man, but he had no such protection from what was to take place in his private life over the next few years.

While Eddie was finally beginning to see the fruits of his efforts in the public sphere in the 1960s, he was at the same time starting to see the ravages of his neglect of his home life. On November 7, 1961, Jewell left.[1] Eddie remembered it as the worst day of his life.

> I came home for dinner at five o'clock one day and my house was deserted. My wife had left me and carried the kids. When I opened the door there was an echo that almost sounded around the world. When I closed the door, the echo just bounced back at me, it was empty. Everything was gone; all the furnishings. Nothing was left in there except the bed, a table I could eat on, and one chair. There was no one there but the housekeeper. I said, "Margaret, what happened?" She said, "I don't know, a truck just backed up here." That took a lot out of my life and stirred me around.

When Margaret was later asked at the divorce trial what Eddie did when he arrived home and found the place empty, she answered with two words: "He wept."

Admittedly, it was not a total shock. Eddie realized they were having problems and had tried unsuccessfully to get Jewell to attend marriage counseling.

> It was not a complete surprise. I knew that the differences were there. I knew that something was happening but I didn't know what. I knew that things were not well but I never expected something so sudden, to come home and there was nothing there. I didn't expect complete and sudden desertion like that.

Social activities were Eddie's escape from his never-ending work and the harsh realities of a segregated society. He was outgoing and loved being with people, always the life of the party. "Around town, his bearish embraces and greetings of 'honey'... led some to call him the 'kissin' physician."[2] All his patients seemed to love Eddie, but the women patients adored him. As one friend noted, "With him, you have to share him with everybody you meet."[3] With all the time Eddie spent on his work and his causes and with his popularity, not much time or emotional energy was left. Living with Eddie could not have been easy for someone like Jewell who was not socially oriented.

All this came to a head in November 1961. Two years later, when it appeared that reconciliation was impossible, Eddie filed for divorce.

This was not to be an easy divorce. Even looking at exceptionally bitter divorces does not prepare one for the "three-ring circus" atmosphere of this case. Eddie remembered how the case dragged on and the bills piled up.

> One time she said she didn't want the divorce and then another time she said she did. Eventually, when I thought it was hopeless, I filed for divorce claiming that she had left me. In this instance, I was the plaintiff and she was the defendant. During this whole turmoil, we had quite a tangled thing with the lawyers and all this. Every time I looked around there were bills and more bills coming in. You have no idea about the price. Nobody cared—it was astronomical!

The drawn-out nature of the trial is partially attributable to Jewell's inability to find an acceptable attorney. As Eddie remembered,

> [f]inally, she couldn't get along with any of the lawyers that she was working with because they had tried to say, "Hey that is not the way you do this." So she dismissed them all, one after another, until finally she said "I'll be my own lawyer." She went to court all alone. She did the whole thing. You are able to do that in America. But it's the kind of a thing, if there is something wrong with your car, are you going to fix it? You can't do it so you take it to a mechanic. If you are sick the best way out is to call a physician. Jewell should have never been her own lawyer.

The trial was very public, with constant newspaper coverage, and some of the disruptions to Eddie's life were major. On February 2, 1964, Margurite Belafonte, the woman whom Eddie was, by that time, seeing on a regular basis, was producing a spring fashion show at the Park Sheraton Hotel in Washington to raise money for the U.S. Nigerian Foundation For the Ojike Memorial Medical Center. Ten children organized by Jewell's friend Mrs. Clara Newkirk Dawson demonstrated outside the hotel in support of Jewell, claiming that "[w]e picketed because Mrs. Mazique is a defendant in a fight involving her children, her property rights, and a divorce action, and we think justice is being rationed to her in the matter."[4] The signs had slogans saying "Let Not Justice Be Rationed to Jewell R. Mazique in Domestic Relations Court" and "Lovely Gowns do Not Conceal the Betrayal of Black Mothers and Children in the District of Columbia."[5] Eddie's sister Maude mentioned in her diary that they also passed out literature.[6]

Mrs. Dawson followed up the picketing with a letter of complaint to the *Washington Afro-American* the following week complaining about the slant the paper put on the protest, indicating it was a Black Muslim organization.[7] She explained that she was part of the Organizing Committee for the "Defense of Mrs. Jewell R. Mazique, the Mazique Children and Husbandless Wives and Fatherless Children," who had banded together to fight for women. Their motto was "Black Women Unite. You Have Your Children to Save."[8]

This was not an isolated incident. Dr. E. Y. Williams, a psychiatrist and one of Eddie's former teachers, became the main confidant for Eddie during this troubled time.[9] He remembered how difficult it was for Eddie to make the break with Jewell and his fear about what would happen with his sons. He told of Eddie's upset about the meetings Jewell disrupted. Dr. Williams's advice to Eddie was to make a clean break since the negative way in which they were interacting over these two years was just hurting both of them. The old phrase from the East Indian patient whom Eddie introduced to Dr. Williams's class, "no blood, no pain," became the passwords from Eddie to his friend and counselor that despite the assaults, he was doing all right.

One of the hardest things for Eddie to deal with was the loss of his children. Nothing could make up for not seeing them each day, but he remembered how he tried to compensate:

> I spent every weekend doing something with them: going to the zoo or going bowling or the Washington Monument, anything that would be outdoors or something of that sort. I never let anything get in the way of those weekends. Any time I went to medical meetings, they came with me. My vacations, they went with me. I always carried them with me wherever I would go. Every August they would take off with me to the NMA conventions. They got into it. To this day they go.[10]

The loneliness, the bills, the public charges, the need to appear for the trial, the demonstrations and disruptions had become a way of life during this time. Eddie tried to pour himself into his work even more than before. That was not enough, however, and he sent for Maude, who was living in Detroit, and she came to be with him. It was she who helped him through these difficult years.

> I sent for Maude to come after the house was vacant for a while. I tried to get along alone by myself for a period of about a year. Maude was my confidant, she always has been. So I told her what was happening and I asked if she could come down and spend some time with me because I couldn't handle the situation alone. She left everything and came here and moved in. That helped a great deal.
>
> She made the home and brightened it up and began to put a lot of junk around in it. I didn't fabulously furnish

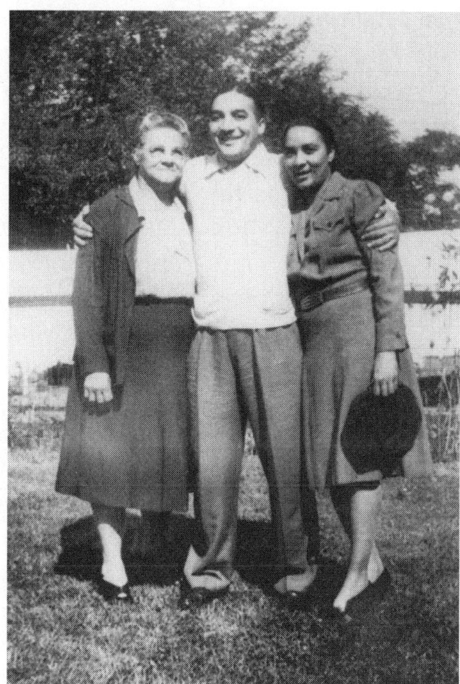

**Fig. 20:** Dr. Mazique poses with his mother, Addie Wilkerson Mazique, and sister Maude Mazique. Photo courtesy of Maude Mazique and Dolores Pelham.

> it but I had a bed, a couch, and a chair put there so that when the door was slammed the sound would be absorbed in the furniture, rugs, and things.
>
> I was a single man for over five years and Maude had to be with me about three or four of those years. She would talk to me about things. She was an immeasurably great source of help during that time. She stuck with me until I married again.

A "Judgment of Absolute Divorce" was issued by Judge John H. Burnett on September 25, 1964. The court found "that on November 7, 1961, without cause, the defendant did desert the plaintiff and the said desertion has been continuous and without cohabitation since said date; and that therefore the court concludes as a matter of law that the plaintiff is entitled to a Judgment of Absolute Divorce."[11]

Over the ensuing months Jewell appealed. On December 21, 1964, the case was argued before a three-judge panel consisting of Chief Judge Hood and two associate judges, Quinn and Myers. The decision was handed down on January 26, 1965. In his concise written decision Judge Quinn stated: "We find her contentions without merit."[12]

Jewell tried throughout the appeals to broaden the scope of the hearings to include such issues as the property rights of wives.

> Citing the Moynihan report which discussed the "deterioration" of the non-white family, as relevant to her case, Mrs. Mazique urged that unless the lower court divorce ruling is reversed, it will place "men in a position to unload families which would return to conditions even worse than slavery."[13]

It was with this broader argument that she attempted to interest the U.S. Supreme Court in her case. She argued that Judge Burnett ignored acts of Congress that protect the property rights of women in the District of Columbia. If Judge Burnett's ruling were allowed to stand, then "marriage annulments can become widespread and wives can have all their properties similarly confiscated."[14]

The divorce case finally came to an end in June when the U.S. Supreme Court refused to review an appeal from Jewell.

Although the trial caused much personal suffering, surprisingly it did little or nothing to damage Eddie's professional life. In fact among one group, the single women, it enhanced his standing. Alma Carter, Eddie's assistant, remembered how the letters and pictures from women he had never met came pouring in after Eddie's divorce.[15] This was one of the facets of Eddie's single life that Maude was especially helpful in controlling. Eddie remembered how Maude took care of his social life at that time:

> I had too much pressure on me, not only immediate pressure for the things that I had to do but outside pressure. I was swamped with a great deal of feminine invasion. I couldn't take care of it. Maude took care of that for me. She would handle the telephone. She would say when I was in and not in. That took care of a lot of the pressure.

Even if Eddie had wanted to wallow in self-pity, he would not have had the time. With the demands of his work, the organizations in which he was involved, and the single women around town, Eddie found himself mercifully occupied. In 1965, Dr. Mazique also had to cope with his

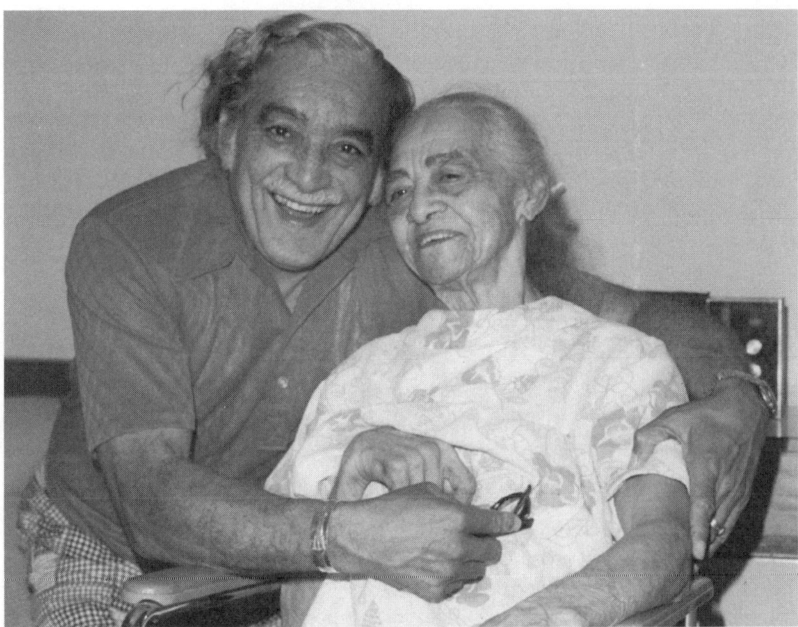

**Fig. 21:** Eddie with his mother on Mother's Day in 1976 when she was ninety-five. Photo courtesy of Maude Mazique and Dolores Pelham.

mother's illness. She was living in Detroit and suffered a severe stroke, the doctors predicting she would not live out the year. Dr. Mazique had her moved to Washington, where she lived with him until 1979, when she died at the age of ninety-eight.[16]

And then there was Margurite. Frances Margurite Byrd was born in Washington, D.C., attended Hampton Institute, where she studied psychology, and then continued her studies at New York University and in Europe. In the late 1940s she married the aspiring singer and actor Harry Belafonte. Before their first child, Adrienne, was born in 1949, there were complications. Margurite was in Washington at the time with her family and her doctor called in a young, up-and-coming doctor with a good reputation for diagnostic skills for consultation. Margurite remembered how terrified she was that day:

> I was pregnant with Adrienne, my oldest daughter, and I came home to Washington for her birth. At the time Harry was going to be on the road. His career was just beginning to catch fire. He didn't want to have to be

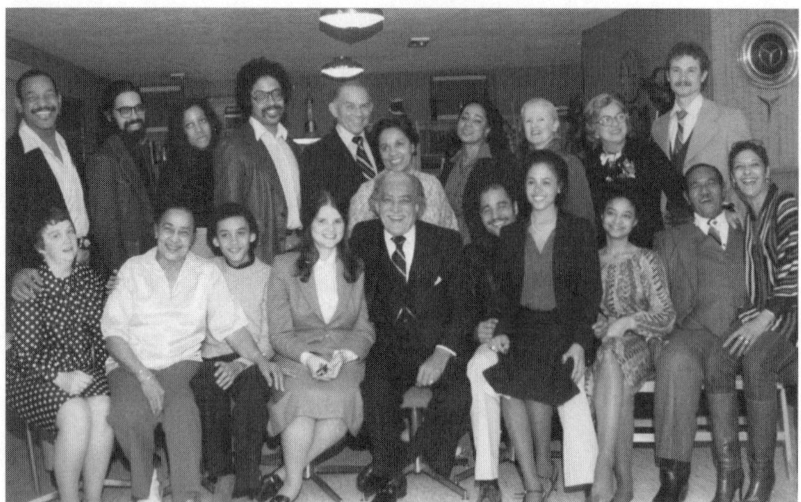

**Fig. 22:** In 1979, the family gathered for the funeral for Addie Wilkerson Mazique. Dr. Mazique (center) poses with some of the family including: sons, Jeffrey (second from left back row) and Edward Houston ("Skip," fourth from left back row); Margurite (behind Dr, Mazique); Maude (second from left in the front row); and brother Alex (seated far right). Photo courtesy of Maude Mazique and Dolores Pelham.

on the road or in the club when I had to go to the hospital. My mother was kind of anxious for me to come home too. I was the first child and she was protective of me. So I came home to have Adrienne and the doctor that I had at that time, who is now deceased, had a private hospital on Ninth Street. That was where I was to go for the delivery. It was something like three months before Adrienne was born when I developed complications. I had very severe pains and my doctor thought I had appendicitis. At that time it was a matter of taking the baby in order to get to the appendix. It was a very upsetting and frightening situation.

The morning I was to go to the hospital, I was sitting in the living room looking out the window, distressed over what might be forthcoming. As I was sitting there waiting for my brother to come and take us to the hospital, a fellow who lived across the street from us drove up and parked in front of our house. He was a

> driver for McGuire Undertakers and he came home for lunch in the hearse. I just went to pieces. I told her, "I am not going. I am going to die at home." My mother called Dr. Adams and told him I was just too upset to put in the hospital. Dr. Adams called Eddie in on a consultation. That was the first time that I met him.
>
> Eddie looked at me and poked around a bit. They left the room to talk; they came back. Eddie came in and gave me injections of penicillin on a regular basis which eventually relieved the pain. What the situation turned out to be was that Adrienne kept on shifting and had created pressure on the kidney. That was the pain and that was the problem. Until this day, he tells Adrienne that she owes her life to him.
>
> After Adrienne was born, I went back to Eddie for a checkup before I went back to New York. I didn't have any contact with him again until after I was divorced.[17]

Margurite became an educational director in early childhood training in New York. In 1957, Harry and Margurite were divorced. From her account in an *Ebony* interview it was a devastating experience. She continued to live in New York with her two daughters, Adrienne and Shari, and in an attempt to put her life back together threw herself into work. She took a job as women's news editor for the *Amsterdam News* and worked at a radio station.

While married to Harry she was relatively unknown, but immediately after her divorce she was "pestered with calls, letters and telegrams from men who wanted to make her their wives [*sic*] . . . Many strange men dropped her letters to inform her that they would be in New York and would like dates."[18] She found herself squired around town by the dapper pastor of the Abyssinian Baptist Church, the Reverend Adam Clayton Powell, whom she met while doing a fashion show to benefit his church. Margurite was in the limelight and she was enjoying it.

Margurite's advice to divorced women was to "get out and meet people and get into a program that will help her fellow man."[19] That is exactly what she did. In 1958 she accepted the cochairmanship of the NAACP Freedom Fund. The purpose of the Freedom Fund was to raise money to underwrite the cost of the legal needs of those involved in civil rights activities. It was a voluntary position but Margurite brought more hard work and determination to the job than some people expected. As she stated then, “I have always been interested in doing something that would help people, and now for the first time I have the leisure and the opportunity to do it.”[20] She cochaired it with such notables as Duke Ellington and Jackie Robinson. One year she even chaired it by herself. Within a five-month period, in 1959, she traveled to sixty-three cities in thirty-eight states. She raised the first million dollars for the NAACP. It is no wonder that in 1960 they decided to offer her a national staff position with the NAACP as director of special projects.[21]

One of Eddie’s attempts to raise funds for the Ojike Memorial Hospital involved trying to interest Harry Belafonte in putting on a benefit concert. Eddie went to New York to meet with Harry but it ended up he was not available. With some unexpected free time Eddie stopped in to see a friend, and it was through this happy coincidence that Eddie spent the afternoon and evening with the former Mrs. Belafonte instead of her ex-husband. Margurite remembered the evening with a chuckle:

> Eddie knew quite a few people, one of whom was a young lady who was in a social club with me. I had just come in town that morning after doing a fashion show benefit for the NAACP and my club was having an afternoon affair that Sunday. I wasn’t really planning to go but what happened was this mutual friend of ours, my club sister, called me and said she had kind of gotten jammed up. Not only had the young man that she had invited to come to this affair come from Connecticut but also her friend from Washington, referring to Eddie, had come up. She wasn’t expecting Eddie. She asked me if I would come go with her and we would make a party of it so she wouldn’t be in too bad of a situation.
>
> She didn’t have a car and I had a brand new one. I went down to her house to pick her and her company up to go to this affair. Eddie decided that I was his date. I guess I was kind of a curiosity, somebody who had just come through a divorce. We went to the party together.
>
> He had a great time. When the party was over way into the night, he was in no state to be put on a plane or the train and sent back to Washington. I thought, what have I got on my hands? I couldn’t leave him so I had to take him home. Fortunately my mother was with me at the time as well as a housekeeper. I brought him home

> and put him on the sofa in the living room. I woke my mother to tell her, guess who I brought home? I didn't want her to get up in the night and see him there. Of course she knew of him because he had been my doctor. She said, "What?" but she understood.
>
> I got him up early in the morning because he was such a stickler about being in his office at a certain time, or being at the hospital at a certain time and he always was. He was very anxious to get back. I got him to the train station and got him back to Washington. Of course, he called that night to say he had gotten home and everything was fine. From that night on he called every night. It was at least a good four or five years until we married but he did not miss a night. His phone bills must have been astronomical. Sometimes he saved phone calls and got on the train or plane and came to New York. Then it reached the point where he was either in New York on the weekend or I was down here.[22]

She was beautiful, intelligent, community-oriented, and a lot of fun. There was no question about it, Eddie was smitten.

In 1964, Margurite, or "Frankie" as Eddie called her, decided to move to Washington and open up a charm school called Belafonte's School of Elegance. Her income was such that she had the funding to undertake whatever business venture she desired. By this time she was earning a large income of her own through her modeling and promotional work with such major companies as American Airlines, American Tourister Luggage, and Ballantine Beer. She had also received a very generous divorce settlement that included a new house, a car, and a lien on all her ex-husband's earnings. Not surprisingly, her choice was to move to Washington where she had her family and Eddie.

The school was such a success that Margurite remembered being overwhelmed by her undertaking:

> I came back to Washington to open this school. It was not a modeling school although it was identified as that. It was really a school to groom young women because I felt that black girls needed it more so than anybody. I opened the school and I had quite a bit of funding because I was doing promotional work and

> personal appearances. Elegance was the name of the school. I tied it in with a number of the junior and senior high schools where the young ladies came over for speech or for grooming. I had dance teachers who taught the basic ballet steps so they could walk. It really took off like a hot fire. It ran away with me. They did not have anything quite like it in the Washington area. It was an attractive building on Twelfth Street, N.E. My brother had built the building; he was the architect for me. That would have been 1963 or 1964.[23]

A constant drain on her energies, Margurite was happy to shut down the school for the summer of 1965 and overjoyed that she had an offer of work in which she could put to use more of the skills that she had learned in her academic training.

> I went to work for the government in June of 1965. I closed the school for the summer. I was so glad to get out of the school. I had the students; I had fantastic teachers but it was really working the living daylights out of me. My name had been submitted to the Justice Department to be a psychological consultant and that job had to do with the "Cities in Crisis." It was just before Watts. We had seven cities that had been identified as being in crisis and that they were likely to blow. They were Los Angeles, Philadelphia, Detroit, Chicago, Rochester, New York, Baltimore, and Washington, D.C. My role was to act as a mediator. I was to get in and talk with key officials both black and white and find out the causes and establish a way of warding it off if we possibly could. That first year, six of the cities accepted the assistance from the federal government to talk and attempt to mediate. California's Governor [Edmund] Brown said they did not need or want any advice from the federal government. They totally refused the federal government's offer of assistance. Watts blew. It just erupted like a fireball. That was the only one that first year.[24]

After the first year, Margurite found she was doing something worthwhile, challenging, and fulfilling and had no desire to leave.

Continued service to the federal government was destined to become a way of life for Margurite. She went on to conduct the HEW Fellows program and later Head Start, where she could dwell on her main interest of working to benefit children.

By early 1964, she and Eddie were already combining their impressive talents. On the afternoon of February 22, Margurite organized the fashion show to benefit the Ojike Memorial Medical Center that was picketed by those who supported Jewell's claims of an unfair trial.[25] This mutual support for public service was to become a way of life after the two were married.

Eddie fit in well with Frankie's family too. Both of her parents had become patients, and Eddie was the only doctor Mr. Byrd would let touch him. Margurite's daughters liked Eddie too, especially Shari, the youngest. Margurite remembers:

> Shari was only two when we divorced. She strongly identified with Eddie as a father figure. Eddie was able to deliver discipline in such a manner that they would not become offended by it. Even after they were grown, they would call, if they knew I was away, to check on Eddie. Adrienne was every bit of a lady and knew how to act and how to behave. I could never count on Shari or Eddie. He and Shari used to get into mischief all the time. They didn't hurt anybody but they were just going to do it their way. Shari has applied a lot of that "go after it and get what you want" attitude of Eddie's. And like Eddie, Shari does it in a jocular way.[26]

In an interview just eighteen months after her divorce, Margurite said she was not ready to put another man in her life. She said she was "more critical than in the past" and "looking for a certain amount of emotional stability."[27] She also stated that the "next time I get married it is going to be an extremely expensive situation," noting that her alimony would stop when she got remarried.[28] In 1967, she and Eddie were both ready for remarriage. Even their wedding, however, was to be surrounded with some controversy.

As Margurite described it,

> [w]e got married on June 24, 1967. That was the same Saturday that his cousin, Charlie Wexler, was getting

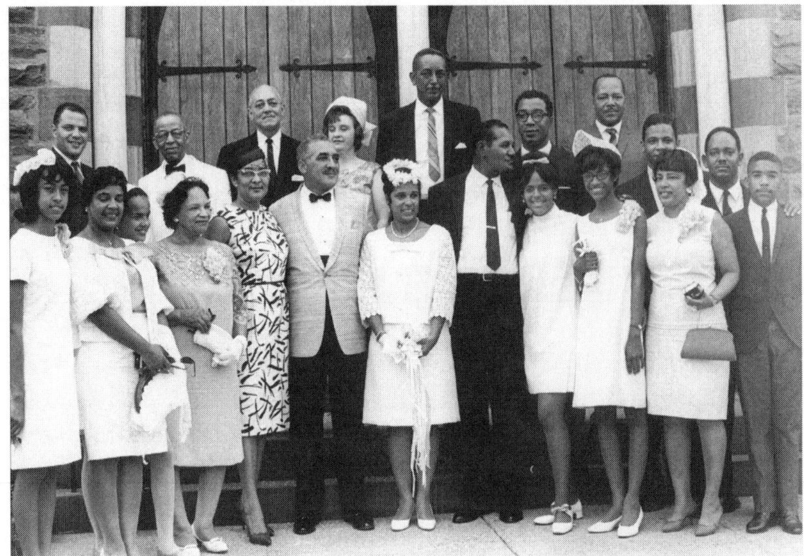

**Fig. 23:** Dr. Mazique and Margurite Belafonte with family and friends on their wedding day, June 24, 1967. Margurite's daughters, Shari Belafonte (third from left) and Adrienne Belafonte (fourth from right), pose with the group. Photo courtesy of Maude Mazique and Dolores Pelham.

> married in Baltimore. Their wedding was in the morning. Eddie took my new car and drove to Baltimore with another cousin. They left the church to start back because they weren't going to the reception because he had to get back for his own wedding. When they were coming back Eddie suddenly realized there were no brakes on the car. The brakes were completely gone! He was moving along at a pretty good clip. By turning the wheels into the curb and skidding along he eventually stopped the car. Some people who were leaving the Wexler wedding and heading back to Washington for his wedding saw him stranded and that is how he got back. This made him late for his own wedding. When they examined the car someone had tampered with the brakes.[29]

In trying to explain the reason for her breakup with Harry, Margurite told an interviewer that initially she put all the blame on Harry. After time passed, however, she started to examine the relationship to see if she could have done things differently. She came to the conclusion that

> [h]e had been made to feel inferior to me. I had the education. I made the money in the beginning. With a shock, I recognized later that he had to resent it. And so I cut down on my activities. I recognized that in order for him to develop to his full talent I would have to take a back seat.[30]

Perhaps her willingness to take a back seat despite her many talents and achievements is what was to make her marriage with Eddie such a success. Eddie's first marriage, with someone who was in some ways competitive with him, had failed miserably. Margurite told the interviewer rather hopefully that "[s]ome people say second marriages work out better."[31] This prediction turned out to be accurate for both Eddie and Margurite.

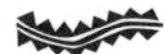

# CHAPTER TEN 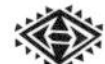

# The Turmoil of the Sixties

> Until a more positive concern is given to the rights and dignity of man, mental disorders will continue to increase. Frustrations will remain with us, and crimes will continue as long as families starve in a land of plenty and abundance; diseases and delinquency will continue to spread, when medical care is not made available to all citizens . . . rejection neurosis will continue to climb, as long as Negro citizens are subjected to second class citizenship . . . psychopathic personalities shall prevail, as long as citizens are subjected to sub-standard housing, inadequate clothing and denials of equal educational and economic opportunities.
>
> — *Edward C. Mazique, Inaugural Address as Incoming President of the American Association of Social Psychiatry, 1961*

If the sixties was a tumultuous time for Eddie personally, the turmoil in the country was even greater. The societal events that were shaking the nation had a tremendous impact on its black citizens. Eddie was very much in sympathy with the underlying conditions that led to the upheavals of the 1960s, and he was involved in some of the major events.[1] Thus, when discussing his life, it was the assassination of Martin Luther King Jr. and the D.C. riots that stood out in his mind when he spoke of the late 1960s.

The bonds of racism were hard to loosen. Laws were being passed and Supreme Court decisions were being made, but enforcing desegregation was not easy. Blacks and sympathetic white supporters were becoming mobilized to fight for civil rights. A tired Rosa Parks refused to give up her seat on the bus to a white man in 1955, sparking the Montgomery bus boycott led by Martin Luther King Jr. Students from North Carolina Agricultural and Technological State University began sit-ins in 1960 after being denied service at a lunch counter. The first integration suit in the North was filed in 1960 as black parents sued and won to end "de facto" segregation in New Rochelle, New York. The Freedom Ride movement began in 1961 challenging discrimination in interstate transportation. The Congress of Racial Equality (CORE) sent thousands of members south to test the laws. New black organizations such as the Student Non-Violent Coordinating Committee (SNCC) and the Southern Christian Leadership Conference (SCLC) were formed to supplement the more established NAACP and Urban League.[2]

Despite the nonviolence of the protest techniques, the country was turned into a battleground as those controlling schools, universities, housing, transportation, and workplaces refused to comply with the new laws. Twelve thousand federal troops were sent to the University of Mississippi campus in 1962 to maintain order as riots erupted in protest over the admission of James Meredith, a twenty-nine-year-old black veteran. In 1963, the black civil rights leader Medgar Evers was assassinated at his home in Jackson, Mississippi, and four black children were killed in the bombing of the Sixteenth Street Baptist Church in Birmingham, Alabama.

By 1963, there was a growing discontent about the lack of progress toward equal rights. The rhetoric of the Kennedy administration had led to rising expectations among the black community but the conditions did not justify the expectations. One and a half million blacks were unemployed in 1963, totaling 22 percent of the jobless population even though they comprised only 11 percent of the work force. A recession that had dried up jobs in manufacturing where blacks had made the greatest inroads was just coming to an end. The economic gap between whites and blacks had actually increased since Kennedy had taken office. Added to this situation was the continued lack of freedom with regard to housing, schooling, voting, and accommodations and the persistence of unequal treatment by legal authorities.

A march was planned to focus the country on the problems facing minorities and the poor. The Urban League and A. Philip Randolph, head of the Brotherhood of Sleeping Car Porters, wanted to concentrate on jobs. CORE, SCLC, SNCC, and the NAACP wanted to attract attention to the issues of civil rights. The stated purpose of the proposed March on Washington was to make the public and the lawmakers cognizant of both issues.[3]

Scenes from Birmingham, Alabama, in April and May 1963 of the police dogs and water hoses used to stop peaceful demonstrators—many of whom were children—were ubiquitous on television screens throughout America. The viciousness of the attacks in Birmingham led to an outcry from across the country for civil rights, giving impetus to a march that up to this point had garnered little enthusiasm.

According to Kennedy's special counsel and biographer Theodore Sorensen, Kennedy moved slowly on civil rights, fearing that a bruising battle that could not be won with the Congress would in the long run do more damage than good. Whatever the reason for the delay, with widespread local demonstrations throughout the country in June, the time was ripe for the Kennedy administration to finally make civil rights a priority. There had also been mounting pressure from within the administration. Secretary of Defense Robert McNamara took a strong initiative, issuing a directive on June 7 to all armed forces bases to oppose any discriminatory practices, not only on bases but also in nearby communities, since such opposition might have an impact on equal opportunity for servicemen and their families. G. Mennen Williams, the former governor of Michigan, who had worked with Eddie in the past for health care reform, was at this time the assistant secretary of state and a Kennedy confidant. He wrote the president in June suggesting "hard hitting administrative actions."[4] Most surprising of all, especially to the liberals who had opposed his inclusion on the presidential ticket, was the push from Vice President Lyndon Johnson, who was emerging as the administration's strongest advocate for a substantive civil rights bill.

In his Civil Rights Address on the evening of June 11, 1963, President Kennedy outlined the events that led that day to the successful integration of the University of Alabama and then went on to make his strongest statement of reform to date. Part of the speech addressed the inherent wrongness and hypocrisy of segregation in a democratic system of government:

> We preach freedom around the world, and we mean it. And we cherish our freedom here at home. But are we to say to the world—and much more importantly to each other—that this is the land of the free, except for the Negroes; that we have no second-class citizens, except for Negroes; that we have no class or caste system, no ghettos, no master race, except with respect to the Negroes?
>
> Now the time has come for this nation to fulfill its promise. The events in Birmingham and elsewhere have

> so increased the cries for equality that no city or state or legislative body can prudently choose to ignore them.[5]

Kennedy's speech went beyond the usual lofty rhetoric and indicated that he was asking Congress for legislation that would ensure all Americans the rights to which he believed they were entitled, including the right to be served in all facilities open to the public, the right to attend public schools, and greater protection for the right to vote.

"Recognizing the call of history, Kennedy [had] made an abrupt turn and accepted the mantel of moral leadership King urged upon him . . . [becoming] the first American President to take the official position that segregation was morally wrong."[6] Other politicians were not so ready for a change in direction. Many southern Senators quickly got together after the speech and vowed to fight the president's proposals. Among them was Senator Eastland, who had withdrawn his son from Sidwell upon learning that Eddie's son was enrolled.[7]

The White House was naturally unhappy about the proposed March on Washington. Fearing violence and a backlash that would hinder the passage of the Civil Rights Bill, Kennedy in a June 22 meeting tried to dissuade the march leaders. Failing to stop the march, the administration tried to gain some control by creating a task force at the Justice Department "to monitor plans for the March and give assistance wherever appropriate."[8]

The mainstream press almost unanimously opposed the March on Washington. The District press was no exception. The *Washington Star* called it "climactic idiocy" that would produce no "happy ending."[9]

Although A. Phillip Randolph became the nominal chairman for the March on Washington, it was Bayard Rustin, a more controversial figure, who was to become the main organizing force behind it. The SCLC's Walter E. Fauntroy was the Washington coordinator.

Walter Fauntroy was born on Westminster Street in Washington, right around the corner from where Eddie was to locate his office on Ninth and S Streets. Walter was a teenager when Dr. Mazique moved his office into the neighborhood near the Bethel Baptist Church, of which Walter was a member and in which he worked while he attended school. Walter Fauntroy remembered how "[t]he church raised funds through dinners sold in the neighborhood to send me to college. Of course, Ed bought many a chitlin dinner."[10] Eddie was the physician for the pastor of the church.

Walter went away to college, graduating from Virginia Union University and Yale University Divinity School. Shortly after he finished his schooling, the pastor of Bethel Baptist Church died and Walter Fauntroy was called upon to become the new pastor. Eddie became his doctor. The amazing thing to Reverend Fauntroy was that Eddie "never charged me a thing."[11]

The March on Washington was to be the first of many of the joint efforts between Eddie and the Reverend Walter Fauntroy. The way Fauntroy remembered it,

> [h]e was valuable to us as a link to the NMA when we were organizing the March on Washington. What I did was put together people who might come to assist me in many of the arrangements. One of the things I relied heavily on Ed for was the provision of emergency medical service. I would credit Ed's participation as being definitive in establishing the cadences to which activist groups have marched since 1963.
>
> Our March in '63 was the largest assemblage to that date of American citizens for the purpose of insuring their First Amendment rights. We had to work out where the first aid tents needed to be and what the plans were for evacuating people in case of a health emergency. Once we had done that for '63, the people over at the National Capital Park Commission who had responsibility for the downtown historic sites and therefore had to be involved, had a plan which they have offered every succeeding group that wanted to do a major demonstration. So you find as the years have unfolded, these demonstrations do not occasion the kind of anxiety and fear that we encountered in '63. It is largely because we know how to do it. And with respect to the division of health and emergency services, that kind of thing was done by the likes of Ed Mazique and the people he pulled together. He was a physician who knew the community and knew medicine and what you could do and how you had to handle it if the problem was heat prostration or getting hit in the head with a bottle.
>
> All I know is I told him, "Look Ed, I can't do everything and I don't know everything." Everybody was asking me if I was all uptight about what could happen. A large gathering like this, people will faint and die just of heart attacks or things. That could be very disorienting, so I asked him to help me to use the people that the

> army was going to give us and the federal government and the district were going to give us to make sure that nobody who needed medical help went without it.[12]

Looking at it in retrospect, the March on Washington was both a huge success and a dismal failure. The crowd was somewhere over three hundred thousand, exceeding all expectations. The march and the program were models of harmony between diverse black and white organizations. There were no disruptive incidents and only three people with previous medical problems needed to be hospitalized; one of them died of a heart attack. It was peaceful and it was dignified, with the uplifting speeches and music tugging at the hearts of all but the most hardened racists. There is little doubt that it played some part in the passage of the Civil Rights Act of 1964.

Yet the March on Washington could not and did not solve all the underlying problems facing Afro-Americans. On the way home from the march, a fight broke out when black youths attempted to use white restrooms, waiting rooms, and a restaurant at a bus depot in Meridian, Mississippi.[13] The weekend after the march, a black family moving into a previously white neighborhood was harassed in Pennsylvania. The very next week in Alabama, Governor Wallace had state troopers surround a public school to prevent court-ordered integration. The bombing of the Sixteenth Street Baptist Church in Birmingham, Alabama, which was to kill four young black girls attending Sunday school, occurred less than three weeks after the march.

It was becoming clear that the Martin Luther King Jr. plea for freedom, justice, and brotherhood "Now" was not going to be achieved without resort to civil disturbance. King had warned in his speech that

> [i]t would be fatal for the nation to overlook the urgency of the moment and to underestimate the determination of the Negro. This sweltering summer of the Negro's legitimate discontent will not pass until there is an invigorating autumn of freedom and equality. 1963 is not an end, but a beginning. Those who hope that the Negro needed to blow off steam, and will now be content will have a rude awakening if the Nation returns to business as usual. There will neither be rest nor tranquility in America until the Negro is granted his citizenship rights.[14]

Although the Civil Rights Act of 1964 and the 1965 Voting Rights Act were passed and signed by President Johnson, they were not enough to quell the unrest. The economic position of blacks was largely unimproved. With huge outlays of money required to support the conflict in Vietnam, the social programs of the Johnson administration became unfeasible. The expectations aroused by the March on Washington could not be met.

A chronology of events related to civil rights for the years 1964 and 1965 produces a picture of ever-escalating violence. Such incidents as the murders of three civil rights volunteers in Mississippi; the clubbing and shooting of a marcher in Marion, Alabama, by a state trooper; and the beating of three Unitarian ministers, leading to the eventual death of one, in Selma, Alabama, while they were assisting in the civil rights drive being directed by Dr. Martin Luther King Jr. are indicative of the amount of force those opposed to segregation were willing to use. Mass demonstrations and marches were held by civil rights advocates in Chicago; Bogalusa, Louisiana; and Selma and Montgomery, Alabama, while the Ku Klux Klan held a memorial march for a white youth slain in racial conflict. Meanwhile black militant groups such as the Black Muslims and Deacons for Defense and Justice were gaining adherents.

The march from Selma, Alabama, to the capital of Montgomery was a fifty-one-mile, five-day trek whose purpose was to make the public aware that blacks had been denied registration to vote in Selma. Governor George C. Wallace fought the participants' right to march every step of the way. First attempted on March 7, the march was stopped by two hundred Alabama state troopers and sheriff's posse men. They charged into the ranks of the 525 black marchers with tear gas, nightsticks, and whips. Sixty-seven marchers were treated for injuries and 17 of them were hospitalized. On March 9, another march on Montgomery was begun with the ranks now swelling to 1,500 and including hundreds of northern clergymen and civil rights workers. By then, a restraining order had been issued by a federal judge and the demonstrators turned back. Finally, on March 17, the same judge upheld the right of the demonstrators to march and Governor Wallace was ordered to provide police protection for the marchers. "Aroused by the events in Alabama, the Federal government brought forth the 1965 Voting Rights Act, one of the most powerful civil rights measures in American history."[15]

Walter Fauntroy, the coordinator for the Selma-Montgomery March, once again consulted Eddie.

> Eddie was my personal physician, so everything I did I checked with him. In 1965, I coordinated the Selma-Montgomery March and asked him to contact as many of

> his colleagues in the medical community as possible both for financial support and for presence. He not only did that but he made the trip with us to Selma for the march.[16]

Tensions did not ease as the sixties progressed. Conditions did improve for some blacks, yet in the poorer sections of the cities the daily plight of the minorities remained largely unchanged. The predominately black section of Los Angeles called Watts, with an unemployment rate of 35 percent, was the first to explode. A six-day spree of looting, burning, and rioting in August 1965 cost the lives of 35 people, with another 883 injured and property and fire damage totaling 221 million dollars. In March 1966, Watts erupted again.

On April 29, 1966, President Johnson sent his third Civil Rights Bill to Congress, and as 1968 began he was still appealing to Congress to pass legislation ensuring the safety of citizens exercising their rights by making the murder of a civil rights worker, a student seeking education, or a person attempting to vote a federal crime punishable by life imprisonment. The Johnson bill also attempted to desegregate schools and public facilities and outlaw discrimination in all housing based on racial or religious grounds.

The year 1966 also saw the shooting of James Meredith and the increase in the appeal of the concept of "black power" as hard-liners continued to struggle to resist changes that would bring equity to the American system. In July, riots broke out in black sections of Chicago and Cleveland. Near rioting ensued at the end of July and into August as Martin Luther King led demonstrations for an "open city" in a white section of Chicago.[17]

The following year "de facto" segregation was ruled unconstitutional in the District of Columbia and total desegregation of District schools was ordered to be completed by the fall. While civil rights advances were thus being made, they were being made all too slowly for most blacks, and in 1967 racial tension was at an all-time high. Over the "long hot summer" Boston, Newark, Buffalo, Detroit, New Haven, Cincinnati, and Cambridge, Maryland, all erupted in violence. At the end of July, President Johnson appointed the National Advisory Commission on Civil Disorder to discover what had happened and why it had happened, and to determine how to keep it from ever happening again.

The Kerner Commission, as it became known, offered no surprises when it described the causes of the civil disorders of the 1960s.[18] Heading the list were pervasive discrimination and segregation that excluded "a great number of Negroes from the benefits of economic progress through discrimination in employment and education, and their enforced confinement in segregated housing and schools."[19] The increased black migration into the northern cities that led to a depletion of already very limited resources and the black ghettos in which poverty and segregation had intersected to destroy hope and opportunity were suggested as the other basic causes of the disorders. The ghettos, with their high crime rate, lack of health facilities, poor municipal services, poor educational opportunity, high unemployment, biased administration of justice, and lack of recreational facilities made for a hopeless situation for most black youths. Meanwhile whites and blacks outside the ghetto had prospered to a degree unparalleled in history. Television and other media flaunted the gains of the majority of the people. Expectations had been raised by the successful legal and political civil rights' battles, yet inner-city blacks were not much better off than they had been before all the marches and protests.

In March 1968, when the Kerner Commission issued its report, Washington, D.C., was still believed by most to be riot-proof. The expanding federal bureaucracy assured jobs and prosperity to many in the nation's capital. A 1966 *Jet* article speaking of the many top positions in government held by blacks under the Great Society said Washington had perhaps "the biggest and wealthiest set of professional Negroes in America."[20] They did not include in their article the lawyers, doctors, and businessmen and women who already made "the nation's capital the city with the highest income for Negroes in the country."[21]

Progress had definitely been made in Washington. The medical society, the hospitals, the YMCA, the restaurants, the schools, in fact all the institutions that Eddie and his colleagues had sought to desegregate were now integrated. Twenty-five percent of the federal employees were black, a large number of them with secure, well-paying jobs. There was a black, Robert C. Weaver, in the Cabinet. Thurgood Marshall sat on the Supreme Court. "In comparative terms, Negroes in Washington are generally better educated, better paid and live in better housing than in any other major city in the Nation."[22] This had been achieved in Washington without the explosive racial turmoil that had proven necessary in many areas of the country.

The door to full equality had been left ajar but not opened wide. One reporter in a 1963 article had called it the "sophisticated discrimination that remains after legal and overt barriers fall."[23] There still remained housing shortages, limited job opportunities, and slums and schools that became resegregated as a result of housing and employment restrictions. Sterling Tucker, executive director of the Urban League, stated the problem and the complaint of professional Washingtonians succinctly:

> We want the stigma of race removed. We're tired of carrying every other Negro on our backs. And every Negro in America carries every other Negro on his back.
>
> The reason Ralph Bunche couldn't get into a white tennis club or Carl Rowan into the Cosmos Club is because from the moment his application came up, he was looked on like every other Negro—whether he be a criminal or poor Mississippi cropper.
>
> His qualifications meant nothing. It adds up to this: Ralph Bunche can't be free until the lowliest Negro share cropper from Mississippi is free."[24]

Even though conditions had improved for many of the black professionals in Washington, there were still pockets of what author Constance McLaughlin Green had called in the 1965 update of her comprehensive study of Washington, the "Other Washington."[25] This was a Washington rarely seen by the capital's numerous tourists. There had been massive changes during the period that Green described, and since her account there had certainly been improvements. Nevertheless, some of the terrible conditions she so comprehensively documented in her book and discussed in the 1965 update still existed in 1968. Although a legally integrated city, Washington still had many areas that consisted of overpriced, congested, substandard housing that was inhabited almost totally by poor blacks. While only about 4 percent of the workforce was unemployed, in the areas that would soon be affected by the riots the rate was more than two or three times higher than in the rest of the city. In these ghetto areas lived the "hard-core" unemployed and many others who were employed below their abilities. Large sections of the city, especially the poorer ones, were without adequate transportation, further limiting job opportunities for those who resided in these areas. The infant mortality rate was still so high in Washington that only Mississippi's was worse. Although there was one "black bank," Industrial Bank of Washington, founded in 1934, access to money and reasonable credit were still problems for many minority inner-city dwellers. Seeing the financial need, Eddie and several friends founded United National Bank of Washington in 1964.[26]

Realizing the unrest in the city, President Johnson pushed a reorganization plan for the District through Congress. A black man, Walter Washington, was appointed as mayor and a black majority was created in the new nine-man city council, including Walter Fauntroy, who served as its vice chairman. Private industry was even beginning to follow the government's lead by opening more than menial jobs to Washington's blacks.

In the spring of 1968, feeling pressured by the war in Vietnam and the black militants to make a major effort to alter the direction in which the country was moving, Martin Luther King Jr. proposed to hold the Poor People's Campaign, "a 'last chance' project to arouse the American conscience toward constructive democratic change."[27] It was to begin in Washington, D.C., with demonstrations that included the poor from all races. Ten cities and five rural areas were chosen, from which two hundred poor people would be recruited and trained in nonviolent techniques. The length of time for the demonstrations was not set, with the understanding that the demonstrators would stay as long as it took to get a response from the nation. While the Selma and Birmingham demonstrations were designed to address political issues, the Poor People's Campaign focused on economic problems. King wanted an "Economic Bill of Rights" guaranteeing jobs to those people who wanted to work—and were able to work. Dr. King believed that if the SCLC could make "the movement powerful enough, dramatic enough, morally appealing enough, that people of goodwill, the churches, labor, liberals, intellectuals, students, poor people themselves [would] begin to put pressure on congressmen to the point that they [could] no longer elude our demands."[28]

In April 1968, in a moving and eloquent article written just prior to his assassination, Dr. King explained his rationale for the Poor People's Campaign:

> The policy of the Federal Government is to play Russian roulette with riots; it is prepared to gamble with another summer of disaster. Despite two consecutive summers of violence, not a single basic cause of riots has been corrected. All of the misery that stoked the flames of rage and rebellion remains undiminished. With unemployment, intolerable housing and discriminatory education a scourge in Negro ghettos, Congress and the Administration still tinker with trivial, halfhearted measures.
>
> ... For us in the Southern Christian Leadership Conference, violence is not only morally repugnant, it is pragmatically barren.... We cannot condone either riots or the equivalent evil of passivity.
>
> ... We believe that if this campaign succeeds, nonviolence will again be the dominant instrument for

> social change—and jobs and income will be placed in the hands of the tormented poor. If it fails, non-violence will be discredited, and the country may be plunged into a holocaust—a tragedy deepened by the awareness that it was avoidable.
>
> ...The discontent is so deep, the anger so ingrained, the despair, the restlessness so wide, that something has to be brought into being to serve as a channel through which these deep emotional feelings, these deep angry feelings, can be funneled. There has to be an outlet, and I see this campaign as a way to transmute the inchoate rage of the ghetto into a constructive and creative channel.
>
> ...I'm convinced that if something isn't done to deal with the very harsh and real economic problems of the ghetto, the talk of guerilla warfare is going to become much more real. The nation has not yet recognized the seriousness of it.... As committed as I am to non-violence, I have to face this fact: If we do not get a positive response in Washington many more Negroes will begin to think and act in violent terms.[29]

Just as they were with Eddie, the medical inequities that existed in the United States were of concern to Dr. King. He emphasized this again in his final article when he pointed out:

> Medical care is virtually out of reach of millions of black and white poor. They are aware of the great advances of medical science—heart transplants, miracle drugs—but their children still die of preventable diseases and even suffer brain damage due to protein deficiency.[30]

Other black leaders were far from enthusiastic about the campaign. Bayard Rustin, the coordinator for the 1963 March on Washington, and Roy Wilkins, the executive secretary for the NAACP, tried to dissuade King. They feared that this time Dr. King would not be able to ensure the peacefulness of all the participants.

On Thursday, April 4, while working in Memphis, Tennessee, on his plans for the Poor People's Campaign, Dr. Martin Luther King Jr. was shot. After the news bulletin that he had died aired at 8:19 that evening, burning and looting erupted in 125 cities across the country. One of those cities was Washington, D.C.

Although the riot seemed to catch many of those in authority off guard, many of the black leaders in Washington had been expecting problems for some time. In May 1963, Rep. Adam Clayton Powell (D-NY) told a Washington audience that the city faced "one of the worst race riots in the history of the United States" if conditions did not improve quickly.[31] The *Washington Afro-American* also made the same prediction.[32] Eddie was among those who felt some kind of conflict was almost inevitable:

> The riots were not really brought about by the death of Dr. Martin Luther King. I think the riots were due to a combination of pent-up feelings among a group that could hardly take any more. They were just sitting on a powder keg waiting for some incident to set it off so they could do something to give vent to their feelings. The death of Martin Luther King was just the spark that caused it to explode. Even if you look just at medical care for blacks: not being able to enter hospitals, not being able to have their own doctors with them, and being given inferior rooms. I think the riots were a combination of the emotions people had been having all these years as a result of various kinds of negative experiences and they couldn't hold it back anymore. Yet they had no weapon and nothing to fight with and they just tried this as one way of fighting back. Then when this thing started there was just no stopping it.

The statistics on the riot make it clear that it was the worst outbreak of racial violence the city had ever seen. By the time it was quelled, the death toll was nine, 1,202 persons were injured, and over 6,000 had been arrested. There were 1,130 fires reported and the final estimate of real property damage, excluding personal property, was set at fifteen million dollars.[33]

As in most cases, the statistics do not tell the whole story of the riot. For Eddie and others I interviewed who had experienced those days in 1968, the riot was much more than statistics. It was a heartbreaking experience.

At the time of the riots, Reverend Fauntroy was Washington bureau director for the SCLC and as such was helping to coordinate the Poor People's Campaign for Martin Luther King Jr. In February, he had come under a congressional attack demanding he either resign his city position or break off with the city's "black militants" who were supporting the campaign. Rep. William J. Scherle (R-IA) had charged that Fauntroy had "placed himself in a contradictory position, and a position which the city cannot tolerate."[34] Fauntroy, who had been appointed by President Johnson, refused to yield to pressure and said the president's silence must be interpreted as support for his position.

Fauntroy prevailed, and on the evening of the riot, he still held his position both with the District and with the SCLC. He had come to the SCLC office adjacent to the People's Drugstore on Fourteenth Street and gone out to try to calm the angry crowd of young men led by Stokely Carmichael as they went along the street asking the businesses to close.[35] "'This is not the way to do it, Stokely, this is not the way,'" Fauntroy said as he gently held Carmichael's arm.[36]

Fauntroy remembered it vividly:

> At the time of Dr. King's assassination, I was working for the Poor People's Campaign in an office at Fourteenth and U Streets North West. I was at the church that evening, conducting a prayer service when I heard he had been shot. I left the church at Ninth and S and went to Fourteenth and U where the campaign headquarters were, to conduct what calls I needed to find out whether he had been seriously injured. When we learned that he had in fact died there was some window breaking downstairs and some activity which caused me to go to the streets to try to calm and dissuade people from violent actions.
>
> At the time, I was vice chairman of the city council. I consulted with the police department and Dr. Mazique. I asked the police to get me either a police vehicle or a motorcycle to get me around to the various TV stations to make appeals to people for calm.[37]

Fauntroy entreated his "'black brothers and sisters' to 'handle our grief in the spirit of nonviolence.'"[38] As one eyewitness recalled, "at each stop, there were tears in [Fauntroy's] eyes, sorrow in his voice."[39]

The violence was under control shortly after midnight, and preparations were being made for problems that might arise Friday night. Police were caught off guard when the riots started early Friday afternoon. By 3 P.M. fires were consuming a large number of buildings on Fourteenth Street north of Euclid Street and as far south as U Street and along the parallel Seventh Street corridor and an H Street strip. With the shift of the major activity to the Seventh Street corridor, the riot moved closer to Eddie's office just two blocks away on Ninth Street.

Once the news of the riot spread, downtown workers piled out of their offices and into their cars to head home, creating one of the worst traffic jams in Washington history.[40] The deputy mayor asked that the release of the government workers be staggered, but it was too late. The intersections became jammed with cars attempting illegal turns, causing some motorists to be stuck for hours. A furniture store on Seventh and Q Streets was gutted by fires set by the looters while the firemen sat hemmed in by the fleeing motorists. Even the first troops called into the city found they could not reach their destination because of the congestion. Eddie's wife, Margurite, caught in the traffic, was fearful for his welfare. Later she realized he was very well protected.

> He was able to get home better than I was. They had scrawled the words "Soul Doctor" on the plate glass windows that surrounded his office and they made it a point to come in and escort him to his car every evening. Everything around him was burned and looted but they didn't touch his office. His office was totally unscathed by the whole thing and you would hear such comments as "You got to save the doctor" or "He's a soul brother." It was really marvelous how they watched out for him in that area. He never missed a day going down there to open his office despite all that was going on around him.[41]

It was this Friday of rioting that Eddie also remembered with the most clarity, but with his proximity to the events his observations were very different.

> That Friday afternoon, it was just like a grand picnic they were having. They were joyful at first. Then as the day began to wear on a bit, they were more restless and finally violent. People began to come out and come by my office carrying all kinds of articles like cartons of cigarettes and liquor.
>
> There was a Jewish fellow named Charlie who owned the store just across the street from me on Ninth and S where my office was. In those days there were Jewish

> stores on almost every corner and that was typical of America.[42] Charlie and I were friendly. He was very good to everybody in the neighborhood. They would come in to get little things they needed. After they had left Seventh and S where they had burned a liquor store down they finally arrived at Charlie's place. In the evening I guess around six or something like that, Charlie came over because they were telling him they were getting ready to get his place next. He came over and asked me if I would come out and stop them. Well I did. They had started a fire at his place and I came out and whatever transpired didn't happen. There was the beginning of a blaze and a couple of the kids went in and snuffed it out. That saved it for that day. Charlie came over very grateful and thanked me for helping but I suggested that he keep awake.

By 3:00 P.M. that Friday, the crowds were out of control. At 4:02 P.M. President Johnson signed an executive order providing for the restoration of law and order in the Washington metropolitan area, thus allowing for the mobilization of the army and the air national guard. The *Washington Post* reported that the looting was "nonstop, except for some places near 7th Street with 'Soul Brother' signs painted in the windows."[43] By 5:00 P.M. there had been more than seventy fires, most arson, reported to the fire department.

That evening Eddie was called to go on the air to try to calm the people:

> I was called by someone from one of the television stations. I forget the name of the station now but the announcer was Norman Ross who was in charge of programs, and Norman called and said some viewer had called the station and asked them if they couldn't get me and someone else to try and talk to the community and try and quiet them down. This was the second day. I called Walter Fauntroy and we went to the TV station.
>
> I bet we stayed on the TV station four or five hours just staying on and talking and talking and trying to quiet the people down in the streets and let them know that we could understand their grievances but there was no reason to burn down the way that they were burning down and that they were only burning themselves out of houses and jobs. We had all kinds of telephone calls and we stayed on

> the air until one or two in the morning. It did some good and it was quieted down some but then the next day they called up the national guard and they were all around the corners, all around the city. There were lots of people who would call or come to the office asking what to do with respect to their kids and how to quiet them down. I guess that whole week I was answering questions dealing with the riots more than with medical problems.

The riot never threatened Eddie personally.

> One of the little kids in the neighborhood, Lamar, he was about eight or ten years old, always adored me and my staff. He came along with an older brother and got Bon Amie and printed on my window. I had nothing but glass windows around my office and he printed on there in big letters, "Soul Doctor." Nobody touched my place; they just went by.
>
> During the riots the patients were there and I continued to work. Into the night this thing raged on. By the time I got through at the office, it was about nine o'clock; everybody was a little worried. Frankie said to me that I shouldn't go a certain way, that instead I should go around another way to come home and my secretary told me the same thing. But I saw no reason for it. I said, nobody is going to bother me because everybody knows me and I knew everybody around there. Instead of coming the long way around, I went the short way and came right on straight down Fourteenth Street where all the activity was. All the blazes, the fires, and taking out stuff and nobody said anything except "Hi, Doc" and nothing happened except I just moved right along. There were fires and sirens from fire trucks and ambulances were going on endlessly throughout the night.

The mayor imposed a night-long curfew from 5:30 P.M. Friday to 6:30 A.M. Saturday that prohibited everyone with the exception of police, fireman, doctors, nurses, and sanitation workers from being on the city streets or in public places.[44] The sale of alcohol, firearms, ammunition, and flammable liquids was prohibited. By the end of the evening there were so many fires burning that the fire department was unable to tabulate the exact total. One source lists the total fires for the rioting by Friday at over five hundred. "By midnight, 6,600 troops had restored temporary order, and were patrolling the streets and enforcing a dusk-to-dawn curfew."[45]

Saturday, April 6, was a calmer day. With the troops concentrated in the worst-hit sections, looting broke out mainly in fringe areas. Fires still remained one of the largest concerns, with 120 blazes set that day.[46] The curfew began at 4:00 P.M. that Saturday and was strictly enforced. There were six hundred arrests for curfew violations between 5:30 and 9:00 P.M. and only ten for looting. At an 11:00 P.M. press conference, Cyrus Vance, who was acting as a coordinator of local and federal anti-riot efforts, announced that "[t]he city is secure."[47]

A cool and sunny Sunday found many of the city's residents venturing out to go to Palm Sunday services as things appeared to be returning to normal. One of these services was conducted by the Reverend Fauntroy where he pastored at New Bethel Baptist Church. In it he quoted a statement made by Dr. King in a telephone conversation they had shared only ten days earlier: "I'm afraid, Walter, this country just isn't ready for nonviolence."[48] Afterward, he and Senator Robert F. Kennedy, who had been in the congregation, walked through the riot-stricken area.

There were scattered incidents of looting on Sunday but they were few compared to the previous days and no new fires were reported. Most of the six hundred arrests were for curfew violations.

As things were quieting down in the District, trouble was coming to a head in Baltimore.[49] On Sunday, federal troops moved into the city to assist the six thousand national guardsmen already in place. Governor Spiro T. Agnew requested further assistance as the fires and lootings increased. The rioting in Baltimore ended on April 9 with six dead and more than seven hundred persons injured.

By Monday, schools in Washington were open for part of the day and federal and District government employees were told to report to work, although they were allowed to leave ninety minutes early so they could abide by the 6:00 P.M. curfew. On Tuesday, April 9, Dr. Martin Luther King Jr. was buried and the stores and schools were closed in his honor. On Wednesday, the Washington Senators played the Minnesota Twins in D.C. Stadium without incident while thirty-two thousand fans watched. Even though things were quiet, a shorter curfew would remain in effect until April 12, when the troops finally began their withdrawal. Finally, on April 15, Mayor Washington officially terminated the state of emergency.

The riot was over but some of the destruction incurred would last until the present, with boarded-up buildings still bearing witness to the devastation that was wrought. The Seventh Street corridor suffered a heavy toll.[50] Although the dollar value of the damage was less ($4.3 million on Seventh Street and $6.6 million along Fourteenth Street), there were nearly twice as many buildings damaged along Seventh Street as along Fourteenth Street. About half of the housing destroyed in the city was along the Seventh Street corridor, where a high proportion of the buildings were of mixed land uses with a store on the bottom and an apartment or two on the top. If the fires in the ground-level stores could not be controlled, the apartments located above were also destroyed. About 36 percent (112 units) of the housing units damaged on Seventh Street were destroyed completely. Most of the apartments were rented by black families, many of whom lost all their possessions as well as a place to live.[51]

The assassination of Dr. King prompted the House to expedite a Senate-passed Civil Rights Bill prohibiting racial discrimination in 80 percent of the country's housing. However, the president's signature on the bill on April 11 and his plea for recognizing "the process of law" did little to quell the continued tension in Washington throughout April and May. Five merchants and one bus driver were murdered during this time, and there were threats to business owners and even some looting and fires.[52] It was estimated that the tourist business fell off from 30 to 50 percent. The announcement in late April that the Poor People's Campaign would proceed was received with dread by the beleaguered city officials and nervous Washingtonians.

# CHAPTER ELEVEN

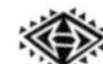

# City of Hope, City of Despair

> Resurrection City has grown rapidly and is composed of inhabitants from all sections of the country representing a contrast in racial and ethnic groups and ages ranging from babies to octogenarians. The only common denominator of these people is poverty. Were it not for the lingering fear following the civil disturbances in April, it would easily be the number one tourist attraction in the Nation. The City is exciting, dynamic changing, and challenging. At this writing the morale is high and spirits elated. The basic philosophy of the people seems to be a firm determination to present to America its poverty, squalor, economic and social inequities. Hence, overcoming physical and environmental hazards becomes a part of their soul-strength and enhances their physical resistance to disease.
>
> — *Edward C. Mazique, 1968*

When Dr. Martin Luther King Jr. conceived of the Poor People's Campaign, he envisioned an encampment in the nation's capital of poor people called the "City of Hope," which he saw as a strong, regularly visible symbol of the poverty in the United States. The purpose of the shantytown would be to dramatize the plight of the urban poor as the down-home mule would be used to point to the rural poverty. Many of the Southern Christian Leadership Conference organizers were opposed to any such encampment and favored having the poor spread around the city in the homes of sympathizers. However, the position prevailed of those who wanted to increase the visibility of the poor by having them all together in one location so that their shantytown could be used as a "poetic springboard from which to launch the nonviolent campaign against the establishment."[1]

Eddie tried to put a good light on Resurrection City with his press releases, but from the beginning it was plagued with problems. Even before Dr. King's death many of the black leaders objected to the campaign for fear there was no way of ensuring its peacefulness. With King's assassination, the prospects for success were even less hopeful.

Dr. Martin Luther King Jr. and Reverend Ralph Abernathy were an effective team. In retrospect historians accord Abernathy a lot of the credit for the successful efforts of the SCLC. However, with Abernathy having to take command and promptly begin the campaign with little time to establish himself as the headman, it had to be expected that there would be even more difficulties than there would have been for Dr. King. Many people had not had sufficient time to accept this new and very different man as their leader, and his personality and background were such that even with time he would not have the rapport with the white liberals that Dr. King had been able to establish.[2]

As expected, southern Senators soundly denounced the proposed campaign and objected to the park permit for Resurrection City. The District officials had to take note of these objections since their finances were still controlled by committees dominated by southerners. City officials let it be known they were better prepared than they had been for the riots, with 8,000 federal troops and 1,800 national guardsmen standing by.

Talks had begun in late April to decide on permits for the use of parkland for Resurrection City. Walter Fauntroy in his role as both vice chairman of the city council and SCLC's Washington representative "became a key figure in the talks, mediating disputes and encouraging practical discussion rather than rhetoric."[3] Finally, a six-page permit was issued on May 10 by the National Park Service to use fifteen acres of West Potomac Park between the Reflecting Pool and Independence Avenue from the Lincoln Memorial to Seventeenth Street. The population of the shantytown was limited to three thousand, and it was agreed the park police would not enter unless they were invited. Firearms, liquor, and open fires were prohibited and garbage had to be removed and sewage and bathing facilities provided.

Plywood and plastic-sheeting huts were to be constructed to house the people, who reached a peak population of 2,600. Eventually, the shantytown had its own dining tent, dispensary, and city hall. The population consisted mostly of poor people who had arrived on bus caravans from the South and from a few northern states.

The problems with the media started with the first press conference on May 13 when Abernathy was scheduled to drive the first stake for the construction of Resurrection City. Abernathy was several hours late, and while the press were waiting they had their first angry encounter with the marshals, who barked orders, blocked any interviews with marchers, and generally attempted to intimidate the reporters. The marshals were largely youths, frequently from tough city gangs, who had been recruited to maintain order and security for the encampment. They were so erratic in their behavior and so antagonistic to the press, many of whom had previously been sympathetic to the campaign, that an older group in their twenties was eventually formed called the "Tent City Rangers" to oversee the marshals. The marshals could not easily be controlled, for they represented the more militant group that the SCLC was anxious to contain within the folds of their nonviolent movement. Presenting a good front to the reporters, while at the same time not openly challenging the militant marshals, was to prove to be an impossible task.

The weather went against a successful campaign. It rained most of the time the marchers were in Washington, repeatedly halting construction and making a mud hole out of Resurrection City. Financial difficulties also plagued the campaign. It was difficult to tell from the information given to the press just how much more money was needed, and different officials gave conflicting accounts at various times. In the meantime, the large demonstration on Solidarity Day had to be postponed until housing could be completed. To present the campaign's demands to various federal departments and to make residents feel involved, some forty small demonstrations and marches, usually involving less than 325 people, were held before Solidarity Day.

This lack of aggressive activity was apparently part of the plan in hopes that the large number of people expected to participate in Solidarity Day would not be frightened off. Strategy or not, however, it left people sloshing through the mud with little to occupy their time. With very few ways to channel their energy, some of the younger residents of Resurrection City began causing trouble. This assault from within the confines of Resurrection City was even more of a threat to the success of the Poor People's Campaign than the assaults from the weather or lack of funding. "While most of the shantytown residents were docile and uncomplaining, a significant number of young 'dudes', many of them urban gang members, were, from their arrival, constantly getting out of hand, drinking, assaulting other residents and outsiders, harassing newsmen, taunting police, and stealing everything that could be lifted."[4]

Finally, on May 22, the leaders sent two hundred of the most troublesome youths, mostly from Chicago and Detroit street gangs, home. The Reverand James Bevel, in making the announcement, stated: "They went around and beat up on our white people. They interfered with the workers and were hostile to the press. We had to get them out."[5]

In the midst of the Poor People's Campaign another blow was struck to poor and black Americans. Their favorite candidate for president, Senator Robert Kennedy, was shot and killed in Los Angeles on June 5. Andrew Young[6] remembered how

> Robert Kennedy's assassination just brought everything to a halt, and I think we began to grieve about Martin in the context of Bobby Kennedy's assassination because Bobby Kennedy had been with us in Atlanta at Martin's funeral. And many of us began to see in him a hope for the future. We kind of transferred a little of our loyalty, a little of our trust and a little of our hope to him, and now he was gone too.[7]

Mrs. Kennedy, along with her husband's remains, was flown to New York by presidential jet the following day. She was accompanied and comforted on the plane by, among others, Mrs. Martin Luther King Jr. and Mrs. Medgar Evers.

Bayard Rustin, although he had been opposed to the Poor People's Campaign and had become much more moderate in his thinking since the 1963 March on Washington, agreed to take command of organizing Solidarity Day. In trying to present the demands of the campaign in some form that he deemed politically feasible, Rustin alienated the leadership to such an extent that they refused to support his statement. On June 6 he announced his resignation; on June 9 it was accepted and he was replaced by Sterling Tucker, the director of Washington's Urban League.

The Rustin resignation seemed to be the final straw for the press. They had been harassed and prevented from doing interviews by the marshals; they had repeatedly been kept waiting for hours at press conferences and then received little information for their trouble; sometimes they received conflicting information due to the disorganization evident within the SCLC ranks; and they were aware of the crimes within Resurrection City. Since there was so little real action going on, the reporters were starting to focus attention on the problems within the campaign, especially the crime situation, instead of on the issues of hunger and poverty. The media were becoming increasingly critical. "By the end of the week [of June 6], the campaign had clearly lost the sympathy of an essential ally [the press], and was thereafter constantly on the defensive."[8]

With the original deadline, June 16, of their park permit rapidly approaching, the SCLC requested a thirty-day extension. They were granted only one week extra, with the new deadline being June 23.

At meetings held in Washington to draw support from the local black community, campaign workers received only half-hearted responses. Not much was happening to inspire support. The small marches that had taken place were rather dull, with little confrontation and few arrests. Unfortunately, the only happenings of any interest taking place within the campaign were negative. The disorganization and violence in Resurrection City and the open quarrels between the various ethnic groups involved were sapping away any support that could be expected from the locals. Even on the day of the Solidarity Day March, a reporter found little interest among the people in the Negro neighborhoods that had been scarred by the rioting a few months earlier. Standing across from the local headquarters of the Poor People's Campaign, a black youth summed up the apparent feelings of many in his neighborhood: "It's just another march that's not going to change a damn thing for black folks."[9]

June 19, Solidarity Day, was the one bright spot of the Poor People's Campaign. "Sterling Tucker and a small volunteer staff had, in the space of only ten days, done their job efficiently and well."[10] For a change it was a clear day, one of the few during the entire campaign. District officials had every available policeman on duty along with 500 police reserves and 1,100 national guardsmen. It was an orderly crowd and they were not needed. The estimates of crowd size ranged from 50,000 to 100,000.

The press accounts of the march almost unanimously noted the difference between the mood of the marchers and speakers that day as compared to the 1963 March on Washington. The hopes were not as high. Some described it as lack of "optimism," "patience worn thin," or "bitter frustration with the government's failure to help the poor."[11] Regardless of the description one chose, it was clear that many felt they had moved the government as much as was possible with nonviolent tactics.

The crowd seemed to mill around and paid little attention to most of the speeches, although Mrs. Martin Luther King Jr. was loudly applauded. She spoke eloquently of the violence perpetrated against the poor:

> Poverty can produce a most deadly kind of violence. In this society violence against poor people and

> minority groups is routine. I remind you that starving a child is violence; suppressing a culture is violence; neglecting schoolchildren is violence; punishing a mother and her child is violence; discrimination against a workingman is violence; ghetto housing is violence; ignoring medical needs is violence; contempt for equality is violence; even a lack of will power to help humanity is a sick and sinister form of violence.[12]

Abernathy spoke last and rather anticlimactically to a much diminished crowd. Of special interest were the nearly six pages of his twenty-nine-page text in which he outlined the concessions the Poor People's Campaign had gotten from the various federal agencies.[13] These included the Department of Agriculture's agreement to introduce federal food programs into more than two hundred of the poorest counties and a promise to increase the quality of federally distributed surplus foods; Housing and Urban Development's guarantee to relocate residents of urban renewal areas until housing could be arranged for them; and a pledge of jobs for one hundred thousand unemployed workers by January 1969 from the Department of Labor. Wilbur J. Cohen, the secretary of Health, Education and Welfare, issued a statement for Solidarity Day in which he listed twenty-one steps that HEW was taking to assist the poor. These included bringing "'adequate and essential health services to the poor' and reduc[ing] radically the death rate among disadvantaged mothers and their infants" and implementing the Supreme Court ruling that having a man in the house could not be used as a reason for a state to deny aid to families with dependent children.[14]

These concessions were of special importance since none of the Poor People's Campaign's six major demands—(l) to end hunger, (2) to end bad housing, (3) to end unemployment and guarantee an income for those unable to work, (4) the provision of adequate health care for all citizens, (5) to provide full equality of educational opportunity, and (6) an end to violence and repression at home and abroad—could possibly be hoped to be achieved by any one political movement. It was these piecemeal agreements from the agencies, not some sweeping demands, that were to be the positive legacy of the Poor People's Campaign.[15]

There were only two criminal incidents reported by the press during the Solidarity Day proceedings: an eighteen-year-old Washington man was arrested near the Reflecting Pool for carrying a loaded gun and a fifteen-year-old received a superficial stab wound from some juveniles

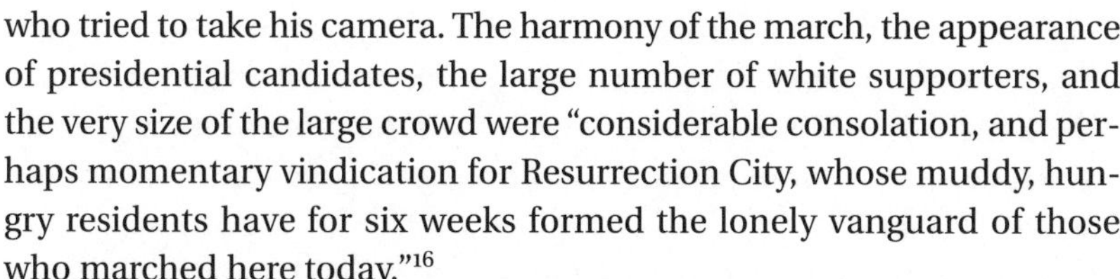

who tried to take his camera. The harmony of the march, the appearance of presidential candidates, the large number of white supporters, and the very size of the large crowd were "considerable consolation, and perhaps momentary vindication for Resurrection City, whose muddy, hungry residents have for six weeks formed the lonely vanguard of those who marched here today."[16]

Resurrection City was much less peaceful. Violence continued through the night in the encampment, with park police claiming they were told of fifteen assaults between the time the Lincoln Memorial program was completed and 9:00 P.M. Given the agreement the park service had reached with the SCLC, the police were not permitted inside Resurrection City to investigate. By 2:00 A.M. the total was listed at seventeen, with one of the incidents resulting in a youth's being taken by ambulance to Freedmen's Hospital for a cut throat and convulsions. Another victim turned out to be a marshal who had been hit over the head with a plank of wood by another marshal.[17]

Alvin Jackson, a black electrician who had been a security marshal at Resurrection City, resigned the day after the Solidarity Day March. In an interview that was carried on the front page of the *Washington Post* he said:

> The reason the population of this city is going down is not mud, poor food, rain or lousy homes. Most of these people come from places that would make this city look good. The reason they leave is that men are getting tired of coming home from a day's picketing to find their belongings stolen or their wife raped. There are rapes, robberies, and cuttings every day, and there is nothing we can do about it even when we catch the guys who did it. If the leaders there don't do something soon this is going to be known as blood city instead of Resurrection City.[18]

Jackson went on to say his fear was that the good of the campaign would be forgotten because of the violence. "This is a great campaign and a just one," he said, "and it has just goals."[19]

SCLC officials tried to put the best possible light on the story by having Abernathy claim that to his knowledge Jackson was not a resident of the city or a marshal. He further argued that Mr. Jackson was planted by some group to subvert the campaign. He did admit there had been some crimes committed.[20] Abernathy stated that "[w]e are poor people and possess all the anxieties and aggressive tendencies of the poor all over America. I would say that we have less crime, far less crime, than other poverty areas of comparable size and we have dealt with it without police and without jail."[21]

The taunting and throwing of things at police and passing motorists, the intimidation and attacks against the press, the assaults on people near as well as those within Resurrection City, the treatment of whites, even those who had come to offer their assistance for a cause in which they believed, was taking its toll on public sympathy for the campaign.[22] No matter what Abernathy would argue, "Resurrection City in its final week was unquestionably a turbulent and dangerous place."[23]

The demonstration at the Agriculture Department the day following Solidarity Day led to a clash with police. Seventy-seven demonstrators were arrested and six campaigners and three policemen were injured. A comment by a policeman ("I've been waiting for this for a long time") and the reported overreaction by other officers ("Several policemen actually went berserk and had to be held back by other officers") seemed to indicate that the police patience with Resurrection City residents was over.[24] The protesters threw bottles, rocks, and sticks at the police, and the police fought back with tear gas. It looked as if a riot situation was developing. Campaign marshals and police conferred and eventually were able to negotiate the campaigners back into Resurrection City while the police withdrew, thus preventing a more serious outbreak.

As with the police, District government officials, representatives on Capitol Hill, and the officials of the Interior Department were also losing patience with the campaign and Resurrection City. Interior's decision not to extend the permit for Resurrection City was leaked to the press on Friday, June 21. That same day the Mexican-Americans, feeling their cause had been slighted, pulled out and three campaigners were arrested on separate robbery charges, including the head of the Tent City Rangers.[25] By Sunday, June 23, an article appeared in the *Washington Post* claiming that while Mayor Walter E. Washington and his aides were still committed to the goals of the campaign, they now regarded the continued occupation of Resurrection City as "menacing."[26] The article made it clear that Thursday's encounter at the Agriculture Department had wiped out any image improvement that had been garnered from the Solidarity Day March.

Even many of those in the SCLC felt that Resurrection City had become a liability to their cause. Allegedly, Mr. Fauntroy privately told some of his city government colleagues that the situation was "out of hand" at the encampment.[27] One report quoted an SCLC official as saying, "It has become a noose around our neck."[28] "What the Organization now concedes privately is that the focus of the Campaign has been allowed to shift from the basic battle against poverty to a defense of life in the city and an attempt to rectify previous mistakes."[29]

In a press conference Friday afternoon, Reverend Abernathy was more eloquent and honest about the violence within Resurrection City than previously.[30]

> I make no excuse for violence, here or anywhere. It is wrong. . . . I do not want the poor people to imitate the lowest form of behavior in a racist society. . . . But there is a greater evil than a few outbreaks in Resurrection City. It is the evil of widespread poverty in America, and I challenge America, I challenge the press and every leader in the power structure which inflicts poverty on millions of Americans to tell me what their excuse is for poverty. . . . I am saying to America, you can blame me for violence in Resurrection City if you wish; I accept it. But who is to blame for the violence of slums, the violence of discrimination, the violence of broken promises and lies to the poor, the violence of unequal and inadequate education, the violence of a punitive welfare system, the violence of cheating American Indians and Mexican-Americans and Appalachian whites and northern and southern blacks?[31]

He summed up the grievances of the poor with one question for which he demanded a public answer from the president: "Why does the United States government pay the Mississippi plantation of a United States Senator more than $13,000 a month not to grow food or fiber, and at the same time why does the government pay a starving child in Mississippi only $9 a month, and what are you going to do about it?"[32] Dr. Abernathy was referring to Senator James O. Eastland, the same Senator who earlier withdrew his son from Sidwell because Eddie's black son was enrolled.[33] If the Poor People's Campaign could have brought this issue to national attention—plantation subsidies to a wealthy Senator while black children in his district were going hungry—they would have clearly drawn support from a wide range of groups. Instead the campaign got bogged down in the mud and violence of Resurrection City. Abernathy's question never even got printed in the *Washington Post* article that referred to this news conference.

Demonstrations were called off over the weekend until SCLC officials could finalize their plans. Trouble started again early Sunday morning (12:30 A.M.) when police, in response to bottle and rock throwing by a small group within the snow fence around the encampment, lobbed more than seventy-five tear gas grenades into the southwest corner of the darkened shantytown. The gas was picked up by the prevailing winds and carried over most of the fifteen-acre campsite. Andrew Young and SCLC official J. T. Johnson went to the southwest corner and pleaded with the police to stop throwing the gas but they were ignored. Nine residents were treated at local hospitals for effects from the gas and many others stumbled around in the darkness crying and choking. "They were a pathetic and moving sight, these people, most of them black, silhouetted in the glare of huge spotlights and looking tiredly down on the White House and gray government buildings visible in the distance behind their own lights."[34]

Reverend Abernathy had pledged not to let the expiration of the permit force the campaigners out of Resurrection City. SCLC officials apparently were divided on where to make their stand: at the Capitol or in Resurrection City. It was feared that "the city, with its suspected stockpile of firearms, ammunition and Molotov cocktails, could erupt into violence if police moved in to make wholesale arrests."[35] As Andrew Young said, "we just couldn't be sure of our troops."[36] On Monday, June 24, Reverand Abernathy and 229 others were arrested on Capitol Hill and 118 were arrested peacefully at Resurrection City. The task of dismantling the camp was completed by the following day.

Hosea Williams[37] said of the city's closing: "We got trapped down in the mud hole. I want to thank the government for getting us out of it. . . . Now that Resurrection City is gone, we can focus on the real problems—with Congress for instance—instead of wasting half our energy trying to keep kids from throwing rocks."[38] Andrew Young expressed similar feelings, stating that "in one sense, whoever ran us out maybe did us a great favor."[39] In a rally on the evening of the closing, Jesse Jackson outlined the next move of the campaign as nationwide boycotts.[40] However, the Poor People's Campaign was in essence over, with only the smaller departmental concessions to show for the effort. One historian summed up the campaign in rather bleak terms: "The Campaign had no momentum; it had failed both as a moral crusade and as entertainment. Solidarity Day and the arrests of Reverend Abernathy were not sufficient to offset the movement's dullness and uncertain virtue. Black Washington was, according to all available evidence, simply indifferent to the movement; to them it was already over."[41]

It may have been over for the majority of black Washingtonians, but for some it was another reason for violence. Later in the day of June 24, gangs of black youths smashed windows, looted, and threw stones and bottles at police. Police fought back with tear gas. The mayor promptly declared a state of emergency and called in the national guard. By 11:00 P.M. the city was relatively calm, with Mayor Washington emphasizing that the disturbances were not major: "the declaration of the curfew should not be taken to mean that we are in the midst of any disorder of the magnitude which occurred in April."[42] A curfew was imposed until June 25, when the guard was put on standby status. This time the city officials were prepared and the police and military responded quickly and decisively. Only twenty windows were broken and three fires started throughout the city; by midnight June 24, the disturbance was over.[43]

Eddie had been very much involved with Resurrection City from the planning stages until its closing. Focusing on him, as Eddie directed his attention to the medical needs of the residents, allows us to see Resurrection City from a different perspective. It adds some depth to our understanding of Resurrection City and to the problems and political intricacies that were involved. To Eddie, the goal was important enough to struggle against the mud, the politicians, the conservative doctors, the city officials, and the odds to keep Resurrection City open.

> There were so many people, especially blacks, in poverty, so many without jobs, so many without chances of education, so many hungry, so many ill with no services. When the word came out of the depths of Mississippi it afforded them an opportunity to unite on a national basis whereas before it had only been local or municipal. When they began to close ranks on a national basis this showed a gain in respect for the black people, for what could be done. So they moved into Resurrection City and they marched.

The residents were mostly poor, some with emotional problems, many of them malnourished, and they had not been recipients of regular or proper medical care. Then there were the problems caused by the almost constant downpours (2.23 inches of rain fell on Resurrection City in twenty-four hours over June 12 and 13, for example) and poor sanitation. Added to these conditions were the violence within the city and the potential violence from outside during the demonstrations, where beatings and tear gas were always a threat. It was to the nearly impossible task of providing quality health care for all the residents, free of charge, that Eddie turned all his talents of organization, persuasion, and management as well as his medical skills. The Health Services Coordinating Committee (HSCC) was established on May 18, 1968, with Eddie as its chairman.

The HSCC was composed of seven charter members: the National Medical Association, the Medical Committee for Human Rights, the Medico-Chirurgical Society of the District of Columbia Auxiliary, the District Medical Society, the National Dental Society, the Robert T. Freeman Society of Washington, D.C., and a representative from the Seventh Day Adventists. Several of these organizations were already providing some services when the HSCC was formed to coordinate the health services into a comprehensive and organized form.[44]

All the needs for on-site medical care were provided, including the structures, machinery, pharmaceuticals, clerical personnel, psychiatric screening, dentists, doctors, nurses, and social workers. The committee arranged that the off-site medical care would be available at Freedmen's Hospital, D.C. General, and D.C. Children's Hospital. Transportation, both for emergency and nonemergency situations, was arranged should hospital care become necessary. They provided or arranged for medical screening programs including tuberculin testing, chest X-rays, and immunizations.

In three different ways the committee strove to meet the various medical needs of the residents of Resurrection City. First, they would provide medical care for acute conditions and medical emergencies that might arise from day to day. Second, they offered a mass medical screening project aimed at giving each inhabitant a general physical exam. Finally, they strove to improve the health of the residents by providing health education. In an attempt to have a greater impact on the plight of the poor, they agreed that information and data would be properly accumulated and assimilated so that it would be made available for medical analysis at some later date. It was hoped that "such health interpretations of scientific data may well serve as a basis for better medical care for the people from the various sections of the country where they reside."[45]

The encampment was covered twenty-four hours a day with the volunteer services of almost four hundred doctors. Two doctors, two nurses, and two medical students were on duty for each six-hour shift, except from 12:00 A.M. to 6:00 A.M. when one doctor and two nurses were on call when available or, at the least, a registered nurse. The dental van had one dentist, two dental students, and one assistant for each shift.[46] A chief officer of the day (O.D.) was assigned to "be in charge of the entire HSCC operation, its personnel and facilities during his tour of duty," which lasted twenty-four hours from 9:00 A.M. one day until 9:00 A.M. the following day.[47] There were ten doctors who acted in this capacity on a rotating basis. Eddie was one of them, serving in this capacity each Wednesday.

Although the HSCC repeatedly stressed their autonomy from any other organization, they worked in a close relationship with the Department of Public Health, Howard University Medical School, and the local hospitals. Having to interact on a regular basis with the Department of Public Health of the District of Columbia did not guarantee a harmonious relationship. Throughout the campaign, conflicts arose and many were never satisfactorily resolved.

The May 18 meeting of the HSCC noted that the Health Department had refused to move their health van into the Resurrection City area and instead kept it a half-mile away. They had held off, claiming they would move it only when adequate plumbing and electricity could be supplied. These facilities were now available and the Health Department was still reluctant to change the van's location. The HSCC decided if the Health Department refused to move the van they should be informed that "unless we can decide where the van stays we will ask them to remove their van from the operation."[48]

By the May 26 meeting, this conflict had still not been resolved. Again, "The committee was united in agreeing that HSCC should not yield under any circumstances to pressures by District officials who favored other locations (particularly peripheral)."[49] As an alternative, it was decided that the Seventh Day Adventist health trailer be used in its stead and be moved to the location of the future health center as soon as possible.

Rather than the HSCC and the Health Department being on better terms by the June 9 meeting, the areas of conflict had increased. The trailer situation had still not been resolved and added to that dispute was the control of the records. A representative from the Health Department had collected all the records from each of the vans and then denied access to the administrator for HSCC. The Health Services Coordinating Committee had agreed to report to the Health Department the number of people seen and the out-going diagnosis but not to hand over records. By taking the records the Health Department was making it impossible for the doctors to do any follow-up work with the patients. It was also feared that the Public Health Department might use the records for their propaganda. "Further, we cannot permit the Dept. of Public Health to use our records for any political machinations of their own."[50] A state of emergency was the only circumstance in which the Health Department would have a legal right to any and all records. It was decided that three steel cabinets with locks would be purchased to prevent any further removal of records.

Added to this situation were the problems the committee was having with D.C. General Hospital and the Public Health nurses. D.C. General had refused to treat patients referred to them and sent the patients back to the site. They were then referred to Freedmen's Hospital where they were accepted for treatment. Although the Public Health nurses were aware that D.C. General had been refusing referrals from the HSCC, they still continued to send patients there.

There was a recommendation made by an HSCC board member "that since we cannot function well within the present situation, we might best sever our relations with the Dept. of Public Health."[51] Instead, an attempt was made to clear things up by sending a committee to meet with Dr. Murray Grant, the director of the Public Health Department. The committee was to request that all records be returned, the trailer be moved to the designated area, and it be made known that the health facilities and program for Resurrection City were under the direction of HSCC with the O.D. in charge and that the Public Health officials and nurses were subject to the O.D.'s authority. It was further decided that if Grant did not accede to these requests, the matter be made public by the issuance of a press release.[52]

With the approach of Solidarity Day on June 19, what had been a private battle for control between the HSCC and the Health Department was made public. The Health Department tried to bypass the HSCC when it made the health services plan for Solidarity Day. In a hard-hitting press release, the HSCC claimed that "[t]he major impediments encountered in delivery of health services have been stumbling blocks placed in our way by the D.C. Department of Public Health, National Park Service and associated organizations."[53] The release went on to say: "In the most important drive for unity and solidarity among poor people of the United States, it is these same organizations which are presenting an artificial facade of concern when in reality they represent the vested interests which have kept the poor, poor."[54]

The Public Health Department was accused of using technical language to "frustrate the purpose and philosophy of the Poor People's Campaign" and to "overshadow the function of the Health Services Coordinating Committee in providing continuity of care."[55] In addition, they claimed that "[t]he blatant by-passing of HSCC in planning the health services for Solidarity Day is further evidence of the malicious divisiveness being employed to widen the gap between those who sincerely care and those whose motives are questionable."[56]

Eddie and the Executive Committee ignored the plans of the Health Department and submitted their own plan for health coverage on Solidarity Day to Sterling Tucker's office. It was a plan that would better meet "the health, spiritual and emotional needs of the Campaign" since it would be implemented "by groups of people and organizations who are sincerely concerned for and understand the plight of the poor."[57]

Eddie and the HSCC won out. "HSCC has been officially designated and authorized by the Southern Christian Leadership Conference to design, coordinate and implement the specific health program for the Solidarity Day March, June 19, 1968."[58] Later in the press release, the point was made again to ensure that no one could misunderstand: "It must be emphasized that the Southern Christian Leadership Conference neither recognizes nor permits any other organization or personnel representing other organizations to participate in the health programs without the specific authorization and permission of HSCC."[59]

The health care coverage was massive. One medical command post and nine medical stations were set up along the route. Eddie served as the general coordinator and headed up the command post. He was joined by Dr. Frederick Heath, the deputy director of the D.C. Public Health Department, and several other doctors, including Dr. John W. Latimer, chairman of the Medical Emergency Disaster Committee. While Red Cross, army, and Public Health Department vans were used, it was clear which organization was in control that day as each of the stations had an HSCC member functioning as the O.D. Some of the trailers were staffed from eight in the morning until eight that evening, while others went straight through until midnight. Eddie's papers show sixty-two physicians participating. Added to this number were Public Health nurses, ambulance drivers, Red Cross personnel, and nurse's aides.[60]

The newspaper reports and other accounts of the march, listing the number of violent incidents as only two, do not reflect the number of medical emergencies. There were 912 patients treated for everything from heart seizures, epilepsy, stab wounds, bleeding ulcers, suspected abortions, and blows to the head. Twenty-nine of the total number of patients were referred to area hospitals and five were admitted.[61]

After the confrontation for the control of health services for Solidarity Day, no attempt was made to cover up the disputes the HSCC had had with the Health Department. In an interview in the *Washington Afro-American,* Drs. Harvey Webb Jr. and Joseph Rhyne, coordinators for the HSCC, quoted the press release that accused the D.C. Department of Public Health as being the major stumbling block to successful delivery of health care services.[62] Reporter Ethel L. Payne, who also served as the head of public relations for HSCC, wrote about the dispute in her column for the *Chicago Daily Defender.* She noted that the HSCC, who had won the behind-the-scenes battle, argued that "at stake was the philosophy of empathy with the poor which was being established with the presence of middle-class black doctors and dentists who were giving time and service voluntarily in a very critical area."[63]

This was not just a black versus white dispute. However, there is no doubt race played some part in the way things developed. The D.C. Public Health Department and other largely white organizations had taken a condescending attitude toward the "poor black folk," and this attitude was intolerable to the area's successful black physicians and dentists and some of the more liberal white professionals.

One of the preexisting organizations that eventually joined with the HSCC was the Medical Committee for Human Rights. This group, headed by Drs. Sidney Wolfe and Philip Askenase, although apparently well intentioned, had not made enough of an effort to include black physicians, nurses, or personnel. The administrator in charge was Mary Holman. Her leadership had apparently been efficient but had led to public criticism from the *Washington Afro-American.* Eddie included excerpts from this article in the minutes to the May 18 meeting of the HSCC:

> Reports have it that the volunteer services of several colored doctors and one nurse for the Poor People's Drive were refused by a white woman from Mississippi who lives in Silver Spring, Md. She is in charge of the medical team.

...Some volunteers are resentful of paternalistic attitudes among some of the white campaign workers. Colored medical volunteers are particularly disturbed and feel they can perform a service if permitted to do so.

The colored nurse who was turned away stressed that her qualifications were acceptable anywhere in the U.S. and foreign countries. She was among top nurses who recently served in Vietnam. A colored medic, who was a member of the medical committee, resigned in protest over the treatment of other would-be volunteers.[64]

At the HSCC meeting Eddie took a firm stand on the recruitment of blacks.

He agreed that an efficiently run organization was important but that other considerations were important because of the nature and purpose of the Poor People's Campaign. He stated that one must appreciate all aspects of the health services operation and not just how well it is run; that in the context of a predominantly black movement it is desirable to have predominantly black leadership in order to avoid a reaction of militancy as well as to project the black image in a favorable, uplifting manner.[65]

The committee, whose members now included Drs. Wolfe and Askenase, agreed unanimously to "endeavor to eliminate or correct situations which would lead to that type of publicity."[66] Dr. Wolfe was to become one of Eddie's favorite members of the committee.

One of the doctors who was very helpful to me was Dr. Sidney Wolfe. He is now working closely with Ralph Nader. Sidney even to this day is very outgoing and liberal and unusual and speaks his mind about things that affect people, health-wise. He was there to help.

Mrs. Holman, who was at this point working with the HSCC, was made a cochairman office administrator with three others. By the June 2 meeting, it could be reported that "Negro participation in the Medical

Trailer was 'improving.'"[67] In an interview reported in the June 15 edition of *U.S. Medicine,* Eddie could honestly state that "the volunteers used included both Negroes and whites. Negroes predominated, however.[68]

Eddie noted that despite the rosy press reports, the HSCC really did not have the help of the conservative D.C. Medical Society: "There were a lot of ultraconservatives who didn't want them here anyway to start this going. We did have the help of the local physicians, mostly black but not of the D.C. Medical Society." Many of the volunteers were young doctors from the National Institutes of Health who were deputized as unpaid employees by the Health Department so they could legally provide help for the marchers. They had to serve on their own time "because conservative congressmen who control NIH purse strings might not take kindly to the PHS [Public Health Service] physicians aiding the marchers on government time."[69]

While the problem of black recruitment was solved, other medical and political problems remained throughout the existence of the encampment. From the beginning, the threat of an epidemic was a real one. Many of the poor people coming to Resurrection City had never been immunized against poliomyelitis, diphtheria, whooping cough, smallpox, or tetanus-typhoid-paratyphoid. The National Medical Association issued a special bulletin, reported in the black press, pointing out the threat and urging those coming to Washington to get their shots at their local health clinic. Eddie had a series of meetings with Dr. Murray Grant of the D.C. Health Department and secured assurance that if they were not done in the local community the immunizations would be done by his department.[70]

Sanitation was a problem from the beginning. The D.C. Health Department came under private criticism from some for not having daily, regularly scheduled sanitation workers on the site.[71] Throughout the existence of Resurrection City, sanitation was a recurring issue and a special area of concern for the doctors, who feared infestation by rats, flies, and mosquitoes, all of which might spread diseases. The HSCC made it their "top priority." Yet the HSCC could do little to solve most of the sanitation problems. Pipes that were to be hooked up for water and sewage were not and garbage collection did not proceed as scheduled.

Dr. Grant had approached Eddie with the suggestion that Resurrection City should be closed because of the "hazardous conditions which posed a threat both to the residents of the city and to the Washington metropolitan community at large."[72] Pointing out that hardships were part of what the residents expected, the HSCC concluded: "It was indicated that it would not be justifiable under any circumstances to evacuate the city for *hypothetical* (rather than real or existent) health problems."[73] Noting that no data had been provided to indicate an epidemic was imminent, they nearly bristled when they added, "Hence, our committee could not be manipulated by non-existent epidemics and unfounded fears."[74]

The doctors of the HSCC shared many of the same fears as the Health Department employees. One of the two health forms in Eddie's files was for Reverend Ralph Abernathy. It showed, among other things, that Reverend Abernathy was, not surprisingly, suffering from physical exhaustion. The only other health form shows a probable diagnosis for an eighteen-year-old man of infectious hepatitis. The possibility of an outbreak of some contagious disease was a reality the HSCC doctors had to face each and every day that Resurrection City existed. Ironically, it may have been the terrible conditions in which the poor residents lived normally that prevented it. Eddie noted in an interview: "They have been putting up with hardship of weather all their lives. . . . And conditions in the shantytown that is Resurrection City are not very different from their home."[75]

As a group sympathetic to the goals of the Poor People's Campaign, however, the HSCC looked at the closing of Resurrection City from a much different vantage point than the Health Department. They were concerned about the sanitary conditions and agreed to convey their concern to Reverend Abernathy the following morning. The problems in mass evacuation, should it be necessary, were also addressed. Yet the doctors felt strongly that any decision to close Resurrection City should come from the SCLC since an "evacuation of the city would constitute the demise of the PPC and their projected plans for a March."[76]

Eddie remembered that the threat of closure was an ongoing one.

> During the whole campaign they attempted more than upon one occasion to close down the City on the basis of health. Walter Washington was the mayor and Julian Bluegart was a special assistant. Anytime they would attempt to close us down, I would go to speak to them to try to keep it open. The one time it was declared that there were drugs, and there were no drugs. Another time there was a claim that there was a hepatitis epidemic. We never had any personal confrontations with people coming in except with city officials, mainly the Health Department. Mayor Washington was not in favor of closing it down nor

> was Julian but he had to have feedback about security and health. They were very patient with us in order to keep it going.
>
> We had contact with the White House through Joe Califano.[77] Joe and I would meet with Julian every morning to make the determination of what was needed to keep this thing from developing into a riot, security and this type of thing. This was before Joe was a cabinet member. We had an open door through Joe to the White House and we managed to keep the thing open.

Interchange with the SCLC was not as well structured as that with the White House. The problem of adequate communication between the SCLC and the HSCC was a topic of discussion at the May 28 meeting. The doctors were having trouble organizing their services to the best advantage since they were not informed ahead of time what the SCLC was planning.

The weather could not have been much worse from a medical standpoint. It rained incessantly, creating mud and additional problems for sanitation. When asked about people's recollections of Resurrection City, they always mention "the mud" first. Joyce Elmore, a nurse and friend of Eddie's who worked at St. Stephen's Church scheduling doctors, remembered that as her most striking image: "The mud, the depth of the mud and how those people survived the rain, the leaks, the mud, the cold and the dreariness."[78]

Margurite remembered having to take the hose to Eddie every evening.

> I hosed him down every night when he came home before he came in the door. All that muck on his boots. He just thought it was the funniest thing—mud up to his knees. I'd get the hose and say, "you're not coming in this house."[79]

At one point in May the rain was so excessive that Eddie and Dr. Murray Grant advised the evacuation of women and children to more secure quarters. Most of the residents went to churches in the area and a few to private homes. The HSCC immediately redirected their health personnel to these churches and homes.[80]

By the June 2 meeting, it looked as if some of the health hazards would be remedied. Garbage collection was to be resumed and the plumbing, water, and electricity were to be hooked up and spraying the ground with DDT to eliminate mosquitoes was to begin by the following day. With the switch to Hosea Williams as the new leader at Resurrection City, it was expected that things would be improving. Other problems, however, were arising. The Reflecting Pool was being used as a swimming pool; a bacteriological count was necessary and some way to make it safer had to be found.

There were enough medical emergencies without the police's overreacting to the small group of youths throwing bottles early in the morning on Sunday, June 23. After treating the victims of the tear gas, the HSCC reacted with a strongly worded press release.

> Early Sunday morning, a minor incident resulted in the use of enough tear gas to saturate the entire area in and around Resurrection City. Consequently, hundreds of people who were sleeping at the time, including large numbers of infants, children and the elderly, were subjected to the dangerous effects of this gas. More than 100 people were treated by volunteer physicians and nurses for the severe irritant effects of the gas on their eyes, skin and upper respiratory passages; approximately twenty were treated for asthmatic attacks which had been precipitated by the gas. There were also 4 elderly persons with heart disease who required intensive medical treatment and prolonged observation after their exposure to the gas. Finally, several people were rendered unconscious by the gas.
>
> Although it is frequently stated that tear gas is harmless, it is potentially lethal when used against a population which includes the elderly, the infirm and infants.
>
> The Health Services Coordinating Committee for the Poor People's Campaign condemns this indiscriminate use of tear gas which clearly involved injury to a great many innocent people. The large number of serious medical problems arising in those who were not even present in the area where the incident occurred is a testimony to the blatant misuse of what is supposedly a riot-control measure.
>
> As health professionals, we strongly urge that saner judgment be exercised in the deployment of such weapons.[81]

The copy of the release in Eddie's files is apparently a draft of the final release. Penned in by hand is an even stronger final statement: "As physicians, we strongly condemn this undisciplined, thoughtless and inhumane action of the police against innocent American citizens."[82]

Resurrection City was dismantled the day following the gassing and the job of the HSCC was over. Whether the Poor People's Campaign was worth the excessive cost is a matter for debate. An article in the *Sunday Star* tried to total up the costs while admitting that "any precise tabulation is impossible."[83] The reporter's estimate was between $1.5 million and $2 million, but this did not include many of the indirect costs such as the time contributed by the doctors and other personnel or the amount of loss to the downtown tourist businesses. Some of this cost was paid by taxpayers, with an estimated $1 million coming mostly out of the District budget. A bill of $71,795 was sent to the SCLC from the National Park Service for dismantling and removing the remains of Resurrection City, but Abernathy refused to pay.[84] In the medical area, the reporter didn't even try to put a figure on the costs: "Without charge, about 500 persons, doctors and other medical personnel served the poor people. Drugs were contributed by major pharmaceutical houses. No attempt has been made to put a price tag on this."[85]

Senator Robert Byrd (D-WV) voiced to the Senate what seemed to be the sentiments of many: "Had the campaign produced substantive results for the poor, these losses might be somewhat less painful."[86] This seems to be the opinion of most of those writing about the campaign.[87] Eddie, as usual, tended to put a more positive light on the results.

> We made it through all right and I think we did a lot of good because we were sensitive to the needs, medically as well as the sociological and economic needs of the poor.
>
> The outgrowth of it was not only the kind of publicity that was received on a national basis as far as the plight of the poor and the blacks but also the cause began to gather momentum not only in the ranks of the blacks but in the ranks of the poor whites, too. At issue here was great participation among the masses.

Although seeing Resurrection City from a different perspective increases our knowledge, it still does not make it possible for us to fully grasp what was taking place. With all its complexities of hope and despair, nonviolent philosophy and violent actions, anger and joy, describing Resurrection City is nearly impossible. Jesse Jackson in speaking of the demolition of Resurrection City said:

> . . . the foundations of Resurrection City were not made by hand. Resurrection City is at best an idea. The real problem that the military had is that it attempted to take its fist and smash the wind. They tried to take a bulldozer and turn around an idea.[88]

When an attempt is made to describe Resurrection City, the problem is the same as in demolishing it. Resurrection City was more than the shantytown. It was the elusive, changing, ethereal dream of a better America where the need for such towns no longer exists.

At least for Eddie and the other physicians, there were some tangible results from their efforts. They had, for a short time, done something to improve the health conditions of the poor. Many were immunized who would not have been, serious and long-neglected health problems were treated, teeth were taken care of, and lectures on medical and dental health, hopefully, would prevent some problems in the future. Open discussion of the status of the people they treated also managed to make the wretched health conditions of the poor a matter of public record.

In an interview reported in the *Washington Post,* Dr. Vinod R. Mody, a tropical disease specialist from India, described the condition of one campaign participant, a fifty-eight-year-old woman from Mississippi. A shocked Dr. Mody stated, "I never would have thought this patient came from the United States. India, maybe. But not the United States."[89] The woman suffered from a partially deformed bone structure, the result of two fractures of the arms that were never treated and that healed improperly, and rickets, a disease of infancy, caused by a lack of vitamin D. "Her rib cage is so thin," Dr. Mody said, "that an easy blow with the hand could crack the bones."[90]

Other patients referred to by Dr. Mody also evidenced illnesses resulting from poor diet and lack of medical care. There was the nine-year-old boy from Alabama with a congenital heart condition. The recommendation of the physician in Alabama, where the mother had taken him, had been to "stop worrying." He also mentioned the seventy-one-year-old man from Mississippi who still had a lead bullet in his foot from a childhood shooting and had sores that would not heal, indicating nutritional problems of long-standing.

A blue-ribbon panel headed by Dr. Benjamin Mays, the former president of Morehouse College, had, earlier in 1968, reported that there were "at least 10 million Americans in 20 states suffering from hunger."[91] They had urged President Johnson to declare a state of emergency and to provide free food for these people. Yet little had been done to alleviate the plight of the poor since the panel findings were made public. The concessions agreed to by the various governmental departments as a result of pressure from the Poor People's Campaign would not begin to meet the extensive needs of the poor.

The first caravans for the Poor People's Campaign made their initial stop in Marks, Mississippi, a town that symbolized the needs that necessitated the march. Marks was one of the nation's poorest towns, with a median income for blacks there of only a little over $500 per year.[92] Touched by the people he had met during the existence of Resurrection City, Eddie found his own way to help.

> We met several people at Resurrection City from Marks, which is one of the poorest towns in Mississippi. Even after the campaign closed down many of the people stayed; they wouldn't go back. They didn't have anywhere to go. So for some reason they kind of made my office a headquarters, a lot of them. They would come down and sit and talk, eat, have their medical needs taken care of, get a little help for overnight and that type of thing.
>
> I can't recall the name of the lady in the forefront, but I recall the name of the man, we called him "Shug." I can't think of his real name. He was the leader of that group from Marks, Mississippi, where he was a native. There also was this little kid whose name was Jimmy. He was so smart and he had so much potential. He could do almost anything yet he was denied doing it and you could see that. Shug and Jimmy got to me as they talked and asked if I would go down to Marks to see if we could set up some kind of health program for the poor people there. They had no medical care and no money.
>
> I said, "All right" and I organized a group and went. We had a dentist and several other physicians and we

> went down there and spent about a week gathering data so we would have some kind of picture to present to the government regarding the health and problems of these people. We spent time examining them; making diagnoses, and saw all kinds of cases. They really lived under horrible conditions: no sewage, no water supply, right on the edge of town just across the railroad tracks. There was no dentist. They had teeth problems and eye problems.
>
> We finally made an entree into the Health Department there and carried the problem to them. They were all white but when we got through going over the problem so that they knew what was going on they agreed to give us an old deserted hospital to fix up. Their attitude was if you want to spare what you can, get your own doctors and bring them on down here, then we will cooperate.

Eddie returned to Washington in March 1969 and promptly wrote a letter to Clifford Hardin, the Secretary of Agriculture, asking for his assistance in relieving the "grave problem of hunger" of the people of Quitman County, Mississippi.[93] The reply received from an assistant deputy administrator stated: "It is this Administration's [Lyndon B. Johnson's] goal to work toward the elimination of hunger and malnutrition wherever it is found to exist in our nation."[94] However, there was no indication that the government would look at the problems the poor of Marks and the remainder of Quitman County faced.

Eddie then attempted to sell the idea of staffing an ongoing health program in Marks to those at the Howard University Medical School.

> We carried the story back to Howard because we needed manpower. I didn't have the time to do it because I had my own practice and a family. I presented the picture to Howard University and they said "All right; it sounds like a good project." I took the position that you are going to be doing your residents a service by providing them with the opportunity to practice and learn medicine. It will let them see what is really happening out there. I had movies and stills. We met at the dental school office and made this presentation.

> When we got through with the presentation, Howard said "We want the project. We'll take it over." I gave it to them and even let them have the pictures, which they said they would give back and never did.
>
> They started the project but it flopped. They worked at it for something like a year or so and then for whatever reason it flopped. It hurt me that it didn't succeed and I really felt it. I used to say that you can get a lot accomplished without stooping. You can still have a lot of pride and get a lot of things accomplished even in what is a difficult situation and still maintain your dignity. But there is a way to do things. The guys would kid me and say, "Mazique, you can say that because you were born and bred in Mississippi and you knew your place." I said, "I understand but I was finding a place for somebody else to get so they would have a place to survive and live and have help." I kinda think that the manner in which you go about accomplishing something as well as an attitude has a lot to do with your achievement whether it will reach fruition or not.
>
> One of the things that hurt me most with that thing was they came back to me to do it again, Shug and the rest of them, but it was too late. The momentum had passed and timing is a great thing. The success of anybody has to do with the timing. When that enthusiasm is gone and what it took to build up that momentum has waned, what are you going to do? The time to strike was then, not three years later to try to come and do it all over again. So it was lost.

At the annual meeting of the National Medical Association in Houston, Texas, in August 1968, Eddie received an Outstanding Achievement Award for the services he rendered at Resurrection City. Eddie had no false modesty when it came to his awards and honors. He thoroughly enjoyed receiving them and was proud of his achievements. No matter what the occasion, Eddie made the most of it, throwing himself into the spirit of the event. The photographs of the presentation show a beaming Eddie being presented the award by the new NMA president, Dr. James Whittico Jr.[95] Although he had received awards from the NMA in 1960, 1965, and 1967, the recognition by his fellow black physicians of his hard work on behalf of the SCLC was especially important to him.

Despite the pleasure in his awards and his own personal achievements, the results, or more accurately the lack of changes, resulting from the Poor People's Campaign made it clear that there was much work left for Eddie and others to do if equal rights for all citizens were ever to be fully realized.

## CHAPTER TWELVE 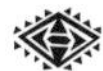

# Continuing Challenges and New Honors

> Discover the organisms that serve as demons of disease through your microscope, but look up and search for sociological ills that may be seen in macrocosm.
>
> — *Edward C. Mazique, address of the retiring president of the medical-dental staff of Providence Hospital, 1985*

Although the riots and the Poor People's Campaign grabbed most of the headlines, many other causes claimed Eddie's attention during the latter half of the 1960s.

On Monday, April 8, 1968, before the federal troops had been recalled from the District of Columbia and prior to the curfew being lifted, a headline in the *Washington Post* already heralded a rebuilding effort.[1] There were many suggestions made during the City Council Public Hearings on Rebuilding and Recovery the following month, but one requisite emerged very clearly from the various viewpoints: "the universal demand for the right of self-determination for the neighborhoods that need rebuilding."[2]

This self-determination was of special concern to the Reverend Fauntroy, who, even before the inception of the riots, had asked Eddie and Marjorie McKenzie Lawson to work with him on a board to develop an innovative plan to improve conditions for the poor inner-city dwellers.[3]

By the 1960s when she came to serve on the board with Eddie, Marjorie McKenzie Lawson already had a most impressive background. She had earned a degree in social work from the University of Michigan and later in law from Columbia University. Her husband, Belford V. Lawson Jr., with whom she shared a legal practice, was involved in many of the prominent civil rights litigations. Mrs. Lawson had served as an early campaign aide to John F. Kennedy and in 1962 she became the first black woman ever appointed to a judgeship by a president. She returned to private practice in 1965, and the next year she and Eddie joined with the Reverend Fauntroy on a project called the Model Inner City Community Organization, or MICCO.

Mrs. Lawson remembered this project as bringing about a close relationship between her and Eddie:

> We really became associated through the urban renewal program that Reverend Fauntroy started before he went to Congress. It was called the Model Inner City Community Organization (MICCO). We started it about 1966 or '67. Reverand Fauntroy was looking about the church area to see what he could do to improve the neighborhood. He began talking to me about housing and I said, "What we need is some urban renewal here." We decided that although urban renewal had a very bad name with black people, if we used it as a tool for ourselves rather than against us, we could turn it around and make it work. We brought together some community leaders and set up a board and we did some study proposals and we went to talk to the District of Columbia Redevelopment Land Agency and told them what we were interested in and asked them to give us an urban renewal program. So they did. Not only that, they funded MICCO so we could be their advisors and assist them with planning.
>
> When the riots started in 1968, we were already in place with a plan and with a message for working with the city to carry it out. We had instant cooperation because we were in place while the city was burning down in places along the Seventh Street and H Street corridors. We had a plan for renewal.[4]

Reverend Fauntroy, seeing the plight of those in the area surrounding his church, came up with a solution that would have input from those people most directly involved. His major concern was to rebuild the neighborhood for those who lived there.

When I returned to the church as pastor in 1959, I became alarmed at what I considered the systematic removal of black and poor people from valuable inner-city land. We had watched Georgetown renewed privately in the years immediately following World War II when blacks had lived there for years. They were either forced out by code enforcement or prices they could not resist for the sale. It had been underway since 1954: something called "urban renewal." In Georgetown where private developers assembled land at market prices, the government entered the business of assembling land by eminent domain and paying a fair price to the owners and then writing down the cost of it to developers consistent with a plan that the government had developed for renewal of the area. The upshot of it all was that on August the 10th, 1960, after a year of studying, I did a speech at the NAACP rally which called urban renewal, urban removal, removing poor and black people from valuable downtown land. As a result, investigations were called for by members of the Congress of these charges and the first Mrs. Mazique was very supportive of me as was Ed. Since Georgetown had been transformed and tens of thousands of blacks and poor people had been driven out of South West, we felt the next was to move us out of what is now called the Shaw area.

In studying what had been done in South West, I came up with a proposal for what I called a new kind of renewal, a renewal with the people, by the people and for the people who live in the community. Eventually, I was successful, through my work in the movement, with the assistance of President Johnson in getting a special grant to enable us to define an area in which we wanted to undertake renewal and do it with, by and for the people. With the people in that the people would be involved in the planning of the renewal. By the people in that to the extent possible the people making money in the process would be people from the neighborhood. For the people in that when it was over we wanted the people to be able to live in the community, unlike what had happened in South West Washington where the relative cost of the

> housing made it impossible for the people who formerly lived there to return.
>
> With that concept I then went about putting together the Model Inner City Community Organization. It was based on the thesis that the people affected by the renewal ought to be involved in the planning of it. That meant not only the people who lived in the houses but also those who delivered services in the area, the professionals, the doctors, the lawyers, the business people who ran establishments, the social service agencies that served the community, the schools both the public and private schools and the Board of Education, and the labor unions that had a stake in the kind of renewal we talked about.[5]

After the riots, there was tension between black and white Washingtonians. Many blacks did not have the capital to rebuild and white businessmen were afraid to rebuild. A coalition of black action groups called the Black United Front (BUF) strongly stated that "black people are going to rebuild this black community."[6] Other organizations were not so diplomatic in their statements. Build Black Incorporated hoped to persuade white merchants to turn over their business sites to blacks for modest fees. Their circulars were headed with "Stop shufflin' and beggin' whitey. Build Black." The literature included statements saying "No more mom and pop stores, slumlords and other exploiters of black people allowed in black communities. No more honkie unions—without black members—and no more honkie owners and contractors without black participation—allowed in black neighborhoods."[7] Reverend Fauntroy and the city council, for their part, "favored helping black businessmen establish themselves in the devastated areas but opposed the 'black only' type of agitation."[8]

Reverend Fauntroy's plan met resistance from those who wanted to exclude all except the black residents. The "liberals" who were trying to organize the poor made an attempt to discredit Mr. Fauntroy and MICCO.

> We put together a board of persons who represented each of those interests. It was a new process but a difficult process because at the same time the poverty program was getting off the ground and that brought the professional organizers to organize poor people for

purposes of participation. We had difficulty with the paid professional organizers who in order to justify and to rationalize their tasks created a "house Negro"—"field Negro" thesis.

I was committed to involve in the planning of renewal all those affected so that if a physician was there, he was part of the community too. If school teachers worked to deliver a service of education, they needed to be involved. If business people ran the establishments, although they lived outside of the community, they needed to be involved.

Ed Mazique was my partner in lending credibility to the so-called "bushies." The liberals who came to run the poverty program were leading the natives to get rid of the "house" ones but they had difficultly with persons like Ed and myself. I was born in the community; I grew up there. I was pastor of a church in the community and everybody knew me. The newcomers were having difficulty trying to explain to them that I was the enemy. And Ed had this office where he had been serving for many years as a physician with a reputation for being not only a good physician but one who would treat people for free if he knew they didn't have any money. So we ended up being very close partners in that regard.

After a bit of that we finally brought the entire community together around the concept that we are in this thing together. All of us have a stake and those who are affected ought to be there to protect their stake. The consequence of it all was that in addition to planning physical renewal with thousands of units of housing that were built on the riot corridors and in addition to providing training as bricklayers and carpenters and electricians and plumbers and the like for the poor about whom we were concerned, we were also, through Ed's expertise and his interests, able to put together a health service delivery package that included something that still exists at the corner of Seventh and R: the Shaw Health Center.

The government acquired land by eminent domain and bought it from its former owners. The government

> would then dispose of the land to nonprofit sponsors from within the community who would gain the ability to, in fact, build and rehabilitate on the land through federal programs so that almost every new housing project in the whole area, thousands of units, was owned by nonprofit sponsors, usually put together by Marjorie Lawson, who knew that field very well.[9]

Ms. Lawson was proud of the results and recalled Reverend Martin Luther King Jr.'s interest in the project:

> The urban renewal plan, in short, really accomplished an awful lot. It built housing, a library, a new junior high school. One of the rallying points was to build a new junior high school, for the existing Shaw Junior High School, which was called "Shameful Shaw" because it was such a terrible school. We have a beautiful new junior high school on Rhode Island Avenue as a result of that effort. At all times, Reverend Martin Luther King Jr. was interested in what we were doing. Of course, he and Reverend Fauntroy were great friends and cohorts. One time we had a parade to emphasize and bring attention to the fact that the new junior high school was needed and King rode in the parade with us. This, of course, was before the riots of 1968.[10]

The permanency of the structures is a testament to the vision of Reverend Fauntroy and the hard work of board members such as Eddie and Marjorie Lawson. As Reverend Fauntroy explains in his verbal tour of the area, they assured that each building would be kept and used for its intended purpose by careful planning on the part of the MICCO board.

> At Seventh and S, there is Lincoln-Westmoreland Apartments—219 units of housing owned by a combination of the Lincoln Temple Church at Eleventh and R and a companion church, a Church of Christ Congregational church in the suburbs, Westmoreland Church. At the corner of Ninth and Rhode Island is New Bethel's 75-unit building called Foster House. Further down at the corner of Seventh Street and Rhode Island

Avenue is the Asbury Dwellings, which belong to the Asbury Methodist Church. It is about 91 units of senior citizen housing in the old Shaw School. You go further down Seventh Street and you see Immaculate Conception Homes, a city block owned by the Immaculate Conception Church there at Seventh and N. Across the street is Gibson Plaza, owned by the First Rising Mount Zion Church. Two city blocks further down it's owned by the House of Prayer.

I mention all that because you must understand that the land in Shaw is the most valuable land in the world. The most valuable residential land in the world is in Washington, D.C. People will pay a price to live that close to the monuments and the points of power. That is why South West went so well. We recognized that unless the ownership of the land was in the hands of people in the community, that you would not be able to hold the land. Accordingly, as a case in point, after it became apparent that this was going to become a secure neighborhood with a subway, we got regular visits from syndicates out of New York wishing to have the churches sell properties. We got offered three times as much as we owed on the property to sell the seventy-five units at Ninth and Rhode Island. Because some syndicates recognize that they could move in, take the building, put a little paint on it, a few bars on the windows, and rent it to people who would like to jog to work rather than spending two hours on the freeway getting into town.

Ed understood all that. With Marjorie Lawson and the rest of us, we put together a process by which those people are anchored in those units. They are anchored because I can say to the people who approached me: "Quite frankly, if I owned the building and you offered me nine million dollars for it and all I owed was three million, I would take it and put a couple million in the bank and live off the interest the rest of my life. Then I would take the other four and travel around the world every year just to see if the world was doing well. But since the Church owns it, what you need to do is go to

> the congregation and ask them if they want to move their members out of their houses."
>
> All of those units are like the trees planted by the river. They shall not be moved because the people who own them have a stake in staying.[11]

At the time the MICCO project was underway, the problems of discrimination in the American Medical Association had still not been resolved. Although Eddie had been admitted in 1952, black physicians were still fighting the battle to fully integrate the American Medical Association and to make it more sensitive to the needs of the poor. While the Poor People's Campaign was in Washington, the AMA was holding its conference in San Francisco. Protestors from the Medical Committee for Human Rights and the Bay Area Poor People's Campaign picketed outside and then disrupted a House of Delegates meeting on June 16, charging the AMA with being the "chief 'culprit' in denying health care to millions of the poor and black."[12] The protestors, many of whom were physicians, blamed the fee system for making health care a privilege instead of a right for many poor citizens. Support for Reverend Abernathy's demands for establishing more health centers, expanding Medicare, and giving the poor a greater voice in health programs was requested. The protestors also charged the AMA with being a racist organization since they had refused to "cleanse its ranks of open racial discrimination."[13]

By the conclusion of the AMA's annual meeting, it was clear that some changes were at least possible in the foreseeable future. The new president and some of the delegates seemed to be moving away from the stand taken by the AMA's 1967–1968 president, who claimed the major problem within the medical profession was "the concept of health care as a right rather than a privilege."[14] The AMA Council on Medical Service stated clearly that good health necessitates ready availability of high-quality health care "without regard" to the ability to pay.[15] Further, there was an admission that the poor were not receiving adequate medical care.

Of utmost importance to Eddie and other black physicians was that the meeting finally produced the first step taken by the American Medical Association toward forcing local medical societies to admit minorities to their ranks. In 1968, most southern chapters of the organization still excluded their fellow black physicians, denying them the right to practice in many of the full-facility hospitals. The June meeting produced a call for changes in the association's bylaws that would "subject any affiliate that denies membership on the grounds of 'color, creed, race, religion or ethnic origin' to dismissal."[16] The AMA amendments committee tried to shelve the resolution, but it was passed almost unanimously by the 242 delegates.

When Eddie's close friend and at that time president of the National Medical Association Dr. Lionel Swan was interviewed about the AMA decision, he admitted that "conditions faced by black doctors—and patients—have improved in recent years."[17] At the same time he pointed out that "Negro doctors are still excluded from hospital-staff membership almost everywhere in the Deep South. In other regions, they are admitted only as token members. Negro specialists rarely receive referrals from white doctors. Black doctors who do manage to achieve staff status almost never move up into administrative positions."[18] Thus despite their grudging acceptance by the members of the local branches of the American Medical Association, black physicians were far from welcome in most places. This was the case in many respects for Eddie and his colleagues in Washington. The problems Eddie and Dr. Spellman had during their first years at Providence, with the segregation of the hospital's patients, were typical of the problems faced by the newly accepted black physicians. The number of blacks admitted to the formerly segregated hospital staffs grew gradually during the 1960s but acceptance as full-fledged colleagues was slow in coming. Eddie, usually in a jovial manner, always tried to speed up this process. Margurite remembered the time she and Eddie attended a District Medical Society dinner.

> He likes challenges. It was instilled in him from his early days. His father would not take no on anything. He identified with his father along this line. His father was a role model for him. His grandfather also. That set the stage.
>
> I recall an event that we went to, a dinner that was given by the D.C. Medical Society. At that time they did not have many black doctors as members. There were enough doctors to make up one table. Just as we were about to sit down, he realized here were ten blacks sitting at this one table. He looked around and said, "The heck with you all, we are going to go over here and sit and get to know some other people." The seats were assigned. I tried to stay but he was insistent. "We want to sit over here, these look like some nice people. Let's sit down here and talk to these people." He sat down

> and opened a napkin up. I went feeling reluctant and embarrassed. I would expect the people to say these seats are taken or we are expecting someone. However, they didn't. As the evening wore on, other people came to the table and Eddie introduced himself. What happened was we had sat down at the table of the president of the society. I think we put him on the spot sitting there. Eddie knew who the president was and purposely chose his table.[19]

By the mid 1970s, it was clear that Eddie was making inroads when he was asked to join the District of Columbia Political Action Committee (DOCPAC). In 1976 he was voted its chairman, doing his job so well that he held the position until his death. P. Douglas Torrence, the director of legislative affairs for the Medical Society of the District of Columbia, remembered how Eddie came in and promptly took over the organization.

> Dr. Mazique was invited as a guest of DOCPAC one evening and within a period of one year, he was elected as chairman of this political action committee that represents all the physicians in Washington.
>
> There will never be a better chairman for this particular political action committee than Ed Mazique because every politician downtown and with all thirteen city council members and the mayor, it's either "Hi, Ed," or "Hello, Eddie," or "Hello, Doc." In many cases he is or has been the personal physician of a number of them. It has always given me a real sense of personal self-satisfaction to go with Dr. Mazique to city council at the District Building when we have to go down and talk about what is going on in the D.C. Medical Society and some of their concerns about legislation. You've always got the entree, not only to see staff people but if a council member is around and they see Dr. Mazique, they just say come on in. It would take me weeks to get an appointment to see someone like that.[20]

Simultaneously, Eddie served as the chairman for the National Medical Political Action Committee, or NMPAC, which was founded in 1979 to act on the behalf of the interests of the National Medical Association.

Throughout the 1960s and the remainder of his life, Eddie continued to work as a representative of the National Medical Association on various government projects, including the Partnership for Health Amendments of 1967 and the President's Committee on Equal Employment Opportunity. In a 1968 brochure outlining a Model Health Centers project, there are pictures of Eddie and others conferring with Vice President Humphrey and President Johnson. A caption under the photograph stated that Dr. Mazique had "worked consistently with NMA, HEW, and HUD on the proposed comprehensive medical care plan."[21]

Comedian and civil rights activist Dick Gregory discussed how Eddie was trusted by both the government and the civil rights leaders:

> The power he had! I don't think there was a president that occupied that White House that didn't have him there for consultation. He was so respected as a human being, above and beyond medicine.
>
> When the people in the civil rights movement would say things to government people, they were suspect because they had to make political decisions. Eddie was someone they could call in who they not only trusted but respected. He had the type of integrity that even if government leaders wouldn't listen to his advice or follow up, the civil rights people knew when he went to see presidents and stuff, he wasn't back there lying. That was the great thing about him—his honesty and integrity.
>
> He really made a difference in a lot of people's lives and made a difference in America. To me, he was always there.[22]

Always one to meet problems head on, Eddie grew and changed with the times. He retained his keen interest and understanding of what was happening in the economic, social, and political spheres and their impact on the medical profession. In an *American Magazine* issue that was dedicated to Eddie,[23] he discussed the entrance of big business into the medical field and the takeover of nonprofit hospitals. His concern was, as always, for the patient if medicine became a business instead of "an art and a science."[24]

Even though he had devoted years of his professional life to fighting for the establishment of Medicare, Eddie was quick to realize when it was headed for trouble. In a guest editorial in a 1985 issue of the *Journal*

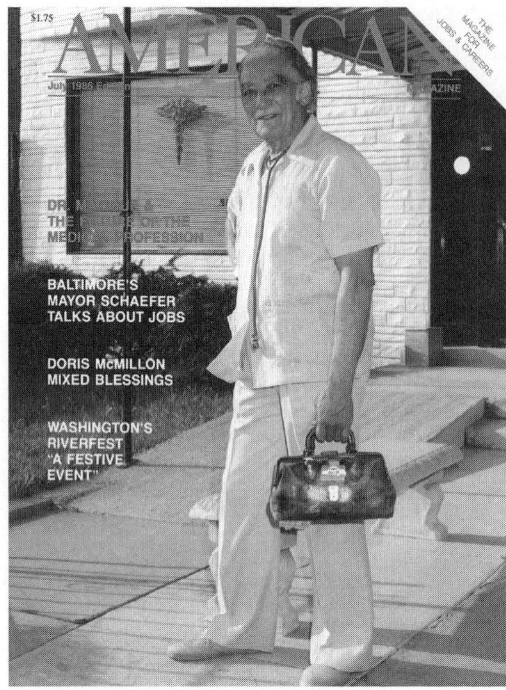


**Fig. 24:** The cover of the July 1986 issue of *American Magazine* dedicated to Dr. Edward C. Mazique for his "50 Years of Excellence." Photo reproduced from *American Magazine.*

*of the National Medical Association,* Eddie discussed "Trends and Transformations in Health Care." His main concerns were the soaring cost of health care and the imminent collapse of the Medicare system. The challenge was new but his concerns and perspective were the same:

> The facts herein presented are designed to stimulate ways and means to cope with today's changes and challenges in medical care. In the conquest of change, the poor, the elderly, and the minorities in our society are usually the neglected and the last to attain financial provisions for adequate medical care.[25]

Over the years, his concern and his dedication to the fight for adequate health care for the elderly, minorities, and the poor never diminished, and his speeches and his affiliations reflected this.

The National Medical Association further honored Eddie when, in 1975, they chose him to be the recipient of the 30th Distinguished Service Medal of the Association. A two-and-a-half-page biography listing his massive achievements was carried in the *Journal.* In the 1980s, Eddie served as president of the Past President's Council of the NMA. The Family Practice Section of the NMA presented Eddie with the Meritorious Service Award, in 1983, for "his many years of continuous, unselfish and dedicated service to the cause of the medical profession and human advancement with foresight, courage and commitment."[26]

In November 1979 Eddie was given the A. H. Robins Award by the D.C. Medical Society for his outstanding service to the community. In 1981, Eddie was named a Life Member of the Medical Society of the District of Columbia (MSDC). This was an honor for those physicians who had been members of the MSDC for forty years. Since forty-year membership would have been impossible for black physicians in 1981, it was also bestowed upon those members who were born in 1911.

Eddie continued to gain acceptance and engender respect among his colleagues at Providence Hospital as well. An indication of his growing social acceptance came in 1977 when he was honored with the "Bull Throwers Award," a once-a-year award. Although it would not rank as a particularly prestigious award in the normal sense, it brought Eddie enormous pleasure because it was a sign of social acceptance from his colleagues at Providence. Margurite remembered how excited he was the night of the banquet:

> They had never named anyone who was not a surgeon as Bull Thrower. The surgeons would be at the hospital early in the morning and they would do all the talking. The doctor who precedes you names the next one. Dr. Sallasi was the one who named Eddie. There is no election. That night you would have thought he was named President of the United States.[27]

Eddie regaled the gathering with memories of his recent trip to Spain and how to be a matador. His evening as a "bull thrower" was a fantastic success. He was so good at it, he was even asked by a colleague, Dr. El Khodary, to assist him to prepare for his presentation the year he was named "bull thrower."[28]

The most striking change in his position as a black physician in Washington came in 1983 when Eddie was elected the president of the medical-dental staff at Providence Hospital, where thirty years earlier he had been denied a staff position because of his color. With his large number of patients and his contacts on Capitol Hill, when funding concerns

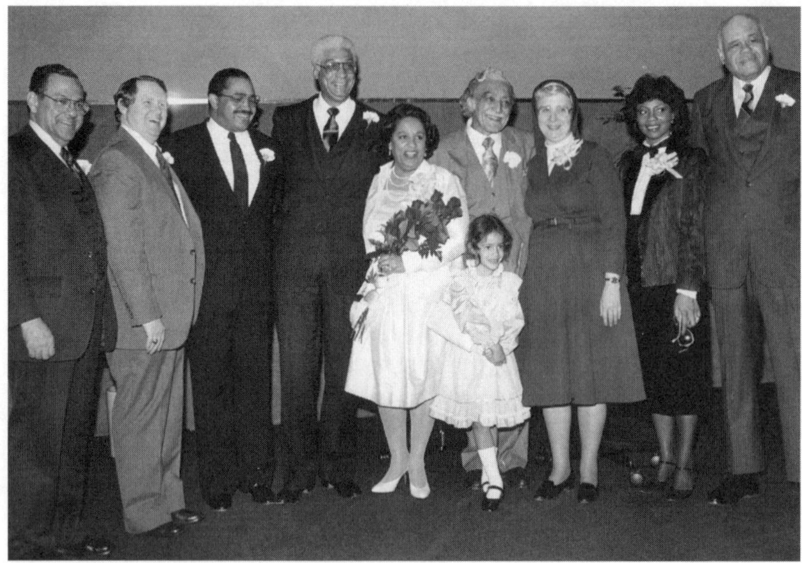

**Fig. 25:** Dr. Mazique and his wife, Margurite, pose with the staff and Sister Irene Klaus (third from right), former president of Providence Hospital. Photo courtesy of Maude Mazique and Dolores Pelham.

arose, Eddie had proven invaluable to Providence. Even so, his election as president was challenged by an element who still could not accept being led by a black man. Eddie remembered his election with pleasure.

> Finally Providence began to ease up and one of the people on the nominating committee called up and said we are going to put your name in. In the early eighties I was put up for election for the president of the medical-dental staff. I was there when the elections came up. The nominating committee presented only one name—mine was the one they came up with. Then there were nominations from the floor.
>
> One of the white guys was sitting next to me and I knew the kind of fellow that he was—one of those diehard conservatives. He was carrying on and said, "Oh, no," and he nominated another fellow from the floor. Then it came down to a vote but it didn't matter; I won the election. I put all my efforts into that for three years. Here was a place that I had to fight to get into.

It was no accident that Eddie was sitting next to that "white guy" at the meeting. Margurite remembered with a laugh how Eddie outfoxed those who wished to defeat him the night of his election to president:

> Eddie would enjoy anything he got into. It spilled over on other people. He could contribute to a situation in a cause but at the same time he could do it in such a manner that it didn't alienate another group. He had that kind of skill. When he had been proposed to become the president of the medical-dental staff over at Providence this was the first time for a black to even be nominated let alone win. He had been very consistent with the hospital and very much a part of the hospital and everyone knew him. They counted on him because he had contacts on the Hill. Eddie was hesitant to run. He did not want to lose—he was a poor loser.
>
> The interesting thing about it was the night that they were having that election, many doctors who had not attended these vast meetings before, came. There was a whole clump there that Eddie hadn't seen at meetings before. They were kind of caucusing in the corner getting their notes together and Eddie went over and took a seat with them. This was the enemy camp! He acted very naïve and very blasé. He chatted and said, "I haven't seen you guys around here before, let me tell you what we have been doing" and what not and they could not get their caucus going because he was sitting in the middle of them.
>
> The night that they were having the election I was involved with a benefit downtown so I wasn't here at the house. He was home at the time I got home, sitting up there at his desk. I said, "Well, how did it go? Did we win?" He answered, "By one vote." I said, "Well, we won."[29]

Eddie served as president-elect from 1983 to 1984, as president in 1984–1985, and this was followed by the position of immediate past president, giving him several years to influence the direction of the hospital. He was an effective leader, as Sister Catherine Norton, president and chief executive officer of the hospital, noted:

> I think Dr. Mazique demands a lot of respect on the part of his colleagues and has lent a lot of leadership, professionally, to the medical staff. He runs a very excellent medical staff meeting. Dr. Mazique doesn't run a tough meeting but he certainly keeps everything right on course. His meetings are usually long enough to allow discussions but he doesn't allow them to deviate from what the meeting is all about. I think he leads the men to make the right decisions.
>
> I think he's very courageous in standing up for what is right. I don't think that he ever backs down from the principles of what is right.[30]

Eddie's priorities while he served as president of the medical-dental staff at Providence were the same he had evidenced throughout his career: a deep caring for each patient as an individual, a special consideration for the poor and the elderly, a continuous battle for equal rights, and a belief that doctors must be concerned about the larger social and political issues, not confined to their own narrow field or even culture. Every speech made and every article that Eddie wrote during this time reflected these concerns. In a 1984 Alumni Day reflection, he summed up what he believed was important to the continued excellence of Providence Hospital:

> Finally, the destiny of Providence is not measured only by our scientific achievements and contributions, but rather by how we practice our profession as an art. The touch of our hands upon the feverish brow of the sick; the sound of our voice to the lonely; the care we reveal for the neglected; the concern we demonstrate for the elderly and homeless; the relief we give to those who suffer in pain; the cheer we give to the disillusioned; the time we give when there is not time; and when we accept and respect differences that are found in each individual and recognize and pursue the good of humanity; not through conflict but through cooperation and love; these are the characteristics that set us apart.[31]

During his tenure as president, Eddie managed educational trips to Canada and in 1984 to the Scandinavian countries. As he had done over the years since his trip to the Communist-bloc countries in 1952, Eddie continued to study other societies to discover how they dealt with their medical and their social problems. An article Eddie authored the following year in the *Journal of the National Medical Association* on "Health Care in Denmark" evidenced once again his continuing concern for the elderly. He focused on how health and social services were linked in Denmark to enable the elderly to stay at home as long as possible. When a nursing home becomes necessary, Eddie noted that it was free of charge, in high-quality buildings, with private rooms and bathrooms, thus providing expensive care but also "reliev[ing] a good deal of the anxiety associated with aging—the fear of abandonment and helplessness, and total loss of dignity."[32]

In his address as retiring president, "Medicine in the Age of Stress and Star Wars," he again emphasized the need to provide for our senior citizens and repeatedly challenged his colleagues to play a part in the social and political changes going on around them.

> There is a wide vacuum between social technology and health. It is ironic that medical science has extended the age of many of our senior citizens, yet we have not shown the vision and fortitude to properly care for them in their declining years.
>
> . . . Let no one set us apart from the rank and file that cares for humanity. Physicians must endeavor not only to understand the socioeconomic aspects of the world in which we live, but must also participate in unfolding new and vibrant ideas to make this a better world in which to live. We dare not hold ourselves aloof from the sweeping stream of history with its economic, social, cultural, and political developments. For medicine is truly in politics. We must continue to carry out the noble ideals of our profession: to work for the good of the whole patient—body, mind, soul and spirit.
>
> . . . We are capable of suturing the fabric of mutual confidence and bonds of brotherhood into one human family. Woven tightly together, we will be able to transmit the right heritage of service and dedication to future generations of the Providence Hospital family.[33]

Eddie's speech as always ended on an optimistic note. He truly believed that though the problems were massive, they were surmountable. Sister

Catherine Norton called Eddie's speech "inspirational" and saw it as reflecting the goals that set Providence apart as a Catholic hospital. "Your call to see the total patient and truly care for him with compassion and respect re-emphasized this hospital's philosophy and mission," Sister Catherine wrote in her letter to Eddie.[34]

Since, as a black man, the respect of his white peers was so hard to win, Eddie's remarks in his retiring address were not exaggerated when he said to his colleagues: "There is no greater satisfaction in the field of medicine than to have gained the confidence, cooperation and respect of one's peers, and to be privileged to dedicate one's life to service, concern, and care of patients."[35] Eddie loved his life's work and to finally rise to the position of president of the medical-dental staff at Providence was perhaps his greatest success in the medical arena. In 1986 Mayor Marion Barry appointed Eddie to the D.C. government's new Board of Medicine, the medical licensing board, to serve as its chairman.[36] The irony was not lost on Eddie. Here was the doctor who for many years was barred from joining the local AMA affiliate and not allowed to practice in many of the District hospitals, heading up the board that controlled who would be licensed to practice in the District of Columbia.

The 1970s and 1980s were filled with well-deserved successes not just in the medical field but in all the areas where he chose to devote his time and effort. One of the most memorable events for Eddie was receiving an honorary degree of Doctor of Science in 1974 from Morehouse and that same year being made a member of the board of trustees. As Eddie recalled, "I was thrilled by it. To me, I thought this was the greatest thing that ever could happen in my life."

Margurite confirmed Eddie's excitement about the honorary degree from Morehouse in telling her version of how Eddie learned of his selection:

> I received a call from Hugh Gloster, the president of Morehouse, saying that they were going to give Eddie an honorary degree. One of the precipitating factors as to why they gave him this degree was when Dr. James Cheek was installed as president at Howard there was a convocation. President Gloster couldn't come and he asked Eddie if he would march in the procession and represent Morehouse College. Eddie went to march and Howard told him that he had to wear the blue and white colors. You wear the colors of

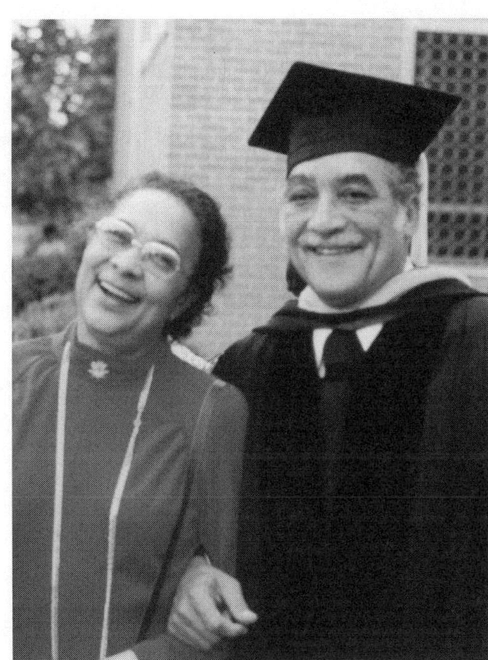

**Fig. 26:** Eddie and Maude when Dr. Mazique was given an honorary doctorate by Morehouse College in 1974. Photo courtesy of Maude Mazique and Dolores Pelham.

the last school where you got a degree. His degree in medicine came from Howard. Eddie wanted to wear Morehouse colors and they told him, "No, he had to wear Howard colors because that was the correct thing to do." He threatened that if he couldn't wear Morehouse colors then he wasn't going to march. I don't think he did.

It was right after that, Morehouse decided because of his contributions and other things they were going to give him an honorary degree. That followed on the back of the fact that he wanted to march in Morehouse colors. I got this call from Hugh telling me that they were going to give Eddie this honorary degree and at the same time he was being named to the Board at Morehouse.

When he would come in for dinner, we would take turns on going first on telling what happened that day. Of course, most of the time he just talked first. That evening when he came in, it was a very chilly evening, I had some soup on. He proceeded to start telling me

> about his day. I said, "No, no, I'm going to talk first. It's my turn and I want to talk first." I said, "I got a very interesting telephone call." I began to string this thing out. "President Gloster of Morehouse College called and he has informed me that the college is going to confer an honorary degree of Doctor of Science on my husband. Plus on top of that he has been named to the Trustee Board." His mouth fell open and I said, "I think that is just fantastic." He dropped his spoon and he was so excited he couldn't eat any more dinner. He just glowed. It was the greatest thing that ever happened.
>
> We were so excited and so delighted; we decided to take the whole staff to Atlanta. Everybody was going to see Eddie get this degree. We were the most excited group![37]

In the midst of the excitement to get ready Eddie neglected to take care of some necessary business, as Margurite remembered well.

> The night before was a Saturday night and we had to go down on Sunday morning for baccalaureate and commencement was on Tuesday. He had to march in the baccalaureate procession. Saturday night was one of his social club nights. I said, "Eddie, don't go tonight because we have to catch an 8:30 plane in the morning. If you go to that club meeting tonight, you are going to be so tired." He had to go. I said, "What about packing? I don't want to stay up all night to pack you." He said, "I'll pack it myself." Now I always do the packing. I said, "Well listen, Eddie, if you go out you will have to do your packing." I thought maybe that would get him to stay, but no, it didn't. He left. Sure enough Eddie came in late. Of course, I was fit to be tied. I said to him, "Don't forget you have to do your packing because you said you would." "I'll do it. I'll do it. You go ahead to bed and get your rest. I'll do my packing." I went on to bed. I tried to hurry him in the morning. We rushed out and jumped in the car. We get to the airport and it was like twenty-nine minutes after eight. His staff was there having a fit trying to hold up the

> plane. I realized only my bag was there. He says, "You didn't pack it?"
>
> He just had a T-shirt on and his jacket. We had to run in because they were trying to hold the plane. We hurried up the steps huffing and puffing and poor Alma was ready to die. I was thinking he had ruined the whole trip. He had on maroon pants. He knew I was angry. He said, "Well I left Morehouse with one pair of pants and I am going back with one pair of pants." I was stifling a laugh.[38]

Eddie stopped at a store on the way to Morehouse and bought a new suit.

> That Sunday on the way from the airport, I saw a K-Mart open. I stopped at the K-Mart and picked up a suit that cost $25 that was black and I got a tie and shirt and put it on there and got there in time for baccalaureate service.

Margurite went to the trouble to have his clothes mailed down for the commencement.

> I had bought him this expensive plaid silk suit. Fortunately my brother was staying at the house and I called him and asked him to send the suit and the tie. The luggage came Sunday night but Tuesday when we went to commencement Eddie had on this $25 suit. And when he got off the platform after receiving his degree, he handed it to me and said, "Here, this is yours." And I said, "Believe me, I have earned it!"[39]

Eddie still preferred his twenty-five-dollar suit since it gave him the opportunity to share the story of arriving at Morehouse with but one pair of pants. Thus, attired in his new suit, Eddie was awarded the honorary Doctor of Science degree on May 21, 1974, in recognition of his "achievements as a medical man" and his "concern for equal status for black physicians and adequate health care for the disadvantaged."[40] As his citation accurately stated, "You have come a long way since you first saw the light of day sixty-three years ago as the sixth of nine children in a black family in Natchez, Mississippi."[41]

Eddie's tenure on the board of trustees continued throughout his life and expanded when it was decided to start a medical school at Morehouse. Eddie was justifiably proud of being one of the founders.

> I've been serving on the board since then. In addition to that we decided that we needed a medical school. We had only two black medical schools: Howard and Meharry. Yet there are 114 medical schools. As a result of inquiry, they finally granted us permission to put up a medical school at Morehouse. I was one of the founders as well as on the board. We started with a small class of twenty-five. It was only two years. Now it is four years and we have thirty-four. It is doing well. So I am on two boards now. The Board of Trustees of Morehouse Medical School as well as Morehouse College.

When support for creating the medical school at Morehouse was at a low, Eddie once again played his role as a facilitator. The president of the Board of Morehouse Medical School, Louis Sullivan, later recalled: "He emphasized that we had made the commitment, we had gone too far to turn back and the mission was too important. He helped jell the opinions."[42]

Eddie's joy at receiving the honorary degree from Morehouse reflected the love he had for his alma mater. Morehouse and its caring faculty had provided the opportunity for a poor country boy to receive an excellent education that would not have been possible in other circumstances. If the administrators had not let him and Douglas work to pay for their room and board, given them scholarships, and even kept them on campus over the summer, Eddie's and Douglas's careers as physicians would have been virtually impossible. When Eddie spoke about Morehouse it was always with love.

> Working with Morehouse has been delightful. I feel I will never be able to entirely repay them the debt of gratitude for even permitting me to develop my full potential. I don't think that without them I would have been able to do it. I know I never could have done it! I feel if I owe real love and allegiance to any institution, it is Morehouse. For that reason I serve in many capacities

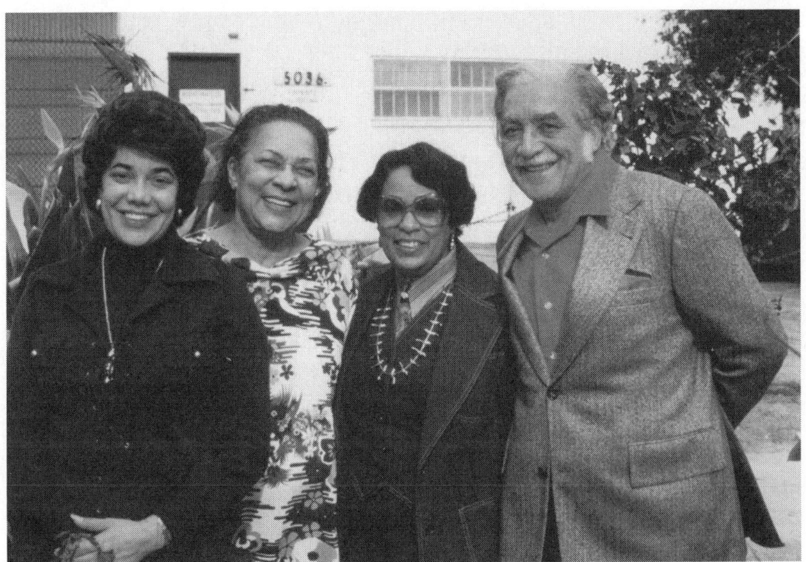


**Fig. 27:** Dolores Pelham (Maude's daughter), Maude Mazique, Margurite Mazique, and Eddie pose for the camera (from left to right). Photo courtesy of Maude Mazique and Dolores Pelham.

> for them. The fact is that I organized the first alumni association here in Washington. We used to meet in my office and my home until it got going.
>
> Another of the highlights of my life was deciding to name a dining hall in honor of my brother Douglas. His death was premature and traumatic in my life because we were so close. He died in 1963 of a coronary. He was a very prominent plastic surgeon, practicing in Chicago. They named a dining hall at Morehouse in his honor—they call it the Douglas Mazique Dining Hall. I have been supporting that dining hall each year to keep it up. We went down there for its dedication.
>
> Beginning last year, I started the Mazique collection of black books for Morehouse. I already have 984 volumes of black literature.

Representative of the many organizations to which Eddie devoted his time is the Boys and Girls Clubs of America.[43] Eddie had started on the board in June 1970 but had not been particularly active until Archie Avedisian became the new executive director in 1972. Mr. Avedisian remembered vividly when he first came to Washington, D.C., to take over the Boys Club:

> Eddie was on the Board of Directors of the Boys Club when I came here. He was not very active with it though. At that time they were on a downgrade. That was one of the reasons why they brought me in here. Right after the riots, they had had a lot of problems with integration; they had a lot of problems with management. The club was mismanaged and went tremendously in the hole. With the problems we had with integration, the staff was not relevant to what was going on.
>
> They were going out of business when I came here. They were one-half a million dollars in debt. We had been kicked out of the United Way. When I came on, the United Way said they would keep us on a month-to-month basis. They had seven directors here in seven years. So they brought me in from Seattle, Washington, to try to turn it around.
>
> Doc was on the board at that time. I worked with the existing board members and found a hard-core group that you have in every board of directors and started working with them to get the operation moving in the right direction and of course Doc was one of the board members who responded. He and I became very close as I am with some of the other board members who have come through that period of time with us.
>
> Right now we are the premier agency in town with the United Way, with funding sources. We serve over 1,700 boys and girls a day here now. We have grown to seven branches. Of course, Doc had played a very important role in that. We have won eighteen national awards in the last twelve years. They only give twelve awards out nationally to 1,100 clubs that compete. So we are probably the club that has received the most awards. When I came here in 1972 we had 1,112 members and today we have close to 5,000. We see 2,051 individuals a day.[44]

Once it was requested, Eddie played a key role in many of the improvements in the organization. Mr. Avedisian recalled how Eddie helped locate a site for establishing a new club as well as securing much-needed grants to enhance their programming.

> We were asked by the local community to come in and open up a club in the Shaw area, which has a very high crime rate and prostitution and drugs. We worked with a small group in a small Baptist church that gave us their facilities. We worked with the local people there and we established a club. Within a year, we totally overwhelmed the church so we just couldn't operate in there. We had too many kids coming in so we started looking for another site.
>
> We were telling Doc about it and we asked him to head up a committee to see if he could locate another site. We were at that time looking at the old Jewish Community Center. He came up with the Family Life Center of the Shilo Baptist Church. They had built a new 5.5-million-dollar facility. We coordinated our efforts and their efforts together where we are now in that facility operating full time. We are handling all of the youth programs and they are handling the older programs and then wherever my staff can assist with the adult programs, we do. The main thrust of ours, of course, is on youth, and so it has helped the people at Shilo Baptist Church get to their goals with being able to cut back on some of their overhead of operations and it has been the same thing for us. We have been able to get in for a lot less and work together with an existing group. I think it is one of the premier examples of coordinating two organizations' efforts into one.
>
> [Another time] we were working on getting a large, $350,000 grant and we had to go through a lot of red tape to get it. You know how it is dealing with the government. I needed some direction or I knew we wouldn't get the funding for it. Doc followed it all the way through for us to make sure he removed those obstacles for us, the potential problems with specific individuals that we saw as we were heading towards that grant.

> There was $423,000 given away nationally out of that particular grant and we got $350,000 of that. That was through his efforts.
>
> His biggest thrust is helping us totally rather than zeroing in on a specific activity. Really going after big things, like helping us with opening doors for getting grants from foundations or from the government, putting us in touch with people we want to get on our board of directors that he relates to and works with on a professional basis. He helps us throughout the total organization.[45]

As with other organizations in which he participated, Eddie's power increased as others became impressed with his demeanor, with what he could accomplish, and with his ability to bring people together. His achievements were respected by his fellow board members, as Mr. Avedisian recalls:

> He's a great motivator of other board members too. Our board highly respects him. What he says and what he thinks weighs very heavily with our board members. As you know there are some power brokers on boards and he is definitely one of them. He believes in what we are trying to do. I think that is why I respect him so much because he is just like having a professional working for you. And it is not only he that works, his staff comes in. I can call the office; whether I talk to Alma or Marcia, and whatever I want to get done they take care of it for me. It's like having a complete staff that is involved. They are all committed to him and the Boy's Club and it is a great connection we have with him.[46]

When Eddie became president of the board, Mr. Avedisian was pleased.

> Doc was also our first black president. I'm sure some board members were thinking, "What kind of leadership is he going to give us?" I had no doubts about him. We have a rule that at the end of three years you have to step down. We rotate them at the end of three years so that we don't overwork anybody.

> The board wanted to change the rule in order to keep him in there longer.
>
> He never cuts back. He is on our area Council Board. He heads up a group and he has never missed those meetings that are down in Richmond or down in the Norfolk area and he will be going in as the president of the Virginia-D.C. Area Council Board of Directors in September. He's also headed up the National Conference Committee when the Boys and Girls Clubs of America National Conference was here and he coordinated the volunteers and got all the people together to put the conference together with the national organization. He welcomed delegates from all over the United States. He did a super job at it—he's a tremendous speaker, as you know. He introduced Vice President Bush and people were still talking about it a year later. I must have received fifty or sixty letters from throughout the United States from Boys and Girls Clubs people telling me what an outstanding job he did as a conference person and as the welcoming person.[47]

Eddie was supportive of expanding the functions of the Boys Club to include much-needed programs for the youth of the Washington metropolitan area.

> You need guys like Doc who are kind of free-will thinkers who are willing to go along with the staff to experiment in some areas that a lot of nonprofit agencies are afraid to get into. Group homes are good examples. We started dealing with family problems and dealing with some broader issues that are crucial to kids that we now serve—getting away from just recreation and things like that. Doc was very instrumental in working with us to get group homes. We have four group homes that we run. They are difficult to run. These are kids who are displaced, who have run away, kids who have been thrown out of their homes. We provide a place in which we set up programs for them and help find them a home. We have between 307 and 325 kids a year with that program.

> The program has been extremely successful for the last couple years and the city is very happy with it because they were having trouble with it. We use a different approach. We have three eight-hours shifts of professional people who work there. I don't personally believe in a "Mom and Pop" operation. We have professional staff there all the time and all the kids are assigned to a club so they get all their activities and all their guidance at their branch. Therefore once they are in a transition into a home, they have some kids they relate to, some adults they feel comfortable with, so they can continue coming to the branches and hopefully cement the relationship they have. It has worked out very successfully. We have a lot of our kids back in school; we've gotten vending licenses so they can go out and make a buck. Yale University has recognized our club as one of the outstanding organizations at providing family support programs.[48]

Eddie also played a role in the much-needed integration of girls into the activities of the Club.

> We also integrated girls into the Boy's Club. He was in on that. Today about 10 percent of the Boys Clubs around the country now serve Boys and Girls, so it was a successful program. We got the first grant. There were other Boys Clubs that ran girls programs historically. We were the first ones who got a grant, during Doc's presidency, to really find out what it is all about to integrate girls into the program. We didn't do it because of any pressure from women's groups or from the law or anything else. We saw that there was a tremendous unmet need in the metropolitan Washington area, especially in the inner city. We were, at that time, trying to generate something. It can't be done overnight. You have to build bathroom facilities and locker and shower areas. You have to completely rehab your building. It has taken us years and years and millions of dollars to do it. On top of that, you have to have additional staff. It is a real undertaking but our Board was committed to

> it and has pulled it off. About 30 percent of our membership every year are girls. About 40 percent of our professional staff are women. This came about under Doc's regime; he was one of the two presidents who were in the driver's seat during this change.[49]

In 1983, Eddie received the Boys Club of America Medallion, "the highest national award that can be given a local board member for unusual devoted service and interest."[50]

Despite his admiration for how Eddie led the board, that was not what impressed Mr. Avedisian the most. It was the same thing that impressed all those with whom Eddie dealt—his warmth, his friendliness, and the way he treated other people. Mr. Avedisian pointed out: "Normally with Board members, it is all business because the board members are in a different financial category and different social scene than the paid professional staff."[51] As was the case with multitudes of others from patients to colleagues to those who only had slight contact with Eddie, Mr. Avedesian's relationship with Eddie was very personal. Ruby Van Croft, director of the Visiting Nurse's Association, felt much the same, as she indicated when speaking of Eddie's relationship with nurses: "They all loved him and enjoyed doing things for him because he treated people with a sense of dignity. Regardless of his station and their station he still had that warmth."[52]

Earlier in his career, Eddie had devoted his efforts to integrating the YMCA. In the 1970s, it was time to use his talents as a skillful negotiator to keep it operating successfully. Kent Cushenberry, a fellow member of a YMCA task force, remembered how Eddie helped to hold things together.

> We worked together on a task force that the mayor put together to try and resolve a very pressing issue of the inner-city YMCA that had to be closed. Due to structural damage and safety hazards they could not allow the building to open and certain community leaders interpreted that as the Y trying to disengage itself from the inner-city community needs.
>
> When the building was closed, certain leaders of the community, particularly the Shaw coalition, were up in arms, vehemently opposed to closing. They did not agree with the logic and developed a coalition of public community groups to protest in the way of demonstrations at

the YMCA at Seventeenth and Rhode Island. They were suing the YMCA and the entire board of directors, a six-and-a-half-million-dollar suit, and just generally being at odds and not communicating. There was non-communication both on the part of the Y and the coalition. The mayor had appointed Sterling Tucker as a consultant to take a look at the situation. He was acceptable to the Y board as well as to the coalition. He made recommendations as to how the situation might be remedied and turned in his report. There was still disagreement between the Y and the coalition as to how the issue could be resolved. That was when the mayor decided to appoint a task force from coalition members, the YMCA, the Anthony Bowen YMCA community, and then some members at large who had proven to be interested citizens. We started out quietly but soon thereafter the meetings became stronger, you might say—much disagreement and not very much communication. Ed proved to be the glue that held the group together for several different reasons. The first two being who he is and the esteem and admiration in which all members of the task force held him and the bridge that he presented from the past to the present. Thirdly, was his ability to get people to work together and to lay down individual differences for the common good. Had he not been on that task force it might well have not succeeded in bringing the parties together, the eventual withdrawal of the suit, to the coming together of all parties and reaching an agreement which still holds.

To watch him work in those meetings! He would sit just looking and observing where different people were coming from. You could see the wheels turning in his head. It didn't matter who was being boisterous or expressing themselves in a violent way or in a quiet way. When he spoke everyone else remained quiet and heard him out and he almost always got agreement. You would get the nodding of the heads and the eventual compromise and we would get over the hurdle. This was interesting because you had the components of the mayor's office, from the Shaw community, from the YMCA both

> from Shaw and the National Board, you had people at large, both white and black, Jew and Christian and Muslim. You had about as diverse a group as you could get from all walks of life, professions, and economic limits. He performed; he acted masterfully.[53]

There was another crisis and Mr. Cushenberry asked for Eddie's assistance again.

> When all hell broke loose over there and the community was in total disarray, and generally being uncooperative, I asked Ed to serve as chairman of the Anthony Bowen YMCA Committee. He has a very busy practice and is involved in many activities but he said, "Yes." Before long he pulled the committee back together again, got people working again, and we honored him with a special luncheon and presented him with a plaque for outstanding services and his wife was with him and the entire community over there turned out for it. It was touching.
>
> It is that kind of thing. When everything is a problem, an issue, and his talents can be used, he finds the time. I find him totally unselfish, farsighted, a deep sense of empathy for others and he just gives unstintingly of his time. We were not the only ones he has supported and helped. I am just amazed. He is a man for all seasons.[54]

Other presidents, directors, and administrators felt much the same as Mr. Cushenberry. Eddie was always there when their organizations needed a boost, a leader or a mediator. The associate executive director of the United Way of the National Council Area, Norman Taylor, initially had his doubts about Eddie's ability to serve as chairman for their fundraising campaign.

> Dr. Mazique agreed to serve as chairman of the D.C. Campaign, which is the largest regional campaign. Here's a guy who is a doctor and I had a little bit of apprehension with him being a doctor and the things that he had to do. Patients were almost sitting on the curb trying to get into his office. You just say to

> yourself, "Gee whiz, can this guy do this? Does he really have time to go to the meetings and really have time to make a call and recruit certain people to be chairmen of certain divisions?" The first meeting was fantastic. "Whatever you need done let me know. Try to give me time so I can try and be there. We're gonna do it and I enjoy it."
>
> He set up his cabinet, met with them, met with the loaned executives. He met with people, encouraged them, and had a little get-together for them. The largest campaign was the D.C. government. You are talking about 40,000 employees of the District Government. He had to make a presentation; he had to kick off a major campaign. If you had a problem you could always call on him.
>
> I would pick him at his house early in the morning and he had his bag, his doctor's valise, and we would go from there. I would take him to the meeting and then after the meeting I would drop him at his office or a hospital. He was off and running for the day. That kind of commitment is just unheard of. At that time, he was involved with Morehouse in getting a medical school started. I think at that time he was also the president of the Boys Club of Washington, which was a big role. Just a fantastic kind of individual! Nothing was too big. He just did a good job. They say when you want a job done, get a busy person. He just keeps going the whole time. It blew my mind. How can you do all this? And he did it all. His wife was just as committed, gave him the impetus to do it. He seemed to kind of grow younger with doing it.[55]

In fact Eddie did such a good job in 1984 that he was asked to do it again. By then Mr. Taylor knew just how well Eddie could do the job.

> The second time he was a pro at it. We sat down; we strategized; we worked it through. He understood the job; he knew what he had to do; he had a commitment to other people, to helping, to reaching out. Whenever you saw him, he had a handshake for you, a smile, and that's the kind of guy he is.[56]

There were many other awards and honors Eddie received and many more organizations he helped with his expertise, his knowledge, his connections, and his ability to get people to work together and to bring compromise where none was seen as possible. Whether it was the Visiting Nurse's Association, the NAACP, the Rotary, the Junior Citizens Corps, the Jim Thorpe Foundation, or the Congressional Black Caucus Subcommittee on the Aged, Eddie served with a dedication and energy few could match. He received awards from the D.C. Chamber of Commerce, the U.S. Department of Health, Education and Welfare, AMVETS, Omega Psi Phi Fraternity, the Council of the District of Columbia, and others too numerous to mention.

With all his awards and all his achievements, it was still the sense of joy that he brought to everything he did that impressed others the most. People were just plain happy to see him. His patients felt better just talking to him, and those with other types of problems could talk and feel he was listening with undivided attention. He turned every experience into fun, whether it was listening to a speech, speaking with a patient, or fishing. His joy was contagious and so people wanted to be around him.

In 1987, Eddie played Santa Claus, as usual, to 104 children in the Parent Child Care Center. After Christmas, Eddie and Margurite along with her sister and brother-in-law went to Barbados for a vacation and a little deep-sea fishing. That Saturday night Eddie had a ball, dancing and carrying on. After retiring, Margurite was awakened from sleep by Eddie making a strange sound. By the time she had run and come back with her brother-in-law, Eddie was dead of a heart attack. He had gone as he would have chosen, quickly and after having had a great time.

Speaking of Eddie when he was still alive, Kent Cushenberry captured the essence of Eddie's contributions and his personal attributes:

> The fact that he is a black physician and comes from the background that he has, is obviously a tremendous accomplishment in and of itself. But he has become a philanthropist, a community activist, and a philosopher of sorts. [He is] a man of many talents and he shares them with others. A lot of people have a lot of talent and achieve a lot but they keep it all close to the vest and don't share it. He is willing to share and he has so much to give and he offers it. If you are receptive you can receive a lot from him and I don't mean material things. I mean morality things.[57]

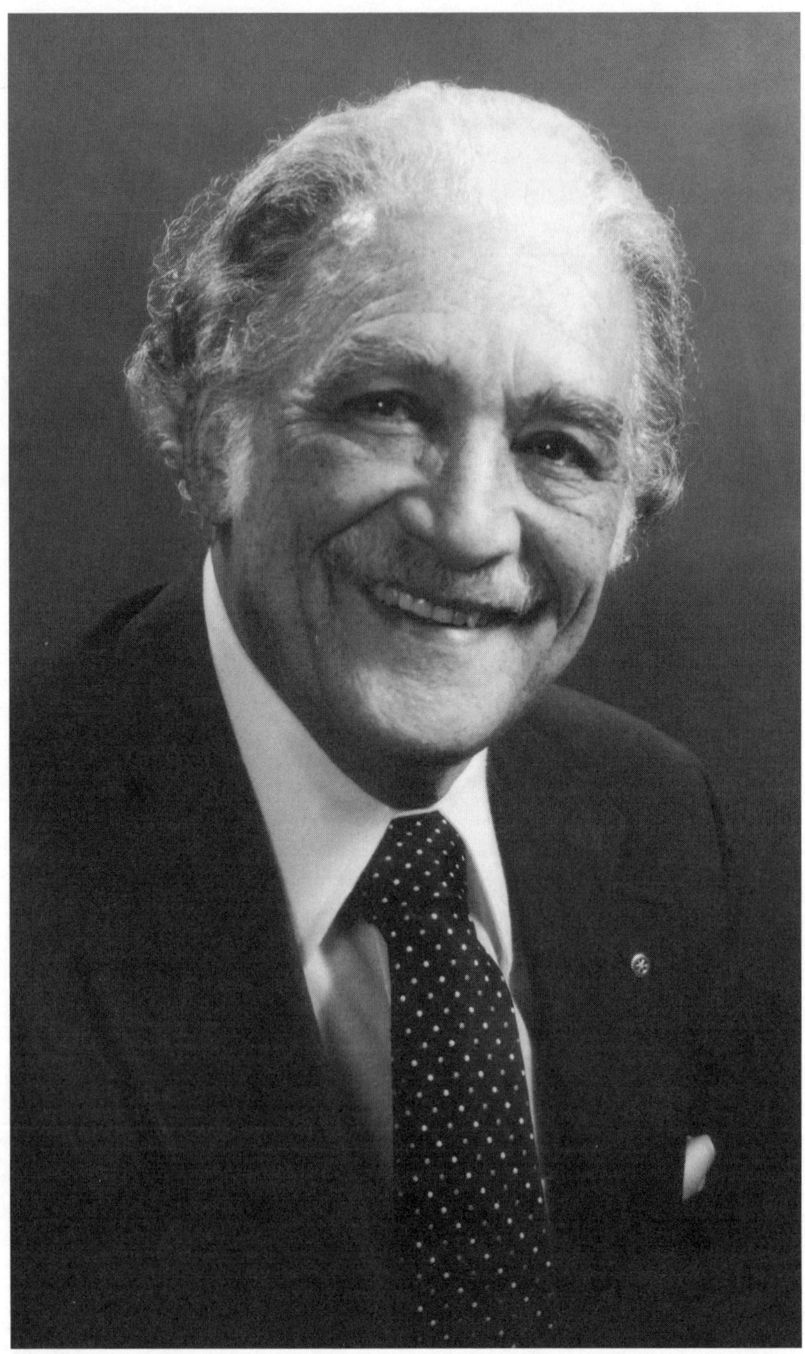

**Fig. 28:** Dr. Mazique in the 1980s. Photo from Edward C. Mazique files.

I don't know anyone that would disagree that [Ed] is a role model personified and has so many attributes that if we can just have one of them, we will be lucky. I don't think that he should only be looked upon as a black role model. I think that he has proven capable of pulling people of all races and ethnic groups and religious backgrounds together and working with them all. It is important for blacks to have black role models. But I think we also should look at it in a larger picture. He is a role model for mankind.[58]

# EPILOGUE 

Last night a bright and shining star
Fell from the heavens above and danced
And taught me the secrets of the Universe
As it guided me to the top rung of the
Miles-long powerful ladder.
I heard nothing as you called my name.
The emotions of only my echo remain.
The sky is clear and blue.
I stand tall; a heavenly voice resounds!
"Come Home Early, Chile."
I'll take you in my arms.
"Come Home Early, Chile!"
— *Edward C. Mazique,*
*"Ode to Owen Dodson"*

Eddie was one of those rare people who is appreciated both during his life and after his death. On the day of his funeral, St. Luke's Episcopal Church was packed with dignitaries, patients, and friends. The mayor and councilpersons of Washington; Vice President Bush's wife, Barbara Bush; Dick Gregory; and many of the physicians in the city were there. The newspaper tributes were extensive, sincere, and flattering. From black press, white press, alumni magazines, medical bulletins, and national magazines poured tributes to Eddie and to the way he had devoted his life to the betterment of others. The lists of the organizations on whose boards he served and the awards he won were massive, far surpassing those mentioned in this biography. But it was not just a series of lists of his affiliations and accomplishments. Many of the writers remembered his special kind of personality: "Dr. Edward C. Mazique will be remembered for his warm, lighthearted, down-to-earth nature. His joy and friendliness brought smiles; his wit brought laughter."[1]

Other articles stressed his tireless efforts to end discrimination in Washington. Eddie's own thoughts from an earlier interview were quoted: "I know I was told more than once, 'Hey, why don't you stick entirely to medicine, keep your nose out of community affairs . . .' but I contend there's not much you can do about combating malaria or TB unless you do indeed do something about the causes of it."[2] It was this philosophy that guided Eddie's life and summed up what he had hoped to achieve. The commentators were unanimous in concluding that he had succeeded.

> By profession he was a physician, a graduate of Howard University's Medical School, but he practiced much more than medicine in his efforts to remove racial barriers in Washington. Dr. Mazique... became an institution in the city, at least in that part of Washington that stood up to be counted for desegregation and integration when these were lonely causes here. In the political and racial spheres as well as the medical, he made a lasting difference.[3]

Yet despite the racial barriers Eddie helped to demolish, racism has not ended. The civil rights movement, with the support of Eddie and countless others, managed to "force the removal of the legal base that supported racial discrimination and segregation, forge a broad-based consensus which believed that overt acts of racism were not morally tolerable in American society, enlist the support of the national government in the pursuit of racial equality, and establish a powerful coalition that brought together the church, labor, intellectuals, idealists, other ethnic groups and the young."[4] The accomplishments of the civil rights movement were remarkable and "accounted for more progress in less time than blacks had made since they first arrived in America in 1619."[5] Despite this progress, "they failed to materially alter the lives of the mass of black people who remained disproportionately poor, badly educated and unable to avail themselves of the opportunities that went to better prepared blacks."[6] Many of the conditions that have prevented blacks from ever bettering themselves still exist in the black ghettos:

> The Movement hardly touched them at all. Unemployment for blacks remained at double the rate for whites, the ghettos continued to deteriorate, crime still plagued black neighborhoods, and the various government programs that sought to address these problems were never funded at the proper level or maintained long enough to make any real difference.[7]

When attacking the problems still facing minorities such as unemployment and the need for welfare reform, better housing, or improved health care, there seems to be little agreement among diverse groups as to the solutions. One source traces the breakup of the consensus back to the riots of the 1960s that "frighten[ed] a number of white people and lessen[ed] their ardor for black-oriented causes."[8] If the whites have lost faith in the black leaders, so too have the disillusioned blacks. Referring to the Miami riots of 1980, author Francis Ward wrote:

> Miami was a dramatic but timely demonstration that they [younger low-income blacks] have little if any confidence in black leadership, local or national. Black leadership has no message for the black dispossessed, no offer of jobs, education or new opportunities it can offer to lure the new generation of surly, angry blacks away from potential violence.[9]

The increase in violence sparked by racial differences has led to the conclusion by some historians that "the rise in the level of activities of various hate groups, the violence in Miami, Howard Beach and Forsyth County were part of something even larger and more disturbing to civil rights leaders and others—the resurgence of racism."[10] Walter Fauntroy apparently concurred in a statement he made while a congressman: "There is a 'new meanness' in human relations in which 'the internal brakes are off.'"[11] A national survey conducted by pollster Louis Harris found that in the late 1980s the nation was still "the haven of much racism and even racial hatred."[12] Housing still remained largely segregated. Statistics from 1980 indicate that 31 percent of blacks lived in neighborhoods that were 90 percent black while six out of ten whites lived in neighborhoods that were completely white.[13]

Later studies have shown no reason to believe there has been improvement since the 1980s. A 1993 Harvard University study on American public schools found that "American public schools are becoming more racially segregated than at any time since the late 1960s."[14] Blacks and Hispanics in metropolitan areas are becoming increasingly isolated in schools with a high ratio of poor children. This is true especially in the Northwest, Midwest, and California—areas where desegregation was not forced. In the Northeast, 76 percent of the black children and 78 percent of Hispanic children attend predominately minority schools. The director of the Harvard Project on School

Desegregation concluded that "[t]he civil rights impulse from the 1960s is dead in the water, and the ship is floating backward toward the shoals of segregation."[15]

Even where schools have been technically integrated, there is no guarantee of any meaningful interaction between the races. A more recent article on the University of Mississippi, the university that James Meredith integrated in September 1962, noted they have a student body that is only 9 percent Afro-American even though in the state of Mississippi Afro-Americans constitute 36 percent of the population. Both black and white students agree that "the two populations exist in parallel universes that occupy the same space."[16] Although such segregation is blamed on more than bigotry, this situation has led the chancellor of the university to comment: "For those of us who have worked all our lives for integration, the re-separation is cause for concern."[17]

An article appearing the same day as the one on the Harvard Project discussed statistics from the federal government's Office of Personnel and Management. The statistics show a marked disparity in the firings of federal workers by race.[18] Although slightly more than one-quarter of the federal employees were minority, more than one-half of those dismissed from jobs in 1992 were minority employees. "This disparity between whites and minorities existed at every pay grade and for every occupational group but was greatest among low-level, blue-collar and clerical workers."[19] Earlier studies in Boston and California have found similar results.

Looking at the current headlines in newspapers any day of the week is enough to convince the reader that segregation, discrimination, and racism are issues that were not solved by the civil rights movement of the 1960s.[20] Whether the younger generations of minorities are attacking the problems as productively as their elders is questionable.

In a thought-provoking article about Eddie written by Courtland Milloy for the *Washington Post,* he took to task the new generation of Washington physicians. Noting the throngs of young black physicians with fancy cars at Eddie's funeral, he indicated they were there partially because of Eddie's work. Stating that Dr. Mazique would have been dissatisfied that so few physicians had picked up his "legacy of activism," he went on to chide them for their lack of community involvement and to criticize the deplorable health conditions in the city.

> How, then, in a town where so many doctors have the privilege of knowing—if not actually working with—such a great man, could health care be in such

> crisis? How could cancer, heart disease, hypertension, drug abuse and AIDS be virtually out of control in the black community?
>
> How could Washington, D.C. with at least 1,100 black doctors—more per square mile than most any place on Earth—have a higher infant mortality rate than Mississippi?[21]

He concluded by saying how disappointed Eddie would be:

> Here was a man who had been born in the poverty of Natchez, Miss., in 1911 but still managed to break down racial barriers 10 times greater than those existing today. Yet, too many of the new doctors, armed with more education and backed by large professional organizations, appear to have fled in the face of adversity, to have turned their backs on the black community.
>
> This was not the Mazique way.[22]

Although consensus may not be found among the different groups as to how to solve the problems confronting the poor, the minorities, and the elderly with whom Eddie was so concerned, there are many trying. The impact Eddie had on others continues even after his death. Some of this influence can be seen in very public ways, such as those Courtland Milloy wrote about in his column written nearly two years after Eddie's death: "Dr. Edward Mazique would be proud. Two years after his death, the legacy of one of Washington's most respected and dedicated physicians lives on impressively."[23]

The two events that Milloy was referring to were the first annual Mazique Scholarship 5k Run and the establishment of one of the nation's first comprehensive parent-child resource centers. The Edward Mazique Memorial Scholarship was established by the Howard University Medical School dean, Dr. Charles Epps, to go to one deserving and needy medical student each year. The 5k run was one method by which funds would be raised each year for the scholarship.

The Parent Child Center was founded in Washington in 1968 and since 1980 had been housed in what is now the Anthony Bowen YMCA. In 1988, the Parent Child Center was renamed in honor of Eddie, their former Santa Claus. From their beginnings in two rooms in the old Anthony Bowen YMCA where they "serv[ed] 70 families they grew to offer a city-wide service to more than 315 low-income families with a budget of more than $1.8 million yearly."[24] In November 1988, the U.S. Department of Health and Human Services announced that the District's Mazique Center would receive $808,302 for the next five years.[25] Ground was broken on the new Edward C. Mazique Parent Child Center in March 1989.

The Parent Child Center is a "community-based agency that provides services to low-income families with young children."[26] Included are services for preschool children, handicapped children, teenaged parents, parents of children with special needs, job training, medical services, nutrition counseling, and referral and intervention services. The new Mazique Center was the first preschool building in Washington designed specifically for the needs of young children.

With this new facility, Courtland Milloy believed, "we can expect that one day there will be additional doctors walking in Mazique's footsteps, carrying on his work in the center that bears his name."[27] There is little doubt that Eddie would be pleased.

Eddie would have also been pleased by the Mazique Family Reunion held in Natchez on April 6–8, 1990. As a matter of fact, he would have been in his glory! Maintaining ties with his family, no matter how distantly related, and with his roots was one of Eddie's great joys in life. Whenever a distant relative arrived in Washington and got in touch, Eddie treated them like a prodigal son.[28] Eddie tried to visit Natchez and his relatives on a regular basis. His "kinfolk" still living in Natchez always enjoyed his visits since, despite his success, he acted like just another member of the family.

It was the dream of Eddie's sister Maude to have a family get-together in Natchez so the younger Maziques could familiarize themselves with their origins and family history. As Maude said in an interview, "I wanted all my brothers' children and families to know their heritage and how to love, live, and be kind."[29] With Maude's encouragement her daughter, Dolores Pelham, choreographed the entire three-day affair and even interested CBS's "Sunday Morning with Charles Kuralt" in featuring it on the show.

Charles Kuralt opened the story of the Maziques, entitled "Going Home," by saying:

> Old Natchez on the bluffs above the Mississippi was the center of a white planter aristocracy before the Civil War. Go there and you still get a feeling for the pride of the Old South—a society built on slavery. You

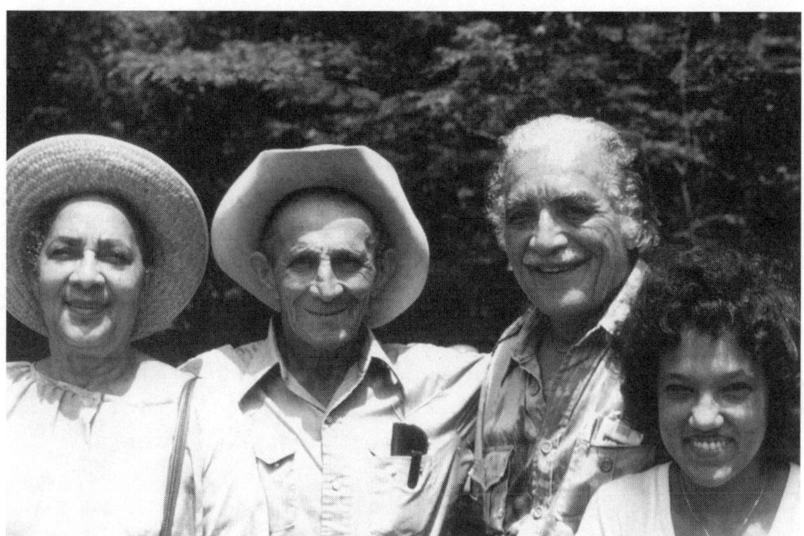

**Fig. 29:** Eddie and his sister Maude Mazique visit with cousin James Boyd Jr. and third cousin Brenda Boyd during a visit to Natchez, Mississippi. Both Eddie and Maude always kept up their contacts with their Natchez roots. Photo courtesy of Maude Mazique and Dolores Pelham.

> wouldn't think there was much for blacks to celebrate in the history of Natchez but, oh, there is![30]

As was evident from the reunion, the story of the slave family whose ambition, intelligence, and hard work made purchasing the plantations belonging to their former master possible was indeed a history to be celebrated.

It was evident from the moment we arrived that Natchez had moved forward on racial integration. The Days Inn that was the headquarters for the reunion boasted a huge sign proclaiming "Welcome Home Maziques." The local newspaper carried two front-page stories about the reunion and one story about Eddie.[31] The reunion included visiting Oakland and China Grove, now in the hands of white owners who could not have been more gracious in opening their homes to the 120 Mazique family members who attended.

Yet the signs of glorifying the segregated past were still in evidence. Every year Natchez presents the Confederate Pageant, a tribute to the Civil War era. We went to see what it was like. The prologue to the program was enough to let the audience know that there were still those who cherished the pre–Civil War times while ignoring the contributions of those whose labor made the "charming way of life" of the plantation owners possible.

> Step into the past tonight with Natchez. Indians, Frenchmen, Britishers, and Spaniards all left their mark on this river city.
>
> But whatever their nationality, whatever their age, the people in early Natchez enjoyed life—at house parties, at garden parties, at dances, at prominent weddings, at the showboat on the river, and before they went hunting.
>
> Little did they know that the year 1861 would change their charming way of life.[32]

The hoopskirts and the pageantry were pretty, but the CBS crew photographing the event found the Mazique party still seated while the others stood at attention when "Dixie" was played.

Despite the offensiveness of some of the old symbols, the reunion was a great success. It had achieved Maude's goals of bringing together the family members and making the younger ones aware of their impressive heritage. Gary Reeves, the announcer for the CBS presentation, concluded by saying, "Maude Mazique and her daughter followed the family tradition. They did something good for the rest. They taught them about roots—the reason the branches of the Mazique family remain so strong."[33]

Many of the ways in which Eddie continues to have an impact on others are less visible but no less real. In an interview with the Reverend Walter Fauntroy after Eddie's death, he discussed a new project in which he was representing Nelson Mandela and the African National Congress. He said, "I am in the process of doing in black South Africa what we did in Shaw. Ed would be very pleased."[34]

Reverend Fauntroy is not the only one who considers whether Eddie would be pleased with what he is doing and failing to do and with the decisions he makes. Eddie had an impact on all of those who knew him. He continues to be a role model influencing the lives of the people who love him.

As Judge H. Carl Moultrie put it while Eddie was living,

> [h]e is one of the greatest guys who ever lived. He has paid his dues. You think of Eddie Mazique in this

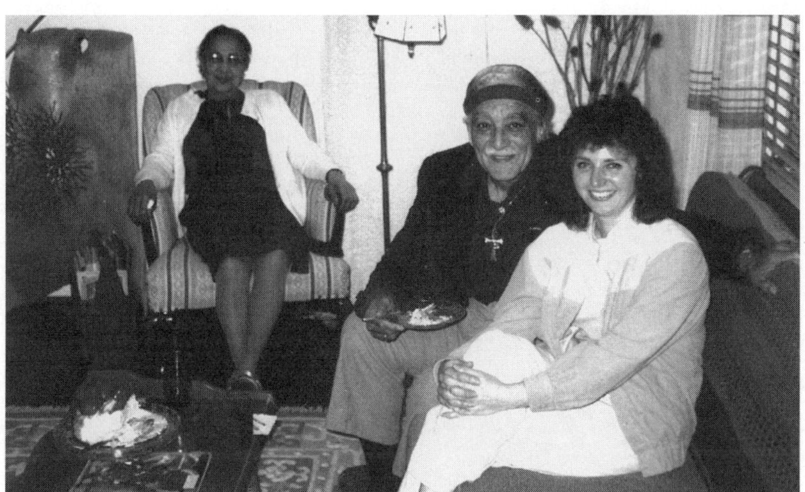

**Fig. 30:** Maude Mazique and Eddie visit with the author in 1984. Author photo.

> city. A lot of people's names you forget, but you won't forget Eddie Mazique's name.[35]

The Morehouse alumni magazine summed up Eddie's life best when it said,

> Dr. Mazique will always be remembered by the persons that were healed and touched by his life's contributions. Friends and loved ones say that he had a special brand of medicine that was used daily: it combined science and social consciousness. One could write endlessly about the achievements of Dr. Mazique.[36]

# NOTES 

## INTRODUCTION

1. The lead quotation is from a transcription of a filmed interview of Dr. Edward Mazique conducted by William A. Elwood of the University of Virginia for the documentary film *The Road to Brown* about the campaign leading to the 1954 *Brown v. Board of Education* Supreme Court decision.
2. This sentiment about how Eddie dealt with people equally and never forgot his roots was reiterated in many interviews. For example, Judge Luke Moore said, "He is easily approached. Nobody is in awe of him. From the very lowest to the very highest, nobody feels that he is condescending" (interview with author, 19 July 1985). Eddie's friend and patient Rip Naylor said, "His best quality is his ability to get along with any and everybody, no matter who it is. No matter how low or how high, he is accepted. He's the same at all times. He's down-to-earth; both feet on the ground. Everybody loves him" (interview with author, 1 March 1985). Samuel Foggie, the president and CEO of United National Bank, which Eddie helped found, put it very well: "That is one thing that is important about him. He is never pretentious and 'put on.' If you meet him at the East Room of the White House or the board room of United National, or you meet him out on the street or at a picnic, he is the same" (interview with author, 16 July 1985).
3. Michel Fabre, *The Unfinished Quest of Richard Wright* (New York: William Morrow and Co., 1973), 1.
4. Benjamin E. Mays, *Born to Rebel* (Athens: University of Georgia Press, 1987), iv.
5. Judge H. Carl Moultrie, interview with author, 15 July 1985.
6. Constance McLaughlin Green, *The Secret City: A History of Race Relations in the Nation's Capital* (Princeton, N.J.: Princeton University Press, 1967), 326.

## CHAPTER ONE

1. *Natchez Tri-Weekly Democrat,* 6 January 1866.
2. Several sources were used for the description of Natchez, including William Banks Taylor, *King Cotton and Old Glory* (Hattiesburg, Miss.: Fox Printing Co., 1977); and Doris Clayton James, *Antebellum Natchez* (Baton Rouge: Louisiana State University Press, 1968).
3. Charles A. Murray, *Travels in North America during the Years 1834, 1835 & 1836,* 2 vols. (London: R. Bentley, 1839), 176–77. The percentage of the population foreign-born was taken from James, *Antebellum Natchez,* 164. The number of Yankees is from *The Seventh Census of the United States, 1850* (Washington, D.C., 1853), 448. The information on the children educated in New England is from Taylor, *King Cotton and Old Glory,* 13. The information on the improvement in Natchez is from William Ransom Hogan and Edwin Adams Davis, eds., *William Johnson's Natchez: The Antebellum Diary of a Free*

*Negro* (Baton Rouge: Louisiana State University Press, 1951), 3; and James, *Antebellum Natchez,* 169.

4. Taylor (*King Cotton and Old Glory,* 14) argued that the regularity with which slaves were freed showed that freeing them elevated the status of the owners. There was an all-time high population of free Negroes in Natchez in 1860.
5. A discussion of the success of the free Negroes is found in various sources, including James, *Antebellum Natchez,* 178; Edwin Adams Davis and William Ransom Hogan, *The Barber of Natchez* (Baton Rouge: Louisiana State University Press, 1954), 240–43; Ira Berlin, *Slaves without Masters: The Free Negro in the Antebellum South* (New York: Pantheon Books, 1974); Larry Koger, *Black Slaveowners: Free Black Slave Masters in South Carolina, 1790–1860* (Jefferson, N.C.: McFarland, 1985); and Michael P. Johnson and James L. Roark, *Black Slavemasters: A Free Family of Color in the Old South* (New York: Norton, 1984).
6. A description of Johnson's accumulated wealth can be found in Hogan and Davis, *William Johnson's Natchez,* 39; of his dealings with the whites in ibid., 53; and of his home in James, *Antebellum Natchez,* 170.
7. *Natchez Free Trader,* 1 June 1858. An excellent discussion of the importance of Robert D. Smith in Natchez history is presented by Mary Warren Miller, "Black History of Natchez, Mississippi," slide presentation for the Historic Natchez Foundation, 25 February 1983.
8. A description of the class distinction among the free Negroes can be found in Hogan and Davis, *William Johnson's Natchez,* 11.
9. For a description of the prevailing slave conditions in Natchez, see Taylor, *King Cotton and Old Glory,* 13. Bishop Green's trip to the Railey plantation is described by him in his account of "Interesting incidents when he visited Natchez." This material was located in the Edith Wyatt Moore Collection. Ms. Moore was an active leader in the WPA Adams County history project. The collection is housed in the Judge George W. Armstrong Library, Natchez, Mississippi.
   Railey's nephew-in-law, Dr. James Green Carson, supported a minister for his slaves and another for Railey's slaves after he became the executor for his Louisiana plantation (John O. Anderson, "Dr. James Green Carson, Ante-Bellum Planter of Mississippi and Louisiana," *Journal of Mississippi History* 18, no. 4 [1956]: 259–60).
10. The contention that Natchez slave owners did everything to improve the lot of their slaves is made by Taylor, *King Cotton and Old Glory,* 13.
11. *Natchez Southern Galaxy,* 9 October 1828.
12. Atrocities committed upon slaves in the Natchez area are recorded in many sources. A northern minister who had spent four years in the "southwest" wrote a letter from Natchez in 1833 describing terrible working conditions, brutal whippings, and even death at the hands of their masters (*American Slavery as It Is: Testimony of a Thousand Witnesses* [1839; New York: Arno Press and the *New York Times,* 1968], 107–8). J. C. Furnas reports an incident in Natchez where a slave was beaten to death with a nail embedded in a picket fence rail and at the inquest it was concluded he died of congestion of the brain (*Goodbye to Uncle Tom* [New York: William Sloane Associates, 1956], 128–29). The conversation between a planter and a new overseer reported by Fredrick Law Olmstead in 1856 captures a common attitude of planters toward their slaves (*The Cotton Kingdom: A Traveler's*

*Observations on Cotton and Slavery in the American Slave States, Based upon Three Former Volumes of Journeys and Investigations by the Same Author,* vol. 1, ed. Arthur M. Schlesinger [New York: Alfred A. Knopf, 1953], 93–94). The owner was explaining that he let his slaves take off a day if they claimed to be sick, even if he did not see definite evidence of their illness. "The overseer replied, 'It's my way, too, now; it didn't use to be, but I had a lesson. There was a nigger one day at Mr. ____'s who was sulky and complaining; he said he couldn't work. I looked at his tongue and it was right clean, and I thought it was nothing but damned sulkiness so I paddled him, and made him go to work; but two days after, he was underground . . . a good eight hundred dollar nigger, and it was a lesson to me about taming possums, that I ain't agoing to forget in a hurry.'" Doris Clayton James (*Antebellum Natchez,* 173) discusses the percentage of the population that was slave and the anxiousness of the owners to control them without incident.

13. William Ransom Hogan and Edwin Adams Davis, eds., *William Johnson's Natchez: The Diary of a Free Negro* (Baton Rouge: Louisiana State University Press, 1951), 345–46.
14. *Natchez Courier,* 20 June 1851.
15. The value of the life of a slave was even less than the free Negro, as can be seen by an ad placed in the *Natchez Free Trader* on 12 February 1838: "Found—A NEGRO'S HEAD WAS PICKED UP ON THE RAIL-ROAD YESTERDAY, WHICH THE OWNER CAN HAVE BY CALLING AT THIS OFFICE AND PAYING FOR THE ADVERTISEMENT."
16. Histories of several families (the Barlands, the Lynchs, and the McCarys) headed by a white male with a black common-law wife are mentioned in the slide presentation for the Historic Natchez Foundation, by Miller, "Black History of Natchez." The McCarys and Barlands are also discussed in various places in William Johnson's diary (Hogan and Davis, *William Johnson's Natchez*). The Lynch family story is told in John Hope Franklin, ed., *Reminiscences of an Active Life: The Autobiography of John Roy Lynch* (Chicago: University of Chicago Press, 1970).
17. A description of the wealth and elegance of the Second Creek neighborhood during the time of the occupation by the Raileys can be found in *The Memento: Old and New Natchez 1700–1897,* vol. 1, rpt. (Natchez, Miss.: Myrtle Bank Publishers, 1984), 12–13.
18. Joseph Holt Ingraham, *The Southwest* (New York: Harper Brothers, 1835), 204.
19. Vernon Lane Wharton, *The Negro in Mississippi: 1865–1890* (Chapel Hill: University of North Carolina Press, 1947), 12.
20. Will Book D, Natchez Courthouse, 153.
21. The good treatment of slaves was apparently the norm in the households of James Railey and his relatives. An account of the freeing of the slaves of his brother-in-law, James Green of Adams County, after his death in 1832 and the role that Railey played as executor can be found in *The African Repository and Colonial Journal* 11, no. 8 (August 1835): 251–52. James Railey was a member of the Mississippi Colonization Society and an officer in the American Colonization Society (Charles Sackett Sydnor, *Slavery in Mississippi* [New York: D. Appleton-Century Co., 1933], 209). See also the unique attitude toward slaves of his nephew-in-law, James Green Carson, whom Railey left as

the executor of his Louisiana property (John O. Anderson, *Journal of Mississippi History* 17, no. 4 [October 1956]: 243–67).

22. James Wilford Garner analyzes the unimportance and lack of participation of Natchez in the Civil War (*Reconstruction in Mississippi* [Baton Rouge: Louisiana State University Press, 1968]). The *New York Times,* 11 July 1866, describes the exodus of planters from the Natchez area after the arrival of the federal army. See also William Charles Harris, *Presidential Reconstruction in Mississippi* (Baton Rouge: Louisiana State University Press, 1967). A personal account of Natchez just after the federal occupation shows how little physical force was needed in Natchez (Annie Harper, *Annie Harper's Journal* [Denton, Tex.: Flower Mound Printing Company, 1983]).
23. Wharton, *The Negro in Mississippi,* 37.
24. Ibid., 38.
25. An account of the conditions on the leased plantations around Natchez can be found in John Eaton, *Grant, Lincoln and the Freedmen, Reminiscences of the Civil War* (New York: Negro Universities Press, 1969), 157–62.

    The most comprehensive historical analysis of blacks during this time period in Mississippi history is presented in Wharton, *The Negro in Mississippi.* An interesting firsthand account of a northern journalist, who crossed the South observing the conditions and not only reported on but actually leased several plantations, can be found in Thomas W. Knox, *Camp-fire and Cotton-field: Southern Adventure in Time of War* (New York: Blelock and Company, 1865). Accounts of the conditions in Natchez were reported on a regular basis in *The National Freedman, A Monthly Journal of the National Freedman's Relief Association,* New York.
26. The "sickness, suffering and destitution" of the Natchez army camp in 1864 were reported by James E. Yeatman, *A Report on the Condition of the Freedmen of the Mississippi* (Saint Louis: Western Sanitary Commission Rooms, 1864), 12–13.
27. James Railey's last will and testament was probated in 1861, Will Book 3, probate box 126, Natchez Courthouse.
28. For a detailed description of the changes in land ownership and the persistence of the "slave holding elite," see Michael Wayne, *The Reshaping of Plantation Society: The Natchez District, 1860–1880* (Baton Rouge: Louisiana State University Press, 1983). Whitelaw Reid, in his travels after the end of the Civil War, observed the animosity toward those who would sell their property to Negroes (*After the War: A Southern Tour* [Cincinnati: Moore, Wilstack and Baldwin, 1866]): "In many portions of the Mississippi Valley the feeling against any ownership of the soil by the Negroes is so strong, that the man who would sell small tracts to them would be in actual personal danger. Every effort will be made to prevent Negroes from acquiring land, and even the renting of small tracts to them is held to be unpatriotic and unworthy of a good citizen" (464–65).

## CHAPTER TWO

1. Excellent descriptions of poor conditions in Mississippi for blacks in the early 1900s can be found in various biographies of Richard Wright. See, for example, Richard Macksey and Frank E. Moorer, eds., *Richard Wright: A Collection of Critical Essays* (Englewood

Cliffs, N.J.: Prentice-Hall, 1984); and Robert Felgar, *Richard Wright* (Boston: Twayne Publishers, 1980).
Natchez had its share of famous black politicians for the newly freed slaves to venerate, including Robert H. Wood, Hiram Rhodes Revels, and John R. Lynch. Robert H. Wood was elected mayor of Natchez, Mississippi, in 1871, winning by a 218-vote margin over his white opponent (George Alexander Sewell, *Mississippi Black History Makers* [Jackson: University of Mississippi Press, 1977], 90–91). He was apparently the only black man ever elected mayor of a city in Mississippi during Reconstruction (Wharton, *The Negro in Mississippi*, 167). Hiram Rhodes Revels was the first black to have served in the U.S. Senate. He settled in Natchez at the end of the Civil War and served in the Senate from February 1870 to March 1871. (See Harry A. Ploski and James Williams, eds., *The Negro Almanac: A Reference Work on the African American* [Detroit: GAR Research, Inc., 1971], 307–9; or Mrs. Charles C. Mosley Sr., *The Negro in Mississippi History* [Jackson, Miss.: Mrs. Charles C. Mosley, 1969], 61–62). John R. Lynch was the first black to preside over a national convention of the Republican Party. In 1869 he was elected to the Mississippi State Legislature. He was elected to Congress from 1873 to 1877 and again from 1881 to 1883 (See *The Negro Almanac*, 317; and Franklin, *Reminiscences of an Active Life*).

2. The descriptions of life at Oakland in this and the following pages are taken largely from interviews with Dr. Edward Craig Mazique and with Alice Boyd Burton (telephone interview with author, 11 December 1984), the daughter of Eddie's aunt Mary Mazique and her husband, James Boyd).
3. Alice Boyd Burton spent much of her early years at Oakland. Oakland still exists although in a somewhat altered state. Therefore, the physical layout of Oakland is taken from the interviews, visits to the site, and records of deeds from the Natchez Courthouse.
The central importance of the family for the Maziques' lifestyle, success, and security comes through in all the stories of Eddie's life in Mississippi. The Mazique family is not unique in the strength of its family life. Recent research has shown that the black family, contrary to the opinions of earlier historians of slavery, stood up well to the attempted undermining during the domination by white slaveholders (Herbert G. Guttman, *The Black Family in Slavery and Freedom, 1750–1925* [New York: Vintage Books, 1976]).
4. Bank loans for which property was mortgaged were recorded in the Deed Books at the Natchez Courthouse. The records show that Alex Mazique, as did most other farmers, frequently mortgaged his property, counting on the forthcoming crops to pay his bills. The story of the lost receipt is one that Grandpa Alex often repeated to Eddie.
5. Roger Williams was a missionary college located in Nashville, Tennessee.
6. Eddie's sister Maude Mazique (born 1904) was the first child of Alex Jr. and Addie Mazique. As the oldest girl, she acted much like a mother to the younger children. This chapter relies heavily on her description of life in Natchez in the early 1900s, where she kept house while the younger children attended Natchez College. Maude Mazique was interviewed numerous times in person and via the telephone from April 1984 to May 1995.
7. Frederick Law Olmstead (*A Journey in the Back Country* [London:

Sampson Low, Son and Co., 1860]) observed and described the depletion of the soil and the misuse of land north of Woodville (see pages 18 through 20). A more detailed description of crop and land problems can be found in Robert L. Brandfon (*Cotton Kingdom of the New South: A History of the Yazoo Mississippi Delta from Reconstruction to the Twentieth Century* (Cambridge, Mass.: Harvard University Press, 1967]), who described the all-time-low cotton crop yield of 1911 as .06 bales per acre. An observer after the Civil War noted that Mississippi land produced between one-half to one bale per acre (Charles Nordoff, *The Cotton States in the Spring and Summer of 1875* [New York: Appleton, 1876], 72).

8. Charles Wexler Jr. and his sister, Kay Wexler, are the children of Charles and Addie Wexler, and second cousins to Edward Craig Mazique on his mother's side of the family. Charlie especially remembers with vivid detail and a certain fondness his early years in Wildsville. They were not born until after Eddie left Wildsville and therefore their memories of Wildsville are of a later time. Charles Wexler, Kay Wexler, and Edward Craig Mazique, interviewed together by author, 20 February 1985.
9. Descriptions of Wildsville and Wexler family are from Charles Wexler, Kay Wexler, and Edward Craig Mazique, interviewed together by author, 20 February 1985.
10. Benjamin Mays in his autobiography (*Born to Rebel,* 22–23) described circumstances similar to those Eddie faced:
There wasn't much going for the Negro in the world in which I was born. The shades of darkness were falling fast upon and around him. The tides of the post-Reconstruction years were being turned deliberately and viciously against him. The ballot was being taken away. Segregation was being enacted into law. Lynching was widespread and vigorously defended. Injustice in the courts was taken for granted whenever a Negro was involved with a white man. . . . When my parents admonished their children, "Be careful and stay out of trouble," they had only one thing in mind: "Stay out of trouble with white people!" My parents were no more cautious or fearful than others; virtually all Negro parents tried in some way to protect their children from the ever present menace of white violence.
11. Julius Rosenwald was a wealthy U.S. merchant and philanthropist. From 1910 to 1925 he served as president of Sears, Roebuck & Company and then moved on to be the chairman of its board. He took a strong interest in black Americans and in 1917 established the Julius Rosenwald Fund to "better the conditions of the Negro through education." The fund succeeded in establishing more than five thousand schools for blacks in the southern states. Rosenwald grants accounted for 15 percent of the money spent on school construction for African-Americans between its inception and 1932.
12. The Reverend William Mazique (born 1910) was a second cousin to Edward Mazique. They grew up together and played together in the Maziques' Natchez home. Grandpa Alex Mazique was a brother to Reverend Mazique's grandfather. Reverend Mazique's comments in an interview conducted by Robert W. Wheeler, Natchez, Mississippi, May 1984, contributed greatly to a description of Dr. Mazique as a youngster and an understanding of what life was like for blacks growing up in Natchez. He very aptly said: "The one thing about Mississippi is there was some things you couldn't do and there was no pretending

that you could." He summed it up well when he said, "I don't think it was the worst place in the world, but it was bad enough." Both these thoughts have been incorporated into the narrative.

13. This lack of segregated neighborhoods was one of the points made by Reverend Stanton in an interview by Robert W. Wheeler, Natchez, Mississippi, May 1984.
14. Mrs. Evelyn Brannon (born 1897) lived across the street from the Maziques on Pine Street. She was the cleaning lady in the post office in Natchez. In Robert W. Wheeler's interview with her (Natchez, Mississippi, May 1984), she discussed the Maziques and described the way things were in Natchez during her early years.
15. Robert W. Wheeler, interview with Evelyn Brannon, Natchez, Mississippi, May 1984.
16. The high caliber of the white residents of Natchez came up in several interviews, including the one Robert W. Wheeler conducted with Michel Dumas (born 1910) in Natchez, Mississippi, May 1984. Michel, a pharmacist, owned a drugstore in Natchez for forty-four years. His father was Dr. Dumas, a well-known and highly respected black physician in Natchez, who practiced at the same time as Edward Mazique's uncle, Dr. James C. Mazique.
    In the Edith Wyatt Moore Collection (Armstrong Library, Natchez, Mississippi), the following statement by Ethel L. Fleming appears in a section entitled "Achievements and Social Conditions of Negroes of Natchez and Vicinity": "It was indeed fortunate for the Negroes of Natchez and vicinity that the highest type of white people settled here. That culture and refinement of the masters and mistresses is still reflected in the lives of the descendents of their slaves as well as in the descendents of the free Negroes who lived here."
17. Working for a laundry was also one of the jobs that novelist Richard Wright held during his youth. Richard Wright, *Blackboy: A Record of Childhood and Youth* (New York: Harper and Brothers, 1945), 73.
18. Maude Mazique, interview with author, Washington, D.C., 23 May 1984.
19. These descriptions of Eddie and Douglas were taken largely from Robert W. Wheeler's interviews with the Reverend William Mazique and with Ms. Janie Haynes, Natchez, Mississippi, May 1984. Ms. Haynes, a friend of the Maziques in school, later became a schoolteacher in Natchez.
20. C. N. McCormick, ed., *Natchez, Mississippi: On Top, Not "Under the Hill"* (Natchez, Mississippi: Daily Democrat Steam Print, 1897).

## CHAPTER THREE

1. The "specialness" of Morehouse and its alumni is a tradition that carries on today. See for example Jacqueline Trescott, "The Men and Mystique of Morehouse," *Washington Post,* 9 November 1987, B-1, B-10; and William Douglas, "Men of 'The House,'" *Atlanta Journal/Atlanta Constitution,* 4 December 1983, 1-F, 7-F.
2. Comprehensive histories of Morehouse including descriptions of the campus and the origins of the college are provided by Benjamin Brawley, *History of Morehouse College* (College Park, Md.: McGrath Publishing, 1970); and Edward A. Jones, *A Candle in the Dark: A History of Morehouse College* (Valley Forge, Pa.: Judson Press, 1967). These descriptions were used to supplement those given in interviews with Dr. Edward C. Mazique and in Dr. Hugh

Gloster's telephone interview with author, 15 June 1985.

3. The statistics on the number of high schools in the South can be found in Herbert Aptheker, *Afro-American History: The Modern Era* (Secaucus, N.J.: Citadel Press, 1971), 175–76. Aptheker includes D.C. and West Virginia in these figures.
4. An excellent analysis of the Niagara Movement can be found in Aptheker, *Afro-American History,* 127–58.
5. W. E. B. Dubois, "Address to the Country," Harper's Ferry, West Virginia, 1906. Quoted in Herbert Aptheker, ed., *A Documentary History of the Negro People in the United States,* vol. 2 (Citadel Press: New York, 1968), 908–9.
6. Similar John Hope quotations can be found in Jones, *A Candle in the Dark,* 131; and Ridgely Torrence, *The Story of John Hope* (New York: Macmillan Co., 1948), 188.
7. Jones, *A Candle in the Dark,* gives a description of the problems Morehouse faced with enrollments and salaries.
8. Benjamin E. Mays, reprinted, *The Morehouse Alumnus,* July 1965, 56.
9. The Barnes incident is reported in Torrence, *The Story of John Hope,* 284–85; and Jones, *A Candle in the Dark,* 110.
10. The Hubert incident is reported in Torrence, *The Story of John Hope,* 318–20; and Jones, *A Candle in the Dark,* 110.
11. The description of this event was taken from a telephone interview by the author with Dr. Hugh Gloster, 15 June 1985.
12. This anecdote was also reported by Jones, *A Candle in the Dark,* 124.
13. The conservative tenor of Morehouse during the 1920s was mentioned in author interviews with Dr. Edward Mazique and Dr. Hugh Gloster. Dr. Hugh Gloster noted in his interview that scholars such as J. Saunders Redding, later of Cornell University, was among those who left because he disagreed with the conservative tendencies of Morehouse.
14. The observations of the Hon. George Crockett were made during a telephone interview with author, 15 June 1985.
15. Howard W. Thurman was known as a great religious orator and educator. He retired in 1965 as the dean of the chapel at Boston University after more than a decade of service. He was also the dean of the chapel at Howard University. His biography was published in 1964: Elizabeth Yates, *Howard Thurman: A Portrait of a Practical Dreamer* (New York: John Day Co., 1964).
16. From an interview Robert W. Wheeler conducted with Mildred Burch, 23 May 1984.
17. George Crockett, telephone interview with author, 15 June 1985. Eddie made such an impression on Morehouse that it was not long after his becoming a doctor that the faculty at Morehouse turned him into a role model for other students. Reverend Jerry Moore, a D.C. city councilman and friend, remembers his days at Morehouse: "He [Eddie] was already a practicing physician and I was made aware of his presence and the work he was doing before I came here [D.C.] by the vice president of Morehouse College, a Dr. C. D. Hubert, who used him as a role model for all those of us who were there in school. He did that through speeches he made and called our attention to what he thought were outstanding personalities who graduated from Morehouse" (Reverend Jerry Moore, interview with author, December 1985).

    Eddie used to have a recruiting poster for Morehouse hanging in his office. It included photos of Martin Luther King Jr., Donn Clendenon, and Eddie, among others. Its theme was "these are Morehouse Men, wouldn't you like to be one of them?"

18. The *Atlanta Daily World* was founded by William A. Scott Jr., who was a 1925 graduate of Morehouse. It was the first Negro daily newspaper.
19. Florence Read's relationship with John Hope and her position at Atlanta University are taken from Torrence, *The Story of John Hope,* 354.
20. The following discussion of the life of Colley Rakestraw Bond was taken from an interview with author, 23 February 1985.

## CHAPTER FOUR

1. Much of the historical discussion of the position of blacks in Washington, D.C., on the following pages, is based on the excellent work by Green, *Secret City.*
2. In 1867, one-fifth of the real estate owners in the District were black. The statistics on the property owned by blacks in Washington are taken from Edward Ingle, *The Negro in the District of Columbia* (Baltimore: Johns Hopkins Press, 1893, 105; Reprint, Freeport, N.Y.: Books for Libraries Press, 1971).
3. For a discussion of the January 1870 antidiscrimination law, see Green, *Secret City,* 96. See also Ingle, *The Negro in the District of Columbia,* 130–33. There is an interesting discussion on the removal of the word white from the District Charter by Edward Ingle on pages 159–60. Legislation for suffrage for black males in the District passed the Congress in 1866 even though in nine loyal states (California, Connecticut, Illinois, Indiana, Iowa, Kansas, Ohio, Pennsylvania, and New Jersey) the right of suffrage was granted only to white males. See a discussion of this issue in Ingle, *The Negro in the District of Columbia,* on pages 156–59.
   Education appears to have always been an important consideration for blacks in the District. In a *Special Report by the Commissioner of Education* in 1871, it was concluded that "it is worthy of observation, also, that in no case has a colored school ever failed for the want of scholars. The parents were always glad to send their children, and the children were always ready to go, even when too poor to be decently fed or clothed. When a school failed it was for want of money, and not for want of appreciation of the benefits of education" (116).
   For a complete discussion of the issues surrounding the 1869 denial of membership to black physicians and the ensuing challenge to the charter through Congress, see W. Montague Cobb, *The First Negro Medical Society* (Washington, D.C.: Associated Publishers, 1939), 11–20. For discussion of this and the 1891 votes on the admission of blacks to the Medical Society of the District, see Ingle, *The Negro in the District of Columbia,* 135–39.
4. For history of the Medico-Chirurgical Society, see Cobb, *First Negro Medical Society.*
5. Green, *Secret City,* 163.
6. In an interview with the author, 27 February 1985, Reverend Albion Ferrell spoke of the Wilson years: "Perhaps the vestiges of segregation and whatnot that people were experiencing in the forties and fifties were really a relic of Woodrow Wilson's presidency. Woodrow Wilson, I think, more than any other president in a hundred years, set back racial progress. It was Woodrow Wilson who practically

segregated the federal government services and made that segregation as official as the government could make it."

7. The discussion of the incident at the House Office Building is in Green, *Secret City,* 167.
8. Membership statistics on the NAACP are taken from Green, *Secret City,* 181.
9. A discussion of the places where segregation did not hold is on page 201 of Green, *Secret City.*
10. According to Green, *Secret City,* 231, 90 percent of blacks held custodial jobs with a top annual pay rate of $1,260; only 9.5 percent held clerical jobs and only forty-seven black men had sub-professional positions. For a more detailed discussion of the Civilian Conservation Corps and U.S. Employment Services practices, see Green, *Secret City,* 232.
11. A more in-depth discussion of the boycotts can be found in Green, *Secret City,* 228–29.
12. The information on Dr. Hildrus A. Poindexter was taken from an interview with the author, Washington, D.C., 27 February 1985.
13. The information about Dr. Paul B. Cornely's reaction to Washington was taken from an interview with the author, Washington, D.C., 25 February 1985.
14. Much of the information on Howard University is taken from Rayford W. Logan, *Howard University: The First Hundred Years, 1867–1967* (New York: New York University Press, 1968).
15. Ibid., 251.
16. Dr. Paul B. Cornely's remembrances of Dr. Mordecai Johnson were taken from an interview with the author, Washington, D.C., 25 February 1985.
17. The discussion of the contribution of Dr. Numa P. G. Adams to the medical school was largely taken from author interviews with Drs. Cornely (Washington, D.C., 25 February 1985) and Joseph L. Johnson (Washington, D.C., 19 February 1985).
18. The figure on the percentage of Negro physicians and surgeons was taken from *Howard University Bulletin,* 1941, 29.
19. The description of Eddie as a student is a composite from author interviews in Washington, D.C., with Eddie's former professors: Drs. Paul Cornely, 25 February 1985; Halston Eagleson, 19 February 1985; Joseph L. Johnson, 19 February 1985; Hildrus A. Poindexter, 27 February 1985; and M. Wharton Young, 22 February 1985.
20. Dr. Hildrus A. Poindexter, interview with author, Washington, D.C., 27 February 1985.
21. Dr. Paul Cornely, interview with author, Washington, D.C., 25 February 1985.
22. Much of the description of what Eddie did in the bookstore was taken from an author interview with Dr. Joseph L. Johnson, Washington, D.C., 19 February 1985.
23. The discussion of the relationship between Howard University and Freedmen's Hospital is taken from Logan, *Howard University,* 40–41 and 372–74.
24. The details on the time Maude Mazique spent in Washington were taken from interviews she did with the author from May 1984 through May 1995.
25. When talking about Eddie's role as a doctor, the people interviewed were unanimous in praising his diagnostic abilities, his love for his

patients, and the way he gave each one his full attention. Architect John Sulton said, "Most of the time, if you have an illness and you go to Dr. Mazique, you wonder whether you should have come because you feel better as soon as you start talking to him" (John Sulton, interview with author, 21 February 1985). Washington, D.C., radio personality Lucille Banks Robinson Miller expressed it this way: "His office is always crowded, to no end. He doesn't have to give much medicine because he gives so much love. He specializes with the senior citizens and they want the love which so many of the doctors don't give" (Lucille Banks Robinson Miller, interview with author, 21 February 1985). Larry Williams, a lawyer and friend of Eddie's nephew Emory, described his abilities this way: "Aside from treating the physiological, he is a master at treating the mental. Without being called a psychologist or psychiatrist, he is probably more effective than 50 percent of the psychiatrists out here practicing today. Just because of his mannerism and the way he does it, his ability to diagnose. He can distinguish between people who have emotional upsets, people who have psychosomatic problems, or people who have physiological problems" (Larry Williams, interview with author, 26 February 1985). Emmie Perkins, a registered nurse, also emphasized that it did not matter to Dr. Mazique if people paid or not: "He always takes time with his patient. Even if they no longer were his patients, if they came under the hospital staff, he would still come and visit them every day. And nobody knew that you were not paying . . . and he took as much time with them as if they were paying" (Emmie Perkins, interview with author, 22 February 1985).

26. The incident between Dr. Mazique and Mrs. Emmie W. Perkins was taken from an interview Mrs. Perkins had with the author, Washington, D.C., 22 February 1985.
27. For interesting discussions of the history of Highland Beach, see "Anne Arundel County Records Uncover Second Mazique Home," *Washington Afro-American,* 19 March 1968, 7; and Deborah Johns Moir, "Highland Beach: A Rich Past with a History Built on a Snub," in "Black History: Historical Sites in Maryland," *Baltimore Sun/Evening Sun,* 13 February 1989, 10.
28. Dr. Herman Stamps, telephone conversation with author, 16 December 1985.

## CHAPTER FIVE

1. Details of the conditions in the District of Columbia in the 1940s through the 1960s are given in Green, *Secret City.*
2. This was the way in which Eddie's professor of anatomy, M. Wharton Young, ended up going to Howard University Medical School. He lived in Missouri, and rather than have to accommodate him in a university there, the state paid for him to attend Howard. As he stated in his interview with the author (Washington, D.C., 22 February 1985), "They said, 'If you would go somewhere else and get out of our face, we will pay your tuition.'"
   The *Missouri ex rel. Gaines v. Canada* case is discussed by Genna Rae McNeil, *Groundwork: Charles Hamilton Houston and the Struggle for Civil Rights* (Philadelphia: University of Pennsylvania Press, 1983).
3. See McNeil, *Groundwork,* 178–84, for discussion of *Hurd v. Hodge.* For further discussion of how his private practice was hindered by

his volunteer work, see McNeil, *Groundwork*, 147–48. William Houston, Charles's father, chided him, saying he spent "all his time 'saving the race' instead of building a private practice and saving money" (ibid., 148).

4. The American Federation of Labor (AFL) and the Congress of Industrial Organizations (CIO) merged in 1955, forming a stronger lobbying unit.
5. Henry Agrad Wallace (1888–1965) was secretary of agriculture during the first two Franklin Delano Roosevelt administrations (1932–1940). In 1940, he was elected vice president and served in this capacity during Roosevelt's third term.
6. Dr. Peter Marshall Murray, on June 27, 1950, was the first Negro elected to the House of Delegates of the American Medical Association. He was a member of the Board of Trustees of Howard University from 1926 to 1951. See Logan, *Howard University*, 309–10. He was also the first doctor to be granted privileges in a white hospital in New York (ibid., 243). Upon his retirement from the House of Delegates of the AMA., he stated, "While I retire from the House, I shall not retire from the fight. I'll be found on the frontline trenches fighting for the ideals of the A.M.A." (Rayford W. Logan and Michael R. Winston, eds., *Dictionary of American Negro Biography* [New York: W. W. Norton and Co., 1982], 466). One of the areas in which he fought the hardest was integration of the health care system.
7. From an author interview with Cleopatra Charlotte Walton, Washington, D.C., 19 February 1985.
8. Samuel Foggie, interview with author, 16 July 1985.
9. The observation that he paid attention to the needs of his patients instead of medicating them was made by his long-time nurse, Alma Carter, in an interview with the author, Washington, D.C., 12 December 1985.
10. Hattie Key, interview with Robert W. Wheeler, Washington, D.C., 23 May 1984.
11. Many of his patients that were interviewed stated how much better they felt when Dr. Mazique simply spoke kind and loving words to them. All his patients indicated they waited for a long time to see him but once it was their turn, they never felt rushed or slighted. Both of these points were mentioned in an interview with Hattie Key conducted by Robert W. Wheeler, Washington, D.C., 23 May 1984, and by Ruby VanCroft in an interview conducted with the author, Washington, D.C., 19 July 1985.
12. Dick Gregory, telephone interview with author, 22 June 1993.
13. Alma Carter, in an interview with the author, commented on the lines at the Riggs Street office, Washington, D.C., 13 December 1985.
14. The account of the treatment of Mr. Hawkins's mother by Dr. Mazique is taken from a document prepared by Mr. Hawkins for the author about his experiences with Dr. Mazique, 20 February 1985.
15. Articles about the Maziques' social life include "Ruth Shipley . . . Chats About . . . D.C.-Baltimore," *Courier*, Washington edition, 45, no. 52 (25 December 1954): 9. Their 1956 reception received widespread publicity, including a description in the "City Life" section of the *Washington Post*, "Yule Party: Two Ambassadors Are Honorees at Supper," 24 December 1956. It was also reported in Lula Jones Garrett, "Dr. and Mrs. Mazique hosts to diplomatic reception,"

*Washington Afro-American,* 29 December 1956, 7. Magazine articles and photographs included *Jet* ("D.C. Society Couple to Present Diplomats," 9, no. 8 [27 December 1956]: 3); *Medicannales* (2, no. 3 [April 1957]); and *Hue* ("Capital Party for Civil Rights Fighters," August 1957, 50–54).

Jewell's articles dealt with such issues as the United Nations' position on freedom for the African nations ("'Freedom for whom?' Real Issue in UN Fight between World Powers," *Washington Afro-American,* 1 October 1960) and a criticism of the education of blacks in the D.C. public school system ("Education—Trends and Development," *Capital Spotlight* 5 May 1961, 2, 8).

Jewell was cited on the AFRO honor roll as a champion for human rights (see "Six Men, Four Women on Honor Roll for '55," *Washington Afro-American,* 31 March 1956; and "Mrs. Hildebrand, 10 Others Honored at Awards Tea, Sunday," *Washington Afro-American,* 19 May 1956).

16. Ralph Matthews, "Jewel Mazique—Ambassador," *Washington Afro-American,* 22 March 1958.
17. The figures on the numbers of professionals are taken from Green, *Secret City,* 250.
18. *New York Times,* 3 February 1948.
19. For a discussion of Truman's initiative, see Green, *Secret City,* 285–86.
20. Green, *Secret City,* 294.
21. "Donahue Sees End of Segregation Here," *Washington Evening Star,* 7 December 1952, A-1. Donohue's comments on Eisenhower were reported in "Authority to End D.C. Segregation Forecast for Eisenhower," *Washington Evening Star,* 9 December 1952, A-2. His beliefs about the school system were reported in "Donohue Says Dual Schools Cost D.C. $5 Million Yearly," *Washington Post,* 9 December 1952, 20.
22. A discussion of the desegregation battle with the Capital City Transit Authority can be found in Green, *Secret City,* 255–60.
23. For a discussion of the differences between Truman and Wallace, see Leonard Dinnerstein, "The Progressive and States' Rights Parties of 1948," in *History of U.S. Political Parties,* vol. 4, *1945–1972, The Politics of Change,* ed. Arthur M. Schlesinger Jr. (New York: Chelsea House Publishers, 1973), 3309–29.
24. See account of McCarthyism in Seymour J. Mandlebaum, *The Social Setting of Intolerance: The Know-Nothings, the Red Scare, and McCarthyism* (Chicago: Scott, Foresman and Co., 1964), 117–76.
25. *Hearings Regarding Communist Infiltration of Labor Unions, Part I* (Washington, D.C.: U.S. Government Printing Office, 1949), 667.
26. *Daily Worker,* 26 April 1949.
27. For a statement of the purpose of the hearings, see *Hearings Regarding Communist Infiltration of Minority Groups, Part I* (Washington, D.C.: U.S. Government Printing Office, 1949), 482.
28. Ibid., 426.
29. For more detail, see the Stokes discussion in ibid., 426, 428.
30. Ibid., 481.
31. In a filmed interview conducted by Dr. William A. Elwood of the University of Virginia, Dr. Mazique elaborated on Charles Houston's laughing about the situation: "He laughed. I never see Charlie laugh much and he was a man short on humor, but one who could recognize

it would play. He knew how to capture any type of inference and how to magnify it. So that it made you feel at ease in the minute he done laughed heartily and said, 'We gonna have fun!'" From page 499 of the transcription of the Edward C. Mazique interview for *The Road to Brown,* a film documentary on the campaign leading to the *Brown v. Board of Education* Supreme Court decision.

32. The account of Dr. Mazique's accompaniment of Henrietta Houston to New York is taken from ibid., 498.
33. Ibid., 497.
34. It was not until October 1954 that the Veteran's Administration declared an end to segregation in all of its hospitals. See Herbert M. Morais, *The History of the Afro-American in Medicine* (Cornwells Heights, Pa.: The Publisher's Agency, 1976), 142.
35. Elwood, *The Road to Brown,* 497.
36. McNeil, *Groundwork,* 193, 206–11, for an account of Charles Houston's death.
37. Excellent general descriptions of integrating the medical societies are given in Morais, *History of the Afro-American in Medicine;* and Dr. W. Montague Cobb, "The Nation's Capital," in *Negroes in Medicine,* by Carl Dietrich Reitzes (Cambridge, Mass.: Harvard University Press, 1958). These works are drawn upon heavily in this section.
38. Program for the "Fifth Annual Charles Sumner Lecture," 26 May 1949, inside cover, Dr. Edward C. Mazique papers.
39. "Memorial of the National Medical Society of the District of Columbia to the Congress of the United States," January 1870, reprinted in Morais, *The History of the Afro-American in Medicine,* appendix F, 220.
40. Morais, *History of the Afro-American in Medicine,* 134.
41. Cobb, "The Nation's Capital," 196.
42. See the discussion of hospital conditions for blacks in ibid., 197.
43. W. Montague Cobb, "The Ruhland Suggestion: Or Must Race Determine Health," *Bulletin of the Medico-Chirurgical Society of the District of Columbia* 6, no. 4 (April 1949): 3.
44. Ibid.
45. Ibid., 4.
46. Ibid., 3.
47. Accounts of the integration of Gallinger are given by Cobb, "The Nation's Capital," 215; and Morais, *History of the Afro-American in Medicine,* 152–53. See "Gallinger Calendar," *Bulletin of the Medico-Chirugical Society of the District of Columbia* 5, no. 3 (March 1948): 3–4 for an outline of the events leading to the integration.
48. Dr. Cobb's account can be found in Cobb, "The Nation's Capital," 215–17. Dr. Mazique's account is from an interview with the author.
49. "Medical Society Board Studies New Appeal by Colored Doctors," *Washington Star,* 1951, in Mazique papers, no page, no date.
50. See "Surprises Dr. Cobb: End of Race Ban by D.C. Medical Society Is Hailed," *Courier,* 3 February 1951, for an account of the decision of the Arlington Country Medical Society.
51. See the following articles with incomplete references from Dr. Mazique's files: "White Medics Vote to Drop Race Bar," 4 May 1952; and "D.C. Doctors Favor Admission of Negroes to Medical Society: Two-to-One Majority in Special Mail Ballot Indicates Sentiment; Action is Not Binding," 4 May 1951. See also "Mazique Seeks Society Membership: White Medicos Drop Color Bar," *Courier,* 5 June 1951;

and John McKelway, "Board Elects Five Negro Doctors to Medical Society," *Washington Star,* 25 September 1952.

52. A newspaper account of the event can be found in "Medical Group Panel Bars Non-Members," *Washington Evening Star,* morning edition, 17 April 1952.

53. The description of the voting and wording of the mandate are taken from accounts in "Doctors Defer Vote on Negro Members," *Washington Post,* 8 May 1952, sec. B, 2; and "D.C. Medical Society to Take New Poll on Negro Membership," *Washington Evening Star,* 8 May 1952.
Discussion of the applications pending can be found in "D.C. Medical Society Ends Racial Bars," *Times Herald,* 1 July 1952; "D.C. Medical Society Votes to Accept Negro Members," *Washington Post,* 16 July 1952; and "Dr. Cobb Cites 6-Year Battle of Med Group," *Washington Afro-American,* 8 July 1952, 22.

54. Accounts of the entry of the black physicians into the District Medical Society are contained in the following newspaper articles: "First in 60 Years: 5 Negro Physicians Admitted to District Medical Society," *Washington Post,* 25 September 1952; "First in Its History: Medical Society Here Accepts 5 Negro Doctors," *Washington Daily News,* 25 September 1952; "D.C. Medical Group Admits Five Negroes: First Members In 60 Years," *Times Herald,* 25 September 1952; and John McKelway, "Board Elects Five Negro Doctors to Medical Society: Are First to Be Admitted by Group Founded in 1817," *Washington Evening Star,* 25 September 1952.

55. Accounts of the incident with the Federation of Citizen's Associations can be found in "Negro Doctors Protest Citizens Federation Action," *Washington Evening Star,* Washington, D.C., 1 July 1953; and "Medical Group Quits Citizens' Federation: Resignation Asked After Acceptance of Negro Doctors," *Washington Sunday Star,* 19 April 1953, A-15.

## CHAPTER SIX

The epigraph is from Edward C. Mazique, *Final Report of the Interracial Practices Committee of the 12th Street YMCA to the Membership of the YMCA of Metropolitan Washington,* December 16, 1957.

1. The discussion in the following paragraphs of the plan to govern the District draws heavily on the account in Green, *Secret City,* 109–18.
2. Eddie served as a member of the Board of Directors of the Washington Home Rule Committee.
3. See account in "D.C. Advisory to Organize, Elect Today," *Washington Post,* 2 July 1952. Accounts of the new council members may be found in "New District Advisors Elect Fleming as Head After Taking Oaths," *Washington Evening Star,* 2 July 1952, A-5; and Richard L. Lyons, "Fleming Heads Advisory Unit, Hints Sessions to be Closed," *Washington Post,* 3 July 1952, 23.
4. J. C. Turner's comments concerning Fleming are taken from an interview with the author, Washington, D.C., 26 February 1985.
5. Mr. Turner's comments concerning fluoridation are taken from an interview with the author, Washington, D.C., 26 February 1985. A discussion of the fluoridation issue may be found in Richard L. Lyons, "City Council Meets in Secret and Openly at First Session,"

*Washington Post,* 16 July 1952, 1, 13; "District's New Citizens' Council at Work: Fluoridation and Licenses Are First Projects," *Washington Evening Star,* 16 July 1952, A-21; and "Fluoridation Report Sees Health Aided," *Washington Post,* 9 August 1952, 13.

6. An account of the integration of the District restaurants may be found in Green, *Secret City,* 295–98.
7. Green, *Secret City,* 298.
8. The discussion of the trip to Gettysburg is taken from an author interview with Father Patrick Nagle, Washington, D.C., 19 February 1985.
9. A mention of Dr. Mazique's opening the meetings to the press can be found in Richard L. Lyons, "D.C. Council Bars Doors; It's Proper to Donohue," *Washington Post,* 13 September 1952, 13.
10. See "Citizens' Council Split on Removing Secrecy from Relief Records," *Washington Evening Star,* 14 November 1952, A-2.
11. "General Davis Gets Appointment to Advisory Group," *Washington Evening Star,* 9 December 1952, B-l.
12. "Honor Roll, 1952," *Washington Afro-American,* 7 February 1953, 15.
13. The 1945 study is reported in Morais, *History of the Afro-American in Medicine,* 141.
14. See the account of the integration of Hadley in Cobb, "The Nation's Capital," 218.
15. See accounts of the efforts of the NAACP to integrate the hospitals in Cobb, "The Nation's Capital," 219, 221; "NAACP in New Offensive: End of Segregation in All Hospitals Urged," *Washington Afro-American,* 18 July 1953, 1–2; "NAACP Asks End of Bias in Hospitals: Dr. Cobb Directs Local Unit in Nation-Wide Drive," *Washington Afro-American,* 18 July 1953, 1–2; "Hospital Bias Radio Topic," *Washington Afro-American,* 25 July 1953; and "Hospital Integration Meeting Here March 8," *Washington Afro-American,* Capital edition, 2 March 1957, 3.
16. For details of the 1954 NAACP campaign to integrate the hospitals, see "NAACP Urges End of Bias in D. C. Hospitals," *Capital Spotlight,* 24 June 1954, 1; and "Two Negro Doctors Added to Staff of Georgetown Hospital," *Washington Evening Star,* 23 September 1954.
17. "D.C. Branch NAACP Spotlights Racial Bias in D.C. Hospitals," *Capital Spotlight,* 24 June 1954, 2.
18. See the following articles on the breakthrough into the private hospitals: "Two Negro Doctors Added to Staff of Georgetown Hospital," *Washington Evening Star,* 23 September 1954; "2 Negroes Join Hospital Staff at Georgetown," *Washington Post and Times Herald,* 24 September 1954; "Dr. Mazique Named to Georgetown Staff," *Washington Afro-American,* Capital edition, 25 September 1954; "G.U., Providence Accept Negro Staff Doctors," *Catholic Standard,* 1 October 1954, 3; and "Patients May Be Admitted Next: D.C.; Hospital Barriers Shaking as Georgetown Accepts 2 Medicos," *Courier,* Washington edition, 2 October 1954.
19. "'A Quiet Transition,' 2 Hospitals Here Lower Race Bars," *Washington Daily News,* 23 September 1954.
20. Ibid.
21. The story about Sibley Hospital was mentioned in an interview conducted by the author with Dr. Mazique and also related by W. Montague Cobb in a newspaper article ("NAACP in New Offensive," 1).
22. George Meany was a labor leader who was elected secretary-treasurer of the AFL in 1939 and held that position until 1952, when he was

elected president. In 1955, when the AFL and CIO merged, he was elected head of the new federation without opposition, a job he held until 1979.

23. Jacqueline Trescott, "Mentor, Mover, Man of Medicine," *Washington Post,* 13 December 1981, K4.
24. The story of how patients brought pressure to bear on the administrators of the hospitals was related to the author in an interview in 1985. The person requested that it not be made public so the names and hospital have been omitted. The information is included in the manuscript because the author felt it was important to show there were people at many levels who played a background but not insignificant role in integrating the hospitals. Dr. Mazique always said, "That is the one who got me into ______ Hospital."
25. Dr. Spellman's comments on this page and the following pages are taken from a telephone interview with the author, 16 August 1991.
26. Dr. Spellman went on to become a well-known physician. When interviewed, he was the dean for medical services at Harvard University Medical School. He was the first black appointed by the District of Columbia Commission on Licensure to the local examining board in medicine and osteopathy since 1897 and only the second in the history of the city. He served as the dean of the Charles R. Drew Postgraduate Medical School of the University of California at Los Angeles and the director of the Kaiser Foundation Health Plan, Inc. and of Kaiser Foundation Hospitals. The information about Dr. Spellman's experiences at Providence Hospital is taken from a telephone interview with the author, 16 August 1991.
27. Information on the Consolidated Parents Group and the Medico-Chirurgical Society contribution may be found in "Doctor's Wives Send CPG Drive 'Over Top,'" *Courier,* 8 August 1953, 1, 4. For a more detailed description of the integration of the District school system, see Green, *Secret City,* 328–34.
28. A Lynn Williams column in the *Courier,* International, on 14 November 1961 ("Rough Going for Senator Eastland") refers to the incident of Woods E. Eastland's removal from Sidewell upon his father's learning of the enrollment of Edward Mazique. See also "Eastland Children Withdrawn from Sidwell School," *Washington Evening Star,* 10 October 1956; and Constance Daniels, "Potomac Parade: All Southerners Are Not Eastlands," *Washington Daily News,* 19 October 1956, 10.
29. The *Catholic Standard* of 27 January 1961 carried an article about Dr. Mazique's speech entitled "First Friday Men to Hear Dr. Mazique." The article listed his many accomplishments in integrating the District Medical Society and the local hospitals. His speech was entitled "Citizens as Doctors" (delivered before The First Friday Club at the Presidential Arms, Friday, May 5, 1961, from Dr. Mazique's papers) and in conclusion stated: "It is impossible to separate the health needs of our Country from its socio-economic, educational and religious problems." This theme of the interrelationship between the different institutions of society was a common thread in his thinking and therefore was reflected in all his speeches.
30. Dr. Mitchell Wright Spellman, telephone conversation with author, 16 August 1991.
31. See Morais, *History of the Afro-American in Medicine,* 143–44; and W. Montague Cobb, "Medico-Chi at Ninety, 1884–1974," *Journal of the*

*National Medical Association* 66, no. 3 (May 1974): 257–58, for more detailed information on the Imhotep Conferences. For general references for the entire commentary on hospital integration, see Morais, *History of the Afro-American in Medicine*, 140–53; and a shorter summary by Cobb, "The Nation's Capital," 191–230.

32. Quoted in Morais, *History of the Afro-American in Medicine*, 144.
33. "'White Citizens Council' Is Organized Here," *Washington Evening Star*, 6 June 1956, A-22.
34. Information on the Anthony Bowen Branch YMCA is from the booklet for the *Anthony Bowen Young Men's Christian Association, Founder's Day Observance, One Hundred Twentieth Anniversary*, Friday March 2, 1973 (Washington, D.C.: Twelfth Street Christian Church).
35. Edward C. Mazique, *Final Report of the Interracial Practices Committee of the 12th Street YMCA to the Membership of the YMCA of Metropolitan Washington, December 16, 1957*, Dr. Mazique's papers, 3.
36. See account of appeal made to the YMCA in "Civic Leaders Appeal to UGF on YMCA Bias," *Washington Afro-American*, 29 December 1956, 6; and Constance Daniels, "Potomac Parade: 'Christian' Association Rejects," *Washington Gaily News*, 21 December 1956.

## CHAPTER SEVEN

The epigraph is from Edward C. Mazique "Doctors and Politics," *Journal of the National Medical Association* 52, no. 2 (March, 1960): 136.

1. The quotation and the voting information come from a written press release in Eddie's private papers apparently designed to promote a speech he was to give at the Capital Press Club. From the tone of the release and the look of the copy, it might have been written by Jewell.
2. For accounts of the event, see the following articles: "Medical, Social Problems Linked," *Milwaukee Sentinel*, 14 August 1958, part 2, 2; and "Hospital Race Bias Attacked by Doctor," *Milwaukee Journal*, 14 August 1958, part 2, 1.
3. The numbers are taken from Robert H. D'Arcy, "NMA Delays Ruling on Health Insurance," *Detroit News*, 14 August 1959, 35; and "Physicians' New Chief Sets Goals," *Detroit Free Press*, 14 August 1959, 9.
4. "In Annual Summer Confabs," *Jet*, 3 September 1959, 7.
5. Accounts can be found in "The Mayor and the Keys to the City: A Parable," *Journal of the National Medical Association* 52, no. 1 (January 1960): 55–56; Jack Pickering, "Negro Doctors Make Peace with Miriani," *Detroit Times*, 14 August 1959, 3; and "Medical Convention Sidelights," *Michigan Chronicle*, 22 August 1959, 1–2.
6. See Edward C. Mazique, "Integration Enters Medicine," *Journal of the National Medical Association* 51, no. 5 (1959): 381–87, for the complete speech.
7. Ibid., 385, 386, 385.
8. Articles that focused on the call for more black physicians and an end to segregation are, for example, Albert Washington, "Doctors Elect Mazique New President of NMA," *Washington Afro-American*, 18 August 1959, 8; Robert H. D'Arcy, "Negro Doctors Hail Detroit's Desegregation of TB Patients," *Detroit News*, 11 August 1959, 10; and "Aspiration with Lavage of Stomach Held Best Treatment of Salicylism," *Scope Weekly*, 26 August 1959, 1, 5.
   Among those articles focusing on Eddie's overall perspective were: Alice B. Dunnigan, "Dr. Mazique to National Medical Association.

New Prexy Tells Medics: 'Go Beyond Race Issue,'" *Pittsburgh Courier,* 22 August 1959; and "'Broaden Outlook,' Prexy Tells Medical Session," *Washington Afro-American,* 15 August 1959, 24. In Eddie's private papers.

9. "Physicians' New Chief Sets Goals," *Detroit Free Press,* 14 August 1959, 9. See also "NMA Head Backs Health Insurance," *Cleveland Plain Dealer,* 13 August 1958, 21; D'Arcy, "NMA Delays Ruling on Health Insurance," 35; "New NMA Head Urges Health Plan," *Washington Star,* 13 August 1959, D-6; and "Aspiration with Lavage of Stomach Held Best Treatment of Salicylism," 1, 5.
10. "NMA's President-Elect Supports Compulsory National Health Plan," *American Medical Association News,* 21 August 1959.
11. "Legislative Policy Urged for NMA," *American Medical Association News,* 7 September 1959.
12. "Group Head Upholds Forand-Type Coverage Plans," *Medical News: A Newspaper for Physicians,* 16 September 1959, 3.
13. Ibid. Eddie's frustration with the "determination of the popular press to ignore our constructive actions" was a theme repeated in many of his speeches. See, for example, Edward C. Mazique, "The Physician's Role in a Changing World or A Medical Strategy in the Atomic Age," a paper delivered to the Norfolk Medical Society, Norfolk, Virginia, 20 April 1960, where this quotation can be found on page 12.
14. Ibid., 3.
15. The discussion in this chapter of the various health care bills and the eventual institution of Medicare is largely taken from Sheri I. David, *With Dignity: The Search for Medicare and Medicaid* (Westport, Conn.: Greenwood Press, 1985). See "Health Bill Seen As Boon to Negro," *Chicago Defender,* 30 April 1949, 1, for a discussion of the Truman federal health insurance plan.
16. David, *With Dignity,* xii.
17. Ibid., 11.
18. U.S. Congress, House, Ways and Means Committee, *Hearings on HR4700,* 86th Cong., 1st sess., 284.
19. See David, *With Dignity,* 12 and 57. It is interesting to note that Eddie was arguing for the formation of a similar committee for the NMA in his "President's Column: Doctors and Politics," *Journal of the National Medical Association* 52, no. 2 (March 1960): 136 and 151.
20. See testimony in support of S.1606 in U.S. Congress, Senate Committee on Education and Labor, *A Bill to Provide for a National Health Program, Part 2, April 16, 17, 18, 19, 22, 23, and 24, 1946, 787–94;* and E. Franklin Frazier, ed., *The Integration of the Negro into American Society* (Washington, D.C.: Howard University Press, 1951). See specifically W. Montague Cobb, "Medicine," in Frazier, *The Integration of the Negro into American Society.*
21. See Montague Cobb's article, "What About Socialized Medicine?" *Chicago Defender,* 30 April 1949, 18–19. The full context of Whittier's address to the NMA can be found in C. Austin Whittier, "President's Address," *Journal of the National Medical Association* 41, no. 5 (September 1949): 229–30.
22. Quoted in Richard T. Ruetten and Donald R. McCoy, *Quest and Response: Minority Rights and the Truman Administration* (Lawrence: University Press of Kansas, 1973), 187.
23. See the account in "N.M.A. Past President Praises National Health

Insurance," *Journal of the National Medical Association* 51, no. 2 (March 1959): 148, for an expansion of Dr. Marshall's views. For more detail on the criticism of the Eisenhower plan by Dr. Cobb et al., see "Medics Hit Ike's Health Proposals," *Washington Afro-American,* Capital edition, 30 January 1954, 28.

24. See the account of the NMA decision to postpone a decision on health care in D'Arcy, "NMA Delays Ruling on Health Insurance," 35.
25. Ibid.
26. Mazique, "Integration Enters Medicine," 386.
27. Mazique, "The Physician's Role in a Changing World or a Medical Strategy in the Atomic Age."
28. Mazique, "Integration Enters Medicine," 386.
29. Ibid., 387.
30. Testimony given in *Hearings Before the Subcommittee on Obscene Literature of the Committee on Post Office and Civil Service of the House of Representatives, 19 May 19 1959, Washington, D.C.,* reprinted in "NMA Activities: Testimony at Congressional Hearings," *Journal of the National Medical Association* 51, no. 5 (September 1959): 409.
31. For a more in-depth discussion of Eddie's views on pornography, see Mazique, "Integration Enters Medicine," 387.
32. This refers to Dr. Paul Cornely, interview with author, Washington, D.C., 25 February 1985.
33. The travelogue was among personal papers given to the author by Edward C. Mazique. Eddie must have made a favorable impression when he was invited to the United Nations, for he was asked again in 1962 by the U.S. representative to the United Nations, Adlai Stevenson, to "learn more about the United Nations and our country's part in it, and to discuss these matters with senior United States officials on the spot." This is taken from a letter from Adlai E. Stevenson to Dr. Edward C. Mazique dated March 12, 1962, which was among the private papers. An account of the Michigan conference can be found in James Robinsin, "Experts Call for Broader Health Care," *Detroit Free Press,* 4 April 1960, 3.
34. Mazique, "The Physician's Role in Changing World," 10–11.
35. Copies of both testimonies are among the private papers given the author by Dr. Mazique: *Hearings on H.R. 10 Before the Senate Finance Committee, 17 June 1959,* reprinted in "NMA Activities: Testimony at Congressional Hearings," *Journal of the National Medical Association* 51, no. 5 (September 1959): 411; and Testimony given in *Hearings Before the Subcommittee on Obscene Literature,* 408–9.
36. See "Annual Interim Meeting," *Journal of the National Medical Association* 52, no. 3 (May 1960): 222–23. See also the article written by Edward C. Mazique, "NMA Backs Fleming: Health Hazards in Foods, Additives Create Legislative Protection Need," *Washington Afro-American,* 27 February 1960, 6.
37. "Annual Interim Meeting," *Journal of the National Medical Association* 52, no. 3 (May 1960): 223.
38. Edward C. Mazique, "Resolution on Chemicals Employed in Food Production and Processing, Resolution Number 1," Interim Meeting—Board of Trustees, National Medical Association, Pittsburgh, Pennsylvania, 8 February 1960, 4, Mazique papers.
39. These facts about the NMA resolution were reported by Eddie in Mazique, "The Physician's Role in Changing World," 8.

40. "NMA Votes Lobbying Unit and Plans Confab," *Pittsburgh Courier,* Southern edition, 20 February 1960, 26.
41. "Recommendations of the President to the Board of Trustees of the National Medical Association at its 65th Annual Convention," Pittsburgh, Pennsylvania, August 1960, 1–2, Mazique papers.
42. "NMA Votes Lobbying Unit," 26.
43. This discussion occurs on pages 7–9 of the address Dr. Mazique delivered in Chicago to the Cook County Medical Association on 27 January 1960. From Dr. Mazique's papers.
44. "NMA President's Testimony on Aid for the Aging. Statement of Dr. Edward C. Mazique," *Hearing Before the Sub-Committee on Problems of the Aging and the Aged of the United States Senate Committee on Labor and Public Welfare, April 12, 1960,* reprinted in *Journal of the National Medical Association* 52, no. 4 (1960): 313.
45. Ibid., 314.
46. Quoted in "Scudder Blood Controversy," *Journal of the National Medical Association* 52, no. 1 (January 1960): 56.
47. W. Montague Cobb, "Blood Transfusion and Race," *Journal of the National Medical Association* 52, no. 4 (July 1960): 281.
48. "Dr. Mazique Denounces Physicians' Recommendation to Separate Blood," reprinted in "Scudder Blood Controversy," 57–58.
49. "Statement of Seven Members of Columbia University Seminar on Genetics and the Evolution of Man," released 14 November 1959, reprinted in "Race and Blood Transfusion: 'Comments on Scudder Thesis,'" *Journal of the National Medical Association* 52, no. 4 (July 1960): 296.
50. For examples of the press coverage, see the following articles: William I. Laurence, "Science in Review," "New Procedure Advocated for Selection of Blood Types in Transfusion," *New York Times,* Sunday, 15 November 1959, sec. 4, 11; "Doctors Denounce Race Blood Theory," *Washington Afro-American,* 19 December 1959; "Mazique Rips into Scudder's Blood Theory," *Pittsburgh Courier,* 28 November 1959; "NMA Prexy Scores 'New Blood' Theory," *Washington Afro-American,* November 1959, 1, 2.; "Scuttling Dr. Scudder's Theory," *Washington Afro-American,* 17 November 1959; "Negro Physician Denounces Blood Theory as Racism," *Washington Star,* 14 November 1959 (this was an Associated Press story). The Arkansas decision was reported in the address Dr. Mazique delivered in Chicago to the Cook County Medical Association on 27 January 1960, 8. From Dr. Mazique's papers.
51. John Scudder and William D. Wigle, "Safer Transfusions Through Appreciation of Variants in Blood Group Antigens in Negro and White Blood Donors," *Journal of the National Medical Association* 52, no. 2 (March 1960): 75–80.
52. The debate was discussed by Eddie during a speech in April 1960. See Mazique, "The Physician's Role in Changing World," 7–8.
53. "Dr. Scudder Now Calls His Remarks on Blood Differences 'Unfortunate,'" *Washington Afro-American,* 30 April 1960, 24.
54. John Scudder, "Practical Concepts in Modern Medicine," *Journal of the National Medical Association* 52, no. 4 (July 1960): 266–77. This was a reprint of the Sixth Annual Charles R. Drew Memorial Lecture at the 48th Annual Meeting of the John A. Andrew Clinical Society, Tuskegee Institute, Alabama, April 23–29, 1960.

55. Cobb, "Blood Transfusion and Race," 282.
56. See the account in "Forand-Type Bill: Negro Doctor's Chief Backs Aid for Aged," *Pittsburgh Press,* 7 August 1960, sec. I, 11.
57. Edward C. Mazique, "Medical Dimensions in the Nuclear Age," Address of the Retiring President, Read at the 65th Annual Convention of the National Medical Association, Pittsburgh, Pennsylvania, August 8–11, 1960, reprinted in *Journal of the National Medical Association* 52, no. 5 (September 1960): 353.
58. Ibid., 358.
59. Edward C. Mazique, "A Package of Legislation for Support by the National Medical Association," 1, Mazique papers. The pieces of legislation listed and described were: a bill outlawing job discrimination for reasons of age; a bill establishing a Senior Citizens Service Training Program; federal grants for medical education; federal assistance for the expansion and construction of medical schools and research; the Keogh Bill for self-employed retirement personnel; a Social Security bill for doctors; mental health; and naturally medical care for the aged. The "package" detailed the present status of bills relating to these matters. Not all of these issues were discussed in the body of the text; only what I considered the most important aspects of his extensive interests were covered. Other issues that Eddie raised with the NMA that have not been discussed were outlined in his "Platform" (also found in Dr. Mazique's papers). These include pushing for Negro detailmen in all the major pharmaceutical houses, a physician placement bureau, and national health funds.
60. Mazique, "Medical Dimensions in Nuclear Age," 354.
61. For an account of Dr. Burney's remarks, see "Burney Addresses National Medical Association: Go Beyond Duties, Doctors Told," *Pittsburgh Post-Gazette and Sun-Telegraph,* 10 August 1960; and "Educators and Interpreters of Health," *National Medical Association Bulletin* 16 (October 1960): 1, 2.
62. "Doctor Lack Called Major U.S. Problem: Surgeon General Cites Need for More without Sacrificing Training Quality," *Pittsburgh Post-Gazette and Sun-Telegraph,* 12 August 1960.
63. For more discussion of Arthur Fleming's position change, see David, *With Dignity,* 49.
64. "NMA Meets in Pittsburgh: Mazique Takes a Strong Stand," *Physician's Forum News Letter* 8, no. 3 (November 1960): 3.
65. Discussion of Governor William's remarks is taken from "Excerpts from an Address by Governor G. Mennen Williams, Read at the 65th Annual Convention of the National Medical Association. Hotel Penn-Sheraton, Pittsburgh, Pennsylvania, 8–11 August 1960," copy among Eddie's private papers, which seems to be a copy of his entire prepared speech.

    It is interesting to note that under the Kennedy administration, G. Mennen Williams was appointed assistant secretary of state for African affairs, once again his interests and concerns dovetailing with Dr. Mazique's.
66. Williams, "Excerpts from an Address Read at the 65th Annual Convention of the National Medical Association."
67. James T. Aldrich, "President's Inaugural Address," read at the 65th Annual Convention of the National Medical Association. Hotel Penn-Sheraton, Pittsburgh, Pennsylvania, August 8–11, 1960, reprinted in

*Journal of the National Medical Association* 52, no. 5 (September 1960): 362.

68. Dr. Montague Cobb described the nature of the early attempts at lobbying by the National Physicians Committee for the Extension of Medical Care, a lobbying group for the AMA, in the following manner:
This group has cast a sad reflection upon the intelligence of the medical profession in the type of propaganda it seems to hold as being the proper level for doctors. This "Committee" has barraged the profession with crude cartoons and cheap vilification smearing national health legislation as communistic and dictatorial. It employed one Dan Gilbert, former associate of hate-mongers Dudley Pelley and Gerald Winrod and an acknowledged race-hating, labor-baiting anti-Semite. His recent letter to doctors throughout the country beginning, "Dear Christian American," has already become notorious. The N.P.C., a registered lobby, has spent over a million dollars in its activities against national health legislation.
Cobb, "What About Socialized Medicine?" 18.
The chairman of the Physician's Forum, Dr. Allan M. Butler, speaking about the AMA's stance against federal health legislation at a later date, was no less critical:
As physicians, we are distressed and ashamed that our principal professional organization should continue its anachronistic and unscientific opposition to the entire Federal social security system. The AMA has and can only resort to political generalities, which were discarded officially by the American people 23 years ago and are now forgotten except by the AMA and a fringe element unresponsive to current American political thought and structures.
Allan M. Butler, "From the Chairman . . . ," *Physician's Forum News Letter* 8, no. 3 (November 1960): 3.1.

69. Mazique, "Medical Dimensions in Nuclear Age," 359.

70. Aldrich, "President's Inaugural Address," 362.

71. The Physician's Forum was an association formed in the early forties by doctors who disagreed with the methods of the American Medical Association. It was comprised of about one thousand physicians, most of whom were associated with the prestigious teaching universities of the East and were well respected but never had the political clout of the AMA. Description of the Physician's Forum taken from David, *With Dignity,* 42.

72. "NMA Meets in Pittsburgh," 3.

73. "NMA Supports Forand-Type Care for Aged," *Medical News: A Newspaper for Physicians,* 31 August 1960, 1, 8.

74. Albert W. Bloom, "Negro Doctor Group Backs Aid for Aged: Convention Also Advocates Mission Be Sent to Congo," *Pittsburgh Post-Gazette and Sun-Telegraph,* 13 August 1960.

75. See the following for various accounts of the conference: "Dr. Aldrich of St. Louis Physician's New President: Community Action Gets Full Support," *Washington Afro-American,* 16 August 1960; and Bloom, "Negro Doctor Group Backs Aid for Aged: Convention Also Advocates Mission Be Sent to Congo."
See Lynn Williams, "NMA 'Conspicuously Silent' on Kennedy Plans: Why Are Negro Doctors Mum on Old Age Care?" *Pittsburgh Courier,* 12 August 1961, 24, for a description of what was done regarding the issue of health care at the 1960 NMA convention.

## CHAPTER EIGHT

The first epigraph is a quote from Edward Peeks, "Doctor Says U.S. Must Act on Health and Discrimination," *Washington Afro-American,* 3 December 1960. The second is from Mazique, "Integration Enters Medicine."

1. "Statement of Edward C. Mazique, M.D., Chairman of Delegation of Physicians of the National Medical to Eastern Europe," 17 September 1960, 1, Mazique papers.
2. Ibid., 1–2.
3. See A. G. Mezerik, ed., *U-2 and Open Skies* (New York: International Review Service, 1960) for an accurate outline of the U-2 incident; and David Wise and Thomas B. Ross, *The U-2 Affair* (New York: Random House, 1962) for a more detailed account.
4. From "Statement of Chairman Khrushchev Preliminary Summit 16 May 1960, USSR Press Release No. 223, Washington, D.C." Cited in Wise and Ross, *The U-2 Affair.*
5. Leroy R. Swift, "Medical Mission to Moscow," *Journal of the National Medical Association* 53, no. 4, (July 1961): 346–51.
6. Larry Still, interview with author, Washington, D.C., 22 February 1985.
7. Ibid.
8. Ibid.
9. Copies of two of Eddie's speeches were among his private papers: "Activities of the National Medical Association," delivered in Warsaw, Poland, September 1960; and "Speech Delivered in Prague, Czechoslovakia, Before the Trade Union of Medical Workers," 9 September 1960.
10. Larry Still, interview with author, Washington, D.C., 22 February 1985.
11. Ibid.
12. Ibid.
13. Ibid.
14. Ibid.
15. Ibid.
16. Ibid.
17. Both quotations contained in "Red-Bloc Medical Care Lauded by D.C. Doctor," *Washington Post,* 17 September 1960, A-8; and "D.C. Doctor Says Reds Lead in Medical Care," *Washington Star,* 17 September 1960. He further stated in the *Star* article that "Capitalist germs are the same as Communist germs. We were able to meet doctors there and talk on the same terms."
18. Ibid.
19. Ibid.
20. "Doctors Differ in Views on Soviet Medicine Gains," *Washington Sunday Star,* 2 October 1960, B-4.
21. Ibid.
22. Larry Still, interview with author, Washington, D.C., 22 February 1985.
23. Ibid.
24. See, for example, the following articles carried in the *Washington Afro-American,* Red Star edition: "Doctors' Trip Abroad Includes Soviet Visit," 16 August 1960; and "NMA Delegation Continues Medical Study Mission," 13 September 1960. See also "U.S. Doctors Visit Famous Heart Clinic," *Washington Afro-American,* 20 September 1960; "U.S. Doctors Spend 10 Days in Moscow," *Washington Afro-American,*

13 September 1960, 1, 2; "Doctors Visit Eastern Europe," *Chicago Defender,* 24 September 1960; and the notices that appeared in *Jet* in the "Medicine" section: "Russian Operation," 22 September 1960, 16; "Poland Asks NMAA Aid on Pre-Natal Clinics," 22 September 1960, 16; and "Medics in Moscow," 29 September 1960, 26.
Reports from Soviet publications did not play up the problems of black physicians in the United States. See for example: "American Doctors Meet Their Soviet Colleagues," *USSR,* January, 1961, 36–37. An Associated Press story from Moscow was titled "U.S. Doctor's Praise Quoted in Russia," *Washington Evening Star,* 30 August 1960, A-8. See also the two reports that appeared in the *New World Review:* "Negro Doctors Visit the Soviet Union," *New World Review,* September 1960, 27; and Murray Young, "West to East—East to West," *New World Review,* October 1960, 7.

25. "U. S. Doctor's Praise Quoted in Russia," *Washington Evening Star,* 30 August 1960, A-8.
26. "Negro Doctors Visit the Soviet Union," *New World Review,* September 1960, 27.
27. Wilbur Cohen was referred to by President John F. Kennedy as "Mr. Social Security." He was a staff member of the Committee on Economic Security (CES) that drafted President Roosevelt's Social Security proposal, which led to the passage of the Social Security Act of 1935. The first employee of the Social Security Board, he served as the chief liaison to Capitol Hill. During President Johnson's administration he was the secretary of HEW.
28. The following discussion of Medicare and Medicaid is based on the account in David, *With Dignity.*
29. Ibid., 42.
30. There is John F. Kennedy for President correspondence from October 3, 1960, among Dr. Mazique's personal papers.
31. *Capital Spotlight,* 26 August 1960.
32. Peeks, "Doctor Says U.S. Must Act on Health and Discrimination."
33. Ibid.
34. See "President's Viewpoint," *Medical Society of the District of Columbia News* 14, no. 12 (December 1981): 3, for a discussion of AMAPAC.
35. Material on the Bay Area Committee is taken from "San Francisco Doctor Who Fought AMA Stand on Medical Care Is Here to Lead Area Physicians," *Washington Post,* 16 July 1961, A-18.
36. Edward C. Mazique, "Statement by Edward C. Mazique, M.D., President, American Association for Social Psychiatry," before the Ways and Means Committee, U.S. House of Representatives, 4 August 1961, reprinted in *Journal of the National Medical Association* 53, no. 6 (September 1961): 652.
37. "NMA Seen 'Duped' in Health Plan Vote," *Washington Afro-American,* 19 August 1961.
38. Ted Poston, "Negro MDs Join Fight on Aid to Aged," *New York Post,* 11 August 1961, 7.
39. "NMA Seen 'Duped' in Health Plan Vote."
40. Ibid.
41. Ibid.
42. See, for example: Lynn Williams, "NMA 'Conspicuously Silent' on Kennedy Plans," *Pittsburgh Courier,* 12 August 1961, 24; and "Why Blindly Follow AMA?" *Washington Afro-American,* 15 August 1961, 4,

which show the support of the black press.

43. "Why Blindly Follow AMA?" 4.
44. See, for example: "NMA Fights Plan of 'Aid to Aged,'" *Washington Afro-American,* 15 August 1961, 1.
45. "National Medical Association Votes for MD Social Security," *Medical Tribune,* 28 August 1961.
46. "NMA Seen 'Duped' in Health Plan Vote."
47. "Afroamerican Doctors Join Fight on 'Aid to Aged,'" *Herald-Dispatch,* 17 August 1961.
48. Ethel L. Payne, "Medical Care Plan for Aged Stirs Community Controversy," *Washington Afro-American,* 12 August 1961.
49. Afroamerican Doctors Join Fight on 'Aid to Aged.'"
50. See for discussion of the sentiment of the delegates: Lynn William, "Mazique Opposes NMA's Stand Against Old Age Medical Care," *Pittsburgh Courier,* 26 August 1961, sec. 2, 5.
51. Larry Still, "What President's Medicare Means to Negroes," *Jet,* 14 June 1962, 16.
52. See chapter 6 in the present work for a discussion of the inception and purpose of the Imhotep Conferences. See Still, "What President's Medicare Means to Negroes," 16–19, for a discussion of the 1962 Imhotep Conference.
53. Still, "What President's Medicare Means to Negroes," 18.
54. Eddie's full testimony can be located in "Statement by Edward C. Mazique, M.D., Representative of the National Medical Association before the Interstate and Foreign Commerce Committee, U.S. House of Representatives, January 30, 1962," reprinted in *Journal of the National Medical Association* 54, no. 2 (March 1962): 270.
55. Edward C. Mazique, "Federal Legislation on Public Health and Welfare," *Bulletin of the National Medical Association,* April 1962, 4–5.
56. For accounts of the sixty-seventh annual convention, see: "NMA Revolts; Backs Medicare," *Chicago Defender,* 18–24 August 1962; "NMA Shifts Stand, Backs Health Plan," *Washington Post,* 18 August 1962, A-2; and "NMA Approves Social Security Plan, Ponders Other Details of Aid to Aged," *Chicago Sun-Times,* 18 August 1962, 26.
57. David, *With Dignity,* 99.
58. Marjorie Hunter, "Johnson Asserts He's 'Just Begun' Aged-Care Fight," *New York Times,* 16 January 1964, 15.
59. E. W. Kenworthy, "Civil Rights Bill Expected to Pass without Setback," *New York Times,* 2 February 1964, 1.
60. See National Medical Association testimony, "H.R. 3920," *Journal of the National Medical Association* 56 (1964): 213–21, for account of the 1964 testimony by the NMA president.
61. "Hearing Before the Committee on Finance United States Senate," 89th Congress, 1st sess. on HR 6675, part 1, April 29, 30 and May 3–7, 1965, 324.
62. "New Medical Complex Proposed," *Washington Post & Times-Star,* 11 August 1965, 13.
63. Mazique, "Integration Enters Medicine," 383.
64. Mazique, "Medical Dimensions in Nuclear Age," 358–59.
65. See for examples of the press coverage of Eddie's proposal of assistance to the Congo: "Negro Doctors' Chief Backs Aid for Aged," *Pittsburgh Press,* 7 August 1960, sec. 1, 11; Albert W. Bloom, "Negro Doctors Support Medical Care for Aged: National Group, in

Convention Here, Also Urges Mission Be Sent to Congo," *Pittsburgh Post-Gazette and Sun Telegraph,* 13 August 1960; "NMA Supports Forand-Type Care for Aged: U.S. Negro Physicians Urged for Congo," *Medical News,* 31 August 1960, 1, 8; and Werner Seims, "Negro Doctor Need Acute NMA Told: Federal Aid Urged by Retiring Head," *Pittsburgh Press,* 9 August 1960, sec. 2, 17.

See also the following articles where aid to the Congo received the headline over Eddie's suggestions on health care legislation: "Send Medical Mission to Africa, Dr. Mazique Urges," *Pittsburgh Courier,* 13 August 1960, sec. 2, 6; "Send Medical Mission to Africa, Dr. Mazique Urges," *Pittsburgh Courier,* 20 August 1960, magazine section, 4–5; and "Congo Aid Asked of Negro Doctors," *Washington Evening Star,* 9 August 1960, A-3.

For more detail, see Mazique, "Medical Dimensions in Nuclear Age," 359.

66. See "Medics Plan Aid in Africa," *Washington Afro-American,* Red Star edition, 13 September 1960, 3, for a discussion on the study commission.
67. See "Negro MDs, Dentists Will Tour Africa in 'Direct Participation' Plan of U.S.," *Medical Tribune,* 20 February 1961; and "On African Trip," *Pittsburgh Courier,* 26 August 1961, 4, for accounts of the trip.
68. National Committee For Ojike Memorial Medical Centre, Minutes of Meeting of November 9, 1962, Progress Report and Financial Statements for the Period July 1, 1962–June 30, 1963, sec. 2, 1, Mazique papers.
69. See A. Oyewole, "Ojike, Mazi Mbonu 1912–1956," in *Historical Dictionary of Nigeria* (Metuchen, N.J.: Scarecrow Press, 1987), 260. A more detailed account of the life of Ojike was found among Eddie's private papers in "Mazi Mbonu Ojike," which, apparently, was prepared for a fundraiser in 1964. See also Eddie's account in "The Ojike Nigerian Hospital Project," *Journal of the National Medical Association* 56, no. 1 (January 1964): 112–14.
70. Dr. Mazique made the tie-in with President Kennedy's "People to People" campaign at a press conference he called on December 15, 1961, to make the formal announcement of the U.S.-Nigerian Foundation For the Ojike Memorial Medical Center. Press release is among Mazique papers.
71. Edward C. Mazique, "Address at the Launching of the National Ojike Memorial Medical Center," Lagos, Nigeria, 11 August 1962, 2, Mazique papers.
72. Mazique, "The Ojike Nigerian Hospital Project," 113. An Irish doctor who had worked in Nigeria in the late 1950s noted that one out of every two children born in Nigeria would die before he or she reached adult life, often suffering great agony as he or she died. See Robert Collis, *African Encounter: A Doctor in Nigeria* (New York: Charles Scribner's Sons, 1961), 193.

Summary accounts of the hospital's progress are included in several documents in Dr. Mazique's papers: an attachment to a letter from K. Ozuomba Mbadiwe to Dr. Edward C. Mazique, dated 26 August, 1963, entitled "A Historical Sketch of the U.S.-Nigerian Foundation For the Ojike Memorial Medical Center Inc. Up To August 19, 1963" and "National Committee for Ojike Memorial Medical Centre,

Minutes of Meeting of November 9, 1962, Progress Report and Financial Statements for the Period July 1, 1962–June 30, 1963."

73. Eddie's files on Ojike contain letters of acceptance for board membership from Martin Luther King Jr., Benjamin Mays, and Thomas Kilgore Jr.
74. Thomas A. Dooley was an American physician who became famous for his medical missionary work in Southeast Asia. MEDICO was organized to sponsor his Asian hospitals and to bring medical care to less developed nations. It ended in 1961 with Dr. Dooley's death at age thirty-four.
75. "Recommendations of the President," 8 August 1965, 3, Mazique papers.
76. Copy of letter from Mr. Robert I. Fleming to Mr. Juan Trippe, 7 October 1963, Mazique papers.
77. "Recommendations of the President," 3.
78. The state of the hospital in 1974 is taken from a letter from Dr. K. O. Mbadiwe and Dr. Edward C. Mazique to All Board Members, U.S. Nigerian Foundation For Ojike Memorial Medical Center, September 30, 1974. Among Dr. Mazique's papers. Information on the dissolution of the foundation is taken from a letter from Juan T. Trippe to Dr. Edward C. Mazique, September 23, 1974. Dr. Mazique and Dr. Mbadiwe's stand on the dissolution is taken from a letter from Dr. K. O. Mbadiwe and Dr. Edward C. Mazique to All Board Members, U.S. Nigerian Foundation For Ojike Memorial Medical Center, September 30, 1974. These were among the Mazique papers.
79. Dr. K. O. Mbadiwe to Edward C. Mazique, 15 July 1982, Mazique papers.

## CHAPTER NINE

1. A massive amount of public documentation exists about the Mazique divorce. Much of the detail has been left out of this chapter because it was not relevant to the main focus of the biography. The actual transcript from the trial in the District of Columbia Court of General Sessions, Domestic Relations, had been routinely deleted by the time I did my research, but the complete record of the appeals was available. Most of the documents from the original trial were submitted for the appeal and the entire proceedings (289 pages) were available on microfiche at the Superior Court of the District of Columbia, Washington, D.C. More details are available in the following publications: "Physician Wins Divorce, But Wife Plans to Appeal," *Washington Afro-American,* 5 September 1964, 1, 2; "Famed D.C. Medic, Mazique, Wins Hot Divorce Battle," *Jet,* September 1964, 23; "Mazique Divorce Case Near End, Appeal Tues.," *Washington Afro-American,* 27 November 1965, 1; "Mrs. Mazique Asks New Divorce Appeal," *Washington Afro-American,* 13 February 1965; and "Supreme Court Action Closes Mazique Case," *Washington-Afro American,* 25 June 1966, 2.
2. Jacqueline Trescott, "Mentor, Mover, Man of Medicine," *Washington Post,* 13 December 1981, K-4, 5.
3. Ruby VanCroft, interview with author, Washington, D.C., 19 July 1985.
4. "Fashion Show Picketed Because of Dr. Mazique," *Washington Afro-American,* 25 February 1964.

5. Ibid.
6. Maude Mazique, personal diary, 28 February 1964, 38.
7. The article about which Mrs. Dawson complained was "Mrs. Belafonte's Show Protested," *Washington Afro-American,* Blue Star edition, 22 February 1964, 1.
8. "Protest Against Story," *Washington Afro-American,* 29 February 1964.
9. The paragraph referring to Eddie's relationship with Dr. E. Y. Williams is taken from an interview of Dr. Williams by the author, Washington, D.C., 20 February 1985.
10. Both of Dr. Mazique's sons, Edward H. Mazique and Jeffrey Mazique, became prominent physicians.
11. All microfiche references in the following citations are from documents filed for the appeal with the Superior Court of the District of Columbia, Washington, D.C. Judgment of Absolute Divorce, Civil Action Number D 2502–63, microfiche no. 0019 0770, 0773.
12. District of Columbia Court of Appeals, No. 3615, *Jewell R. Mazique, Appelant v. Edward C. Mazique, Appellee,* Appeal from the District of Columbia Court of General Sessions (Argued December 21, 1964 Decided January 26, 1965), Jewell R. Mazique pro se, Charles K. Brown Jr. for Appellee before Hood, Chief Judge, and Quinn and Myers Associate Judges, microfiche no. 0019 0826.
13. "Political Pressures Charged in Mazique Divorce Appeal," *Washington Afro-American,* 4 December 1965, 14.
14. "Seek Review of Judge's Verdict in Mazique Case," *Pittsburgh Courier,* 21 May 1966, 1.
15. Discussion of the response from women after Eddie's divorce is taken from an author interview with Alma Carter, Washington, D.C., 12 December 1985.
16. His mother and Margurite's father died on the same November day. See "Double Tragedy Hits Mazique Family," *Washington Afro-American,* 10 November 1979, 1–2.
17. Margurite Mazique, interview with author, 31 May 1991.
18. "Margurite Belafonte Tells—The Tragedy of Divorce," *Ebony,* August 1958, 29–30.
19. Ibid., 30.
20. Ibid., 31.
21. See "Mrs. Margurite Belafonte Joins NAACP Staff," *The Crisis,* October 1960, 540–41, for extra details on this. Some material also taken from an author interview with Margurite Mazique, Washington, D.C., 31 May 1991.
22. Margurite Mazique, interview with author, 31 May 1991.
23. Ibid.
24. Ibid.
25. For more information see "Fashion Show Picketed Because of Dr. Mazique," and the more in-depth account earlier in this chapter.
26. Margurite Mazique, interview with author, 31 May 1991.
27. "Margurite Belafonte Tells—The Tragedy of Divorce," 30.
28. Ibid.
29. Margurite Mazique, interview with author, 31 May 1991.
30. "Margurite Belafonte Tells—The Tragedy of Divorce," next-to-last page.
31. Ibid., last page under photograph.

## CHAPTER TEN

1. There are many interesting incidents in the 1960s in which Dr. Mazique played some part that have not been included here because of space limitations. When I first met comedian and civil rights activist Dick Gregory, he asked, "Did Eddie tell you how he saved my life when the _____ poisoned me?" It was something that Dr. Mazique had never mentioned. Mr. Gregory told me how, while at a meeting in Washington with some high-level political figures, he had been poisoned. After making his exit, Mr. Gregory promptly called Dr. Mazique, who had him proceed directly to the hospital. Dr. Mazique met him there and had his stomach pumped. When I questioned him, Dr. Mazique confirmed that he had found a great deal of poison in Mr. Gregory's stomach contents. Mr. Gregory attributes the saving of his life to Dr. Mazique's quick action. (More in-depth accounts of this incident are taken from a later telephone interview with Dick Gregory, June 1993, and from Edward C. Mazique.)
2. See Harry A. Ploski and James Williams, eds., "Chronology: A Historical Review" and "Civil Rights Organization and Black Power Advances—Past and Present," in *The Negro Almanac: A Reference Work on the African American,* 5th ed. (Detroit, Mich.: GAR Research, 1959); and Thomas Gentile, *March on Washington: August 28, 1963* (Washington, D.C.: New Day Publications, 1983), chap. 1, for more background on what was taking place in the United States during the early 1960s. Much of the background material in this chapter on the March on Washington relies on the Thomas Gentile work.
3. See chap. 18 on "The Fight for Equal Rights" in Theodore C. Sorenson, *Kennedy* (New York: Harper and Row, 1965), 470–506.
4. G. Mennen Williams's Memos: RFK papers, JFK Library, 15 June 1963. Reported in Gentile, *March on Washington,* 28.
5. "President Kennedy's Rights Address," *New York Times,* 12 June 1963, 20.
6. Lerone Bennett Jr., *What Manner of Man: A Biography of Martin Luther King, Jr.* (Chicago: Johnson Publishing Co., 1968), 157.
7. See Williams, "Rough Going for Senator Eastland"; "Eastland Children Withdrawn from Sidwell School"; and "Potomac Parade: All Southerners Are Not Eastlands."
8. Gentile, *March on Washington,* 39.
9. *Washington Star,* editorial, 21 June 1963.
10. Walter E. Fauntroy, telephone interview with author, July 1993.
11. Ibid.
12. Ibid.
13. For the recounting of these events closely surrounding the march, see Gentile, *March on Washington,* 258–59.
14. Martin Luther King Jr., "I Have a Dream," reprinted in James Melvin Washington, ed., *A Testament of Hope: The Essential Writings of Martin Luther King, Jr.* (San Francisco: Harper and Row, 1991), 218.
15. Stephen B. Oates, introduction to *Selma 1965: The March That Changed the South,* by Charles E. Fager (Boston: Beacon Press, 1985), xiii.
16. Walter E. Fauntroy, telephone interview with author, July 1993.
17. More detailed accounts of the civil rights struggles of the 1960s can be found in Ploski and Williams, "Chronology."
18. See Ben W. Gilbert, *Ten Blocks from the White House: Anatomy of the*

*Washington Riots of 1968* (Washington, D.C: Washington Post Company, 1968), for the most complete description of the riots and the conditions surrounding them. This section draws heavily on this material.

19. *Report of the National Advisory Commission on Civil Disorders* (New York: Bantam Books, 1968), 203.
20. E. Fannie Granton, "Rise of New Money Class in Washington, D.C.: Husband, Wife Working Teams in D.C. Earn as Much as $50,000," *Jet* 29, no. 16 (1966): 20.
21. Ibid.
22. Robert E. Baker, "Covert Segregation Galls D.C. Negroes," *Times Herald,* 18 August 1963, A-l.
23. Ibid., A-30.
24. Ibid.
25. See Green, *Secret City,* 8–12, for a discussion of this "Other Washington" phenomenon in Washington.
26. See Jan Nugent Pearce, "Burgeoning Black Banking," *Washington Post,* 14 June 1970, 1ff., Business & Finance section, for a discussion of the need for minority banking services; and Caroline E. Mayer, "Small Banks for Minorities Shift Focus: Deregulation Increases Need to Attract Broader Customer Base," *Washington Post,* 24 June 1985, lff., Washington Business section, for a more current look at minority banking in the District.

    The United National Bank (UNB) was another highly successful business venture for Eddie. In the 1979 "Notice of Annual Meeting of Shareholders," 2, Eddie is listed as the largest stockholder. According to the above-mentioned Caroline E. Mayer article in 1985, UNB was the minority bank with the next to the largest assets and the largest profits (Mayer, "Small Banks for Minorities," 27). Because of a mandatory age for retirement for board members Eddie had to retire from the Board of Directors at age seventy-two. He was replaced by his wife, Margurite.

    The first president and CEO of UNB, Sam Foggie, was talked into the job by Dr. Mazique. He remembered how Eddie cemented the group together: "Almost any board meeting there were problems to be solved. Any time the decision-making process was bogged down, Eddie Mazique would always come up with a solution that seemed to satisfy everybody. He was the cohesive element on the board. If there was a problem, he would listen and go around the table and have everybody give their input. He would sift out the best of what was said and he would come up with the proper solution and we would move on forward" (Samuel L. Foggie, interview with author, Washington, D.C., 16 July 1985).

    Success in this venture was far from guaranteed. In a tribute to Eddie upon his retirement, Dr. William Collins recalled some of the difficult times. In 1967 when the bank's losses were close to one million dollars, a bank examiner suggested they quit operations. It was Eddie who refused to accept defeat. "The stability of the directors, championed by Eddy [*sic*] and encouraged by him, ignored the contempt which had been expressed for our venture into this novel type of bank. We bent our shoulders to the wheel, and recouped our losses." (From a copy of the tribute in Mazique papers.)
27. Quoted in Charles Fager, *Uncertain Resurrection: The Poor People's*

*Washington Campaign* (Grand Rapids, Mich.: William B. Erdmans Publishing Co., 1969), 16–17.

28. Martin Luther King Jr., "Showdown for Non-violence," *Look* 32, no. 18 (16 April 1968): 24.
29. Ibid., 23–25.
30. Ibid., 25.
31. Baker, "Covert Segregation Galls D.C. Negroes," A-30.
32. The position of the *Washington Afro-American* under the editorial direction of C. Sumner Stone was reported in Baker, "Covert Segregation Galls D.C. Negroes," A-30.
33. Estimates on the deaths and fires are consistent. The arrest figures vary from 7,600 in Gentile, *March on Washington,* 32, to 6,306 in Steven D. Price, ed., *Civil Rights, Volume 2* (New York: Facts on File, 1973), 243. For additional statistics on the riots, see also "Report of City Council Public Hearings on the Rebuilding and Recovery of Washington, D.C. from the Civil Disturbances of April, 1968" (Washington, D.C.: City Council, 10 May 1968).
34. Price, *Civil Rights, Volume 2,* 318.
35. See also Gilbert, *March on Washington,* for more detail of Fauntroy's role in attempting to quell the angry crowds and for a complete account of the riots.
36. "14th Street Sealed Off: Fires Set," *Washington Post,* 5 April 1968, A-3.
37. Walter E. Fauntroy, telephone interview with author, July 1993.
38. "14th Street Sealed Off," A-3
39. Gilbert, *Ten Blocks from the White House,* 22.
40. For a more detailed discussion of the traffic problem, see Gilbert, *Ten Blocks from the White House,* 71–74.
41. Margurite Mazique, interview with author, Washington, D.C., 31 May 1991.
42. Eddie's statement about the large number of Jewish-owned businesses at that time in the city is substantiated by others. See, for example, Ben Gilbert's section on "The Merchants" in *Ten Blocks from the White House,* 178–94. Speaking of the damage done to businesses during the riot, he states: "It was generally the white businessmen who suffered—in a large number of cases, the Jewish businessmen. There are no hard figures on the percentage of white businesses in the inner city owned by Jews, but the total is substantial" (179).
43. "14th Street Sealed Off," A-3.
44. See Willard Clopton, "Curfew Imposed as Roving Bands Plunder and Burn," *Washington Post,* 6 April 1968, A-l, A-14, for an account of the fires. Gilbert, *Ten Blocks from the White House,* on page 85, listed the total fires at over five hundred.
45. Gilbert, *Ten Blocks from the White House,* 89.
46. See Willard Clopton Jr. and Robert G. Kaiser, "Fires Dying Out, Looting Declines, Curfew Continues," *Washington Post,* 8 April 1968, A-l, 9.
47. Gilbert, *Ten Blocks from the White House,* 111.
48. Quoted in Clopton and Kaiser, "Fires Dying Out, Looting Declines, Curfew Continues," A-9.
49. See Jack Eisen, "U.S. Troops Called to Baltimore as Fires, Looting Rise," *Washington Post,* 8 April 1968, A-l, 2; and also Price, *Civil Rights, Volume 2,* 232–34, for a more detailed description of the riot in Baltimore.
50. Information on the damage to Seventh Street is taken from *National Capital Planning Commission: Civil Disturbances in Washington,*

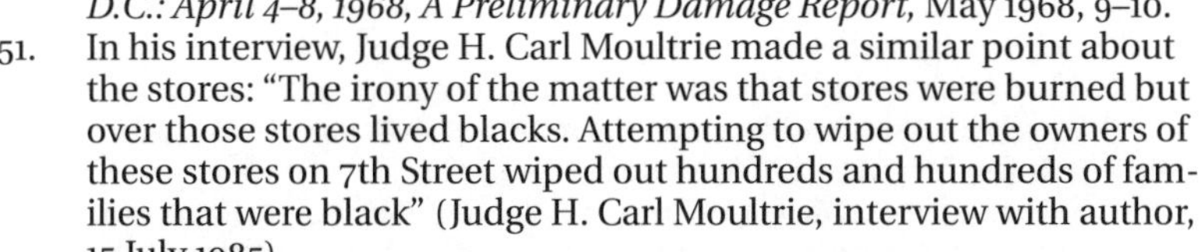

*D.C.: April 4–8, 1968, A Preliminary Damage Report,* May 1968, 9–10.

51. In his interview, Judge H. Carl Moultrie made a similar point about the stores: "The irony of the matter was that stores were burned but over those stores lived blacks. Attempting to wipe out the owners of these stores on 7th Street wiped out hundreds and hundreds of families that were black" (Judge H. Carl Moultrie, interview with author, 15 July 1985).

52. The bus driver's death was the culmination of a series of nighttime bus robberies by blacks. It resulted in a wildcat transit strike. See Fager, *Uncertain Resurrection: The Poor People's Campaign in Washington D.C.;* and Gilbert, *Ten Blocks from the White House,* for a discussion of the uneasiness among Washingtonians, especially whites, during this time.

## CHAPTER ELEVEN

The epigraph is taken from Edward C. Mazique, "Health Services and the Poor People's Campaign," 15 June 1968. This was most likely a press release that Eddie issued as chairman of the Health Services Coordinating Committee for the Poor People's Campaign. It was among Eddie's private papers in a file marked "Poor People's Campaign."

1. Robert C. Maynard, "A Symbol—How it Changed," *Washington Post,* 22 June 1968, A-13.
2. See discussion of the role of Abernathy in Fager, *Uncertain Resurrection,* 19–27. See ibid., 29, for description of the lack of rapport between Reverand Abernathy and the white liberals. The discussion in this chapter of the general details of the Poor People's Campaign relies heavily on three sources: Fager, *Uncertain Resurrection;* Price, *Civil Rights, Volume 2,* 317–32; and Gilbert, *Ten Blocks from the White House,* 195–207.
3. Gilbert, *Ten Blocks from the White House,* 196.
4. Fager, *Uncertain Resurrection,* 51.
5. Quoted in Price, *Civil Rights, Volume 2,* 324.
6. Andrew Young was the executive director of the Southern Christian Leadership Conference who helped draft the Civil Rights Act of 1964 and the Voting Rights Act of 1965. He later served as a three-term congressman, U.S. ambassador to the United Nations (1976–1979), and mayor of Atlanta, Georgia.
7. Quoted in Henry Hampton and Steve Fayer with Sarah Flynn, *Voices of Freedom: An Oral History of the Civil Rights Movement from the 1950s through the 1980s* (New York: Bantam Books, 1990), 479–80.
8. Fager, *Uncertain Resurrection,* 64.
9. Earl Caldwell, "For Demonstrators a Chance to Do Their Thing," *New York Times,* 20 June 1968, 30.
10. Fager, *Uncertain Resurrection,* 75.
11. The first description is from "Protest Asks End of War: Abernathy Vows to Stay Past Deadline," *Washington Post,* 20 June 1968, A-8; the second from Robert B. Semple Jr., "Mood of Marchers: Patience Worn Thin and a Feeling This Is the Last Chance," *New York Times,* 20 June 1968, 31; and the third from Jean M. White, "The March 5 Years Later: Frustration Replaces Hope," *Washington Post,* 20 June 1968, A-9.
12. Quoted in Fager, *Uncertain Resurrection,* 78.
13. See Fager, *Uncertain Resurrection,* 81–82, for a complete list of

concessions that Abernathy claimed he was able to get from the federal agencies.

14. "Protest Asks End of War," A-8.
15. See ibid., 83, for a list of the six major demands.
16. Semple Jr., "Mood of Marchers," 31.
17. See incident reports in "Protest Asks End of War," A-8; and Ben A. Franklin, "Protestors Call for Sharing of Nation's Affluence by All," *New York Times,* 20 June 1968, 30.
18. David A. Jewell and Paul W. Valentine, "Resurrection City: A Community Concerned by Growing Violence," *Washington Post,* 21 June 1963, A-22.
19. Ibid.
20. See accounts of the violence in "Protest Asks End of War," A-8; and Paul W. Valentine, "Police, Poor Clash Outside Tent City," *Washington Post,* 20 June 1968, A-1, 8.
21. "Abernathy Denies Violence Charge," *Washington Post,* 21 June 1963, A-22.
22. The poor treatment of those whose sympathies were strongly with the Poor People's Campaign is exemplified in the case of Drew Pearson Arnold, the twenty-year-old grandson of the famous columnist Drew Pearson. He was headed for the main gate of Resurrection City, on the Tuesday before Solidarity Day, to volunteer to work. He was attacked by youths near the Reflecting Pool. After the incident, he continued on his way and did sign up. See account in Valentine, "Police, Poor Clash," A-l, 8.
23. Fager, *Uncertain Resurrection,* 86.
24. The first quotation is from "Police, Protesters Clash; 77 Arrested at Agriculture," *Washington Post,* 21 June 1968, A-23. The second is from Fager, *Uncertain Resurrection,* 90.
25. See Fager, *Uncertain Resurrection,* for greater detail on the Mexican-American position in the campaign and pages 96ff. for details on their pullout. See "Police Arrest 2 in Protest at Agriculture," *Washington Post,* 22 June 1968, A-13, for description of the arrests of the three campaigners.
26. Carl Bernstein, "Resurrection City Wears Out D.C. Officials' Welcome," *Washington Post,* 23 June 1968, A-10.
27. Ibid., A-10.
28. Maynard, "A Symbol—How It Changed," A-13.
29. Ibid., A-13.
30. See ibid. for a discussion of the news conference.
31. Quoted in Fager, *Uncertain Resurrection,* 99.
32. Ibid.
33. See note 29 in chapter 6 for an account of the Sidwell affair.
34. Fager, *Uncertain Resurrection,* 108. See also the account in "Abernathy Demands Probe of Tear Gas," *Washington Post,* 24 June 1968, A-3.
35. Paul W. Valentine, "Marchers Plan Capitol Protest," *Washington Post,* 24 June 1963, 1.
36. Fager, *Uncertain Resurrection,* 113.
37. Hosea Williams was the Southern Christian Leadership Conference official who led the March on Selma (March 7, 1965). After that march, Williams and Dr. Martin Luther King worked closely together on all projects. Hosea Williams was a few feet away when Martin Luther King was assassinated.

38. Fager, *Uncertain Resurrection,* 118.
39. Paul W. Valentine, "343 Arrested at Capitol, Resurrection City: No Resistance," *Washington Post,* 25 June 1968, A-10.
40. See Robert C. Maynard, "The Next Step: Boycotts in 40 Cities," *Washington Post,* 25 June 1968, A-11, for a discussion of the SCLC boycott plans.
41. Fager, *Uncertain Resurrection,* 124.
42. Valentine, "343 Arrested at Capitol, Resurrection City: Tear Gas Used," A-l.
43. See accounts of the violence and the ending of the violence in Robert L. Asher and William N. Curry, "City Calm as Curfew Is Ended," *Washington Post,* 26 June 1968, A-1, 6; "Speed, Gas Swept Peril Off Streets," *Washington Post,* 26 June 1968, A-l, 6; and Gilbert, *Ten Blocks from the White House,* 195ff.
44. The information in this and the following paragraphs, on the goals of the Health Services Coordinating Committee and how they functioned, is taken from Edward C. Mazique, "Health Services and the Poor People's Campaign," 15 June 1968; "Proposal for Health Facilities for Poor People's Campaign," 9 May 1968; "Meeting of the Health Services Coordinating Committee, May 18, 1968"; "300 MDs Volunteer for 3,000 Poor," *Medical World News,* 21 June 1968, 22–23; "Medical Care for Resurrection City," *Health Services World* 3, no. 7 (July–August 1968): 14–15; and some undated press releases, Mazique papers.
45. Edward C. Mazique, "Health Services and the Poor People's Campaign," 15 June 1968, 4, Mazique papers.
46. The information on the dental van was taken from an undated press release in Dr. Mazique's files.
47. "Meeting of the Health Services Coordinating Committee, May 18, 1968," 13, Mazique papers.
48. Ibid., 11.
49. "Minutes of the Meeting of the Executive Committee of Services Coordinating Committee of Sunday, May 26, 1968," Mazique papers.
50. "Minutes of the Meeting of the Executive Committee of the Health Services Coordinating Committee of Sunday, June 9, 1968," 3, Mazique papers.
51. Ibid., 4.
52. Ibid., 5.
53. Press Release #4, no date, 1, from Dr. Mazique's files.
54. Ibid.
55. Ibid.
56. Ibid., 2.
57. Ibid.
58. "Health Services Coordinating for Solidarity Day March June 19, Committee (HSCC) Health Care Program 1968," no date, 1, Mazique papers.
59. Ibid.
60. Information on the staffing for Solidarity Day was taken from a list entitled "Physicians June 19th," "Health Services Coordinating Committee Medical Care & Public Health Program for Solidarity Day March June 19, 1969," and "Medical Care & Public Health Assignments for Solidarity March June 19, 1968," all among Dr. Mazique's papers.
61. The figures for medical activity during Solidarity Day are taken from "Report of Medical Aid Activity—Solidarity Day, 6/19/68," in Dr.

Mazique's papers.

62. See Lilian Wiggins, "They Cared Enough to Open Their Hearts with Aid: Support for the Poor Came from Women and Men Alike," *Washington Afro-American,* 22 June 1968, 9, for Drs. Webb and Rhyne's statement.
63. Ethel L. Payne, "So This Is Washington," *Chicago Daily Defender,* 22–28 June 1968, 24.
64. "Mary E.," *Washington Afro-American,* Blue Star edition, Stratford, 18 May 1968, 18.
65. "Meeting of the Health Services Coordinating Committee, May 18, 1968," 5, Mazique papers.
66. Ibid., 6.
67. "Minutes of the Meeting of the Executive Committee of the Health Services Coordinating Committee of Sunday, June 2, 1968," 3, Mazique papers.
68. "MDs Seek Insight into Illnesses of Poverty," *U.S. Medicine,* 15 June 1968, 38.
69. "300 MDs Volunteer for 3,000 Poor," 22.
70. See "Poor Peoples March Warned on Medical and Health Hazards," *National Medical Association,* from Dr. Mazique's files; and "Warn Poor People on Health Hazards," *Washington Afro-American,* 21 May 1968, for accounts of the immunizations.
71. See the minutes from the "Meeting of the Health Services Coordinating Committee, May 18, 1968," for criticism of D.C. Health Department for inadequate provision for sanitation. See the "Minutes of the Meeting of the Executive Committee of the Health Services Coordinating Committee of Sunday, May 26, 1968," 2, for a discussion of the importance of sanitation.
72. "Minutes of the Interim Meeting Executive Committee," Tuesday, May 28, 1968, 1, Mazique papers.
73. Ibid.
74. Ibid.
75. "300 MD's Volunteer for 3,000 Poor," 23.
76. "Minutes of Interim Meeting Executive Committee Health Services Coordinating Committee," Tuesday, May 28, 1968, 2, Mazique papers
77. Joe Califano was a lawyer who at this time was serving as Lyndon Johnson's special assistant who designed his anti-poverty programs. From 1977 to 1979 he was secretary of HEW.
78. Joyce Elmore, telephone interview with author, 17 November 1993.
79. Margurite Mazique, interview with author, 31 May 1991.
80. See "300 MDs Volunteer for 3,000 poor," 22; and Edward C. Mazique, "Health Services and the Poor People's Campaign," 15 June 1968, 3, Mazique papers, for a discussion of the evacuation.
81. Press Release #6, no date, from Dr. Mazique's files.
82. Ibid.
83. James Welsh, "Adding up the Costs: Tent City and Campaign Involved Millions," *Washington Sunday Star,* 30 June 1968, 12. This article was reprinted in its entirety in *U.S. Congress, House, Committee on the District of Columbia, Civil Disturbances in Washington* (Washington, D.C.: U.S. Government Printing Office, 1968).
84. Abernathy's refusal to pay the bill submitted by the National Park Service is recounted in Price, "Poor People's Campaign," 330.
85. Welsh, "Adding up the Costs," 12.
86. Quoted in ibid.

87. See Fager, *Uncertain Resurrection;* Price, *Civil Rights, Volume 2,* 317–32; and Gilbert, *Ten Blocks from the White House,* 195–207, for authors' discussions of the lack of substantive results from the Poor People's Campaign.
88. Robert C. Maynard, "The Next Step: Boycotts in 40 Cities," A-l.
89. Stuart Auerbach, "Doctor Finds Ailments of Poor Caused by Malnutrition," *Washington Post,* 22 June 1968, A-13.
90. Ibid.
91. "Land of the Rich, Hungry," *Washington Afro-American,* 30 April 1968, 4.
92. See Fager, "Poor People's Campaign," 321, for a discussion of Marks, Mississippi.
93. Edward C. Mazique to The Honorable Clifford Hardin, Secretary of Agriculture, U.S. Department of Agriculture, 3 March 1969, from Dr. Mazique's papers.
94. Samuel C. Vanneman, Assistant Deputy Administrator, Consumer Food Programs, United States Department of Agriculture, to Edward C. Mazique, 19 March 1969, from Dr. Mazique's papers.
95. See the following sources for photographs of Dr. Mazique receiving the award: "Honored by Fellow M.D.s," *Capital Spotlight,* 12 September 1968, 1; *Jet,* 29 August 1968, 45; and "NMA Annual Meet Seen as Most Outstanding," *Washington Afro-American,* week of 7 September 1968.

## CHAPTER TWELVE

1. "District Starts Rebuilding Job," *Washington Post,* 8 April 1963, A-l.
2. *Report of City Council Hearings on the Rebuilding and Recovery of Washington, D.C. from the Civil Disturbances of April, 1968, May 10, 1968* (Washington, D.C.: Government of the District of Columbia), 3.
3. For more information on Marjorie McKensie Lawson, see her biographical sketches in W. A. Low and Virgil A. Cift, eds., *Encyclopedia of Black America* (New York: McGraw Hill, 1981), 499; and Ploski and Williams, *The Negro Almanac,* 1386. For more background on her accomplishments, see "Kennedy Names Race Woman," *Pittsburgh Courier,* 20 August 1960, 10; and Sandy Fagans, "As a Judge, She's an Angel, Lawyer and Social Worker," *Washington Afro-American,* Blue Star edition, 22 February 1964, 1, 21.
4. Marjorie McKenzie Lawson, telephone interview with author, 13 December 1985.
5. Reverend Walter E. Fauntroy, telephone interview with author, July 1993.
6. Quoted in Gilbert, *Ten Blocks from the White House,* 217.
7. Ibid., 216.
8. Ibid., 215.
9. Reverend Walter E. Fauntroy, telephone interview with author, July 1993.
10. Marjorie McKenzie Lawson, telephone interview with author, 13 December 1985.
11. Reverend Walter E. Fauntroy, telephone interview with author, July 1993.
12. Victor Cohn, "AMA Meeting Disrupted by Protest Group," *Washington Post,* 17 June 1968, A-3.
13. Ibid.
14. Quoted in Victor Cohn, "AMA Cautiously Looks to Future,"

Washington Post, 23 June 1968, A-17.

15. Ibid.
16. "Medicine—Eliminating the Color Bar," *Time,* 28 June 1968, 61.
17. Ibid.
18. Ibid.
19. Margurite Mazique, interview with author, Washington, D.C., 31 May 1991.
20. P. Douglas Torrence, interview with Robert W. Wheeler, Washington, D.C., 23 May 1984.
21. "The National Medical Association's Proposed Model Health Centers," January 22, 1968 (Washington, D.C.: National Medical Association), Mazique papers.
22. Dick Gregory, telephone interview with author, June 1993.
23. The editorial for the July 1986 edition of *American Magazine* contained the following quotation as an explanation of the issue's being dedicated to Dr. Mazique:

    We are pleased and proud to bring to American Magazine a humanitarian who has devoted his life toward the betterment of mankind. He is an exceptional role model for the nation. As we pay tribute to this giant among members of the medical profession in particular and among mankind in general, let us all rejoice that we have men of such high calibre as Dr. Mazique.

    There are never enough good words to describe someone like Dr. Mazique—there is a warmth, tenderness, and caring about him that defies the dictionary and all its words. (*American Magazine,* July 1986, 6)

    The magazine cover featured Dr. Mazique, and the issue included many tributes to Dr. Mazique from organizations and individuals, including the then-current president of the National Medical Association. It also contained an article about Dr. Mazique's accomplishments, several pages of photographs, a partial reprint of his address as the retiring president of the medical-dental staff of Providence Hospital, two pages of Dr. Mazique's quips, and a lengthy interview with Dr. Mazique on the future of the medical profession.
24. "The Future of the Medical Profession: A Diagnosis by Dr. Edward C. Mazique," *American Magazine,* July 1986, 35.
25. Edward C. Mazique, "Trends and Transformations in Health Care," *Journal of the National Medical Association* 77, no. 5 (1985): 368.
26. Quoted from "Meritorious Service Award to Dr. Edward C. Mazique," among Dr. Mazique's papers.
27. Margurite Mazique, interview with author, Washington, D.C., 31 May 1991.
28. Discussion of Dr. Mazique's speech the night of the "Bull Throwers Award" and his assistance to Dr. El Khodary is taken from Dr. Ashraf El Khodary, interview with author, Washington, D.C., 25 February 1985.
29. Margurite Mazique, interview with author, Washington, D.C., 31 May 1991.
30. Sister Catherine Norton, telephone interview with author, 18 February 1985.
31. Edward C. Mazique, "A Physician Reflects on Alumni Day," *Providentially Speaking,* August/September 1984, 11.
32. Edward C. Mazique, "Health Care in Denmark," *Journal of the National Medical Association* 77, no. 1 (1985): 53.
33. Edward C. Mazique, "Medicine in the Age of Stress and Star Wars,"

reprinted in *Journal of the National Medical Association* 78, no. 3 (1986): 238.

34. "Dr. Mazique Completes Term," *Providence Hospital Memo* 18, no. 4 (memo not dated): 3.
35. Mazique, "Medicine in the Age of Stress and Star Wars," 237.
36. See "Six Nominated to Board of Medicine," *Medical Society of the District of Columbia News* 19, no. 7 (July 1986): 1, for more detail on Dr. Mazique's nomination to the Board of Medicine.
37. Margurite Mazique, interview with author, Washington, D.C., 31 May 1991.
38. Ibid.
39. Ibid.
40. From the citation accompanying the conferring of the Degree of Doctor of Science from Morehouse for Dr. Mazique, May, 21, 1974, Mazique papers.
41. Ibid.
42. Trescott, "Mentor, Mover, Man of Medicine," K-5.
43. At the time Eddie started on the board, it was called the Boys Clubs of Greater Washington. It was under his leadership that the membership came to include females.
44. Archie Avedisian, interview with Robert W. Wheeler, 22 May 1984.
45. Ibid.
46. Ibid.
47. Ibid.
48. Ibid.
49. Ibid.
50. "Honors for Dr. Edward Mazique," *Capital Spotlight* 29, no. 43 (28 July 1983): 1.
51. Archie Avedisian, interview with Robert W. Wheeler, 22 May 1984.
52. Ruby Van Croft, interview with author, Washington, D.C., 19 July 1985.
53. Kent Cushenberry, interview with author, Washington, D.C., 12 December 1985.
54. Ibid.
55. Norman Taylor, interview with author, Alexandria, Virginia, 19 July 1985.
56. Ibid.
57. Elaine Jenkins, a friend and patient, made a similar point about his sharing of what he has achieved. "He's a pioneer. He doesn't hold on with any possessiveness to what he has done. When he has done it, you can take it from him and call it your own. He has that inner kind of assurance" (interview with author, 27 February 1985).
58. Kent Cushenberry, interview with author, Washington, D.C., 12 December 1985.

## EPILOGUE

1. "Edward C. Mazique: An Alumnus of Many Callings," *Alumnus: The Morehouse College Alumni Magazine,* spring 1988, 34.
2. Ibid.
3. "Edward Craig Mazique," *Washington Post,* 30 December 1987, A-22.
4. "Civil Rights Organization and Black Power Advocates—Past and Present," in Ploski and Williams, *The Negro Almanac,* 248.
5. Ibid.
6. Ibid.
7. Ibid.

8. Ibid.
9. Quoted in ibid., 250.
10. Ibid., 251.
11. Quoted in ibid., 252.
12. From "The Unfinished Agenda of Race in America," *The NAACP Defense and Educational Fund,* quoted in ibid., 252.
13. Ibid., 259.
14. "Segregation in Schools Widespread, Worsening, National Study Says," *Dallas Morning News,* 14 December 1993, 1-A.
15. Ibid., 10-A.
16. Nancy Kruh, "Ole Miss, New Times: University Struggles with Southern Heritage in an Age of Inclusion," *Dallas Morning News,* 13 December 1993, 16-A.
17. Ibid.
18. See "Racial Disparity Seen in Firings of Federal Workers: Data Show Minority Dismissal Rate More than Twice That for Whites," *Dallas Morning News,* 14 December 1993, 1-A, 22-A, for a discussion of these other studies.
19. Ibid., 1-A.
20. The previous three examples of discrimination and segregation are taken from the *Dallas Morning News* over a two-day period. The ease with which one finds articles referring to racism in any newspaper on any given day is indicative of the recurring problems.
21. Courtland Milloy, "The Legacy of Dr. Mazique, A Physician of Many Callings," *Washington Post,* 5 January 1988, D-3.
22. Ibid.
23. Courtland Milloy, "The Memory of Dr. Mazique Lives on in Help for Infants and Their Families," *Washington Post,* 2 November 1989, C-1.
24. Askia Muhammad, "New Center Honors Famed D.C. Doctor," *Capital Spotlight,* 30 March 1989, 18.
25. Marcia Slacum Greene, "HHS Gives D.C. Group Family Services Grant," *Washington Post,* 1 November 1989.
26. Ibid.
27. Milloy, "The Memory of Dr. Mazique," C-1.
28. Charlene Hardnett (Sukari), whose great grandfather and Eddie's mother were brother and sister, remembered how once she got to know Eddie her life in Washington changed:

    When I first moved to D.C., I really didn't know anybody up here. Then after I met Uncle Eddie, it was like my whole world changed because I had family here. At the time, I was applying to different law schools and so many people told me that you really need someone on your side. I was really depressed because I had called Howard University and tried to get interviews with different people to find what special things I might need or what might help me along in terms of getting in. I didn't have any luck. So I called Uncle Eddie and told him I was applying to law school but I really didn't know anybody up there. I said Howard was my first choice. He asked, "Where are you now?" I gave him the number. He said he would call back in an hour. Uncle Eddie called me back in twenty minutes or less. He said, "You have an interview at two o'clock" and told me the man's name and said, "Don't be late."

In the South, we were always raised to be very close to our family, not just the immediate family. I find that northerners are close to their immediate family. We were raised to be close to all our relatives and extend hospitality to our relatives, even relatives who we never met. That is the same kind of reception that Uncle Eddie and Jeff and Skip extended to me. They were like brothers and adopted father for me. (Charlene Hardnett, interview with author, Washington, D.C., 28 February 1985)

29. Keith Britt, "Maziques Come Home," *Natchez Democrat,* 8 April 1990, 11-A.
30. "Going Home," *Sunday Morning with Charles Kuralt,* CBS television, 1990.
31. See Keith Britt, "Strong Roots Return Mazique Descendants to Natchez," *Natchez Democrat,* 6 April 1990 1-A, 3-A; Britt, "Maziques Come Home," 1-A, 11-A; and Joe Dumas, "Family Spirit Exhibited by D.C. Doctor: 'Eddie' Never Forgot Where He Came From," *Natchez Democrat,* 8 April 1990, 6-C.
32. "Step into the Past with Natchez," *The Confederate Pageant,* City Center Auditorium, 6 April 1990.
33. "Going Home."
34. Reverend Walter E. Fauntroy, telephone interview with author, July 1993.
35. Judge H. Carl Moultrie, interview with author, 15 July 1985.
36. "Edward C. Mazique: An Alumnus of Many Callings," 35.

# BIBLIOGRAPHY 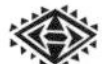

## INTERVIEWS


Avedisian, Archie. Interview by Robert W. Wheeler, 22 May 1984.
Beard, Thelma. Interview by Robert W. Wheeler, May 1984.
Bond, Colley Rakestraw. Interview by author, 23 February 1985.
Boyd, Susie. Interview by Robert W. Wheeler, May 1984.
Boyd, Wilbur and Brenda. Interview by Robert W. Wheeler, May 1984.
Brannon, Evelyn. Interview by Robert W. Wheeler, May 1984.
Burton, Alice Boyd. Telephone interview by author, 11 December 1984.
Burch, Mildred. Interview by Robert W. Wheeler, 23 May 1984.
Campbell, Robert H. Telephone interview by author, 20 February 1985.
Carter, Alma. Interview by author, 12 December 1985.
Conyers, John. Interview by author, 12 December 1985.
Cooper, William H. Interview by author, 28 February 1985.
Corneley, Paul B. Interview by author, Washington, D.C., 25 February 1985.
Crockett, George. Telephone interview by author, 15 June 1985.
Cushenberry, Kent. Interview by author, 12 December 1985.
Dumas, Michel. Interview by Robert W. Wheeler, May 1984.
Eagleson, Halston. Interview by author, 19 February 1985.
Edwards, Minnie. Telephone interview by author, 20 February 1985.
El Khodary, Ashraf. Interview by author, 25 February 1985.
Elmore, Joyce. Interview by author, 17 November 1993.
Eugene, Jonathan. Interview by author, 20 February 1985.
Fauntroy, Walter E. Telephone interview by author, July 1993.
Ferrell, H. Albion. Interview by author, 27 February 1985.
Foggie, Samuel. Interview by author, 16 July 1985.
Gee, Baxter. Telephone interview by author, 26 February 1985.
Gloster, Hugh. Telephone interview by author, 15 June 1985.
Gregory, Dick. Telephone interview by author, 22 June 1993.
Hardnett, Charlene (Sukari). Interview by author, 28 February 1985.
Haynes, Janie. Interview by Robert W. Wheeler, May 1984.
Houston, Charles Hamilton Jr. Interview by author, 23 April 1985.
Jarvis, Charlene Drew.Telephone interview by author, 27 February 1985.
Jenkins, Elaine, Howard Jenkins, and Larry Jenkins. Interview by author, 27 February 1985.
Johnson, Forest. Interview by Robert W. Wheeler, May 1984.
Johnson, Joseph L. Interview by author, 19 February 1985.
Keehan, Sister Carol. Interview by author, 26 February 1985.
Kendrick, R. E. "Ike". Telephone interview by author, 15 July 1985.
Kenney, John A. Interview by author, 25 February 1985.
Key, Hattie. Interview by Robert W. Wheeler, 23 May 1984.
Kurtz, Lewis. Telephone interview by author, 27 February 1985
Lawson, Marjorie McKenzie. Telephone interview by author, 13 December 1985.
Mackel, Augustine Boyd Rogers. Interview by Robert W. Wheeler, May 1984.
Mackel, Esther. Interview by Robert W. Wheeler, May 1984.

Mazique, Anna. Interview by Robert W. Wheeler, May 1984.
Mazique, Edward C. Interviews by author, 1984–1987.
———. A filmed interview conducted by Dr. William A. Elwood of the University of Virginia for the documentary film *The Road to Brown.*
Mazique, Edward Houston. Telephone interview by author, 1989.
Mazique, Emory. Telephone interview by author, 1989.
Mazique, Mamie Lee. Interview by Robert W. Wheeler, May 1984.
Mazique, Margurite. Interview by author, 31 May 1991.
Mazique, Maude. Interviewed by author numerous times in person and via the telephone from April 1984 to May 1995.
Mazique, William. Interview by Robert W. Wheeler, May 1984.
Miller, Lucille Banks Robinson. Interview by author, 21 February 1985.
Moore, Jerry Jr. Interview by author, 11 December 1985.
Moore, Luke. Interview by author, 19 July 1985.
Moultrie, H. Carl. Interview by author, 15 July 1985.
Nagle, Father Patrick. Interview by author, 19 February 1985.
Naylor, Rip. Interview by author, 1 March 1985.
Nazdin, Leo. Interview by author, 18 February 1985.
Norton, Sister Catherine. Telephone interview by author, 18 February 1985.
Perkins, Emmie W. Interview by author, Washington, D.C., 22 February 1985.
Pelham, Dolores. Interviewed by author numerous times in person and via the telephone from April 1984 to May 1995.
Poindexter, Hildrus A. Interview by author, 27 February 1985.
Quash, Joseph. Interview by author, 26 February 1985.
Scarletter, Raymond. Telephone interview by author, 8 March 1985.
Scott, Gail and Jerry Scott. Interview by Robert W. Wheeler, May 1984.
Smith, Marcia. Interview by author, 18 February 1985.
Spellman, Mitchell Wright. Telephone interview by author, 16 August 1991.
Stamps, Herman. Telephone interview by author, 16 December 1985.
Stanton, Robert L. Interview by Robert W. Wheeler, May 1984.
Still, Larry. Interview by author, 22 February, 1985.
Strudwick, Warren J. Interview by author, 11 December 1985.
Sulton, John D. Interview by author 18 February 1985.
Swann, Lionel. Interview by Robert W. Wheeler, May 1984.
Sweeney, Al. Interview by author, 28 February 1985.
Taylor, Norman. Interview by author, 19 July 1985.
Toles, Mary Lee Davis. Interview by Robert W. Wheeler, May 1984.
Torrence, P. Douglas. Interview by Robert W. Wheeler, 23 May 1984.
Turner, J. C. Interview by author, 26 February 1985.
Van Croft, Ruby. Interview by author, 19 July 1985.
Walton, Cleopatra Charlotte. Interview by author, 19 February 1985.
Wexler, Charles, Kay Wexler, and Edward Craig Mazique. Interviewed together by author, 20 February 1985.
White, Leon. Interview by Robert W. Wheeler, May 1984.
Williams, E. Y. Interview by author, 20 February 1985.
Williams, Ernestine. Interview by Robert W. Wheeler, May 1984.
Williams, Larry. Interview by author, 26 February 1985.
Young, M. Wharton. Interview by author, 22 February 1985.

## BOOKS AND ARTICLES

"300 MDs Volunteer for 3,000 Poor." *Medical World News,* 21 June 1968, 22.
Aldrich, James T. "President's Inaugural Address." *Journal of the National Medical Association* 52, no. 5 (September 1960): 361–62.

"American Doctors Meet Their Soviet Colleagues." *USSR,* January 1961, 36–37.
*American Magazine.* July 1966 issue dedicated to Dr. Mazique.
*American Slavery as It Is: Testimony of a Thousand Witnesses.* 1839. Reprint, New York: Arno Press and the *New York Times,* 1968.
Anderson, John O. "Dr. James Green Carson, Ante-Bellum Planter of Mississippi and Louisiana." *Journal of Mississippi History* 17, no. 4 (October 1956): 243–67.
"Annual Interim Meeting." *Journal of the National Medical Association* 52, no. 3 (May 1960): 222–23.
"Annual Summer Confabs." *Jet,* 3 September 1959, 7.
Aptheker, Herbert. *Afro-American History: The Modern Era.* Secaucus, N.J.: Citadel Press, 1971.
———. *A Documentary History of the Negro People in the United States.* Vol. 2. New York: Citadel Press, 1968.
Bennett, Lerone, Jr. *What Manner of Man: A Biography of Martin Luther King, Jr.* Chicago: Johnson Publishing Co., Inc., 1968.
Berlin, Ira. *Slaves without Masters: The Free Negro in the Antebellum South.* New York: Pantheon Books, 1974.
Brandfon, Robert L. *Cotton Kingdom of the New South: A History of the Yazoo Mississippi Delta from Reconstruction to the Twentieth Century.* Cambridge, Mass.: Harvard University Press, 1967.
Brawley, Benjamin. *History of Morehouse College.* College Park, Md.: McGrath Publishing, 1970.
"Capital Party for Civil Rights Fighters." *Hue,* August 1957, 50–54.
Cobb, W. Montague. *The First Negro Medical Society.* Washington, D.C.: Associated Publishers, 1939.
———. "Blood Transfusion and Race." *Journal of the National Medical Association* 52, no. 4 (July 1960): 280–82.
———. "Mazique 1975 NMA Distinguished Service Medalist." *Journal of the National Medical Association* 67, no. 6 (November 1975): 475–76, 443.
———. "Medicine." In *Papers Contributed to the Fourteenth Annual Conference of the Division of the Social Sciences,* May 3 and 4, 1951. Washington, D.C.: Howard University Press, 1951.
———. "Medico-Chi at Ninety, 1884–1974." *Journal of the National Medical Association* 66, no. 3 (May 1974): 257–58.
———. "The Ruhland Suggestion: Or Must Race Determine Health." *Bulletin of the Medico-Chirurgical Society of the District of Columbia* 6, no. 4 (April 1949): 3–6.
Collis, Robert. *African Encounter: A Doctor in Nigeria.* New York: Charles Scribner's Sons, 1961.
David, Sheri I. *With Dignity: The Search for Medicare and Medicaid.* Westport, Conn.: Greenwood Press, 1985.
Davis, Edwin Adams, and William Ransom Hogan. *The Barber of Natchez.* Baton Rouge: Louisiana State University Press, 1954.
"D.C. Society Couple to Present Diplomats." *Jet* 9, no. 8 (27 December 1956): 3.
"Dr. Mazique Completes Term." *Providence Hospital Memo* 18, no. 4 (not dated): 3.
Eaton, John. *Grant, Lincoln and the Freedmen, Reminiscences of the Civil War.* New York: Negro Universities Press, 1969.
"Edward C. Mazique: An Alumnus of Many Callings." *Alumnus: The Morehouse College Alumni Magazine,* spring 1988, 34.
Fabre, Michel. *The Unfinished Quest of Richard Wright.* New York: William Morrow and Co., 1973.

Fager, Charles E. *Selma 1965: The March That Changed the South.* Boston: Beacon Press, 1985.

———. *Uncertain Resurrection: The Poor People's Campaign in Washington, D.C.* Grand Rapids, Mich.: William B. Eerdmans Publishing Co., 1969.

Felgar, Robert. *Richard Wright.* Boston: Twayne Publishers, 1980.

Finley, Robert S. "Late Expedition from New Orleans." *The African Repository and Colonial Journal* 11, no. 8 (August 1835): 250–52.

Franklin, John Hope, ed. *Reminiscences of an Active Life: The Autobiography of John Roy Lynch.* Chicago: University of Chicago Press, 1970.

Frazier, E. Franklin, ed. *The Integration of the Negro into American Society.* Washington, D.C.: Howard University Press, 1951.

Furnas, J. C. *Goodbye to Uncle Tom.* New York: William Sloane Associates, 1956.

"The Future of the Medical Profession: A Diagnosis by Dr. Edward Mazique." *American Magazine,* July 1986, 34ff.

Garner, James Wilford. *Reconstruction in Mississippi.* Baton Rouge: Louisiana State University Press, 1968.

Gentile, Thomas. *March on Washington: August 28, 1963.* Washington, D.C.: New Day Publications, 1983.

Gilbert, Ben W. *Ten Blocks from the White House: Anatomy of the Washington Riots of 1968.* Washington, D.C: *Washington Post* Co., 1968.

Green, Constance McLaughlin. *The Secret City: A History of Race Relations in the Nation's Capital.* Princeton, N.J.: Princeton University Press, 1970.

Guttman, Herbert G. *The Black Family in Slavery and Freedom, 1750–1925.* New York: Vintage Books, 1976.

Hampton, Henry, and Steve Fayer, with Sarah Flynn. *Voices of Freedom: An Oral History of the Civil Rights Movement from the 1950s through the 1980s.* New York: Bantam Books, 1990.

Harper, Annie. *Annie Harper's Journal.* Denton, Tex.: Flower Mound Printing Co., 1983.

Harris, William Charles. *Presidential Reconstruction in Mississippi.* Baton Rouge: Louisiana State University Press, 1967.

*Hearing Before the Committee on Finance United States Senate, 89th Congress, First Session on HR. 6675, Part 1.* April 29, 30, and May 3–7, 1965. Washington, D.C.: U.S. Government Printing Office, 1965.

*Hearings Regarding Communist Infiltration of Labor Unions, Part I.* Washington, D.C.: U.S. Government Printing Office, 1949.

*Historical Dictionary of Nigeria.* Metuchen, N.J.: Scarecrow Press, 1987.

Hogan, William Ransom, and Edwin Adams Davis, eds. *William Johnson's Natchez: The Diary of a Free Negro.* Baton Rouge: Louisiana State University Press, 1951.

"H.R. 3920." *Journal of the National Medical Association* 56 (1964): 213–21.

Ingle, Edward. *The Negro in the District of Columbia.* Baltimore: Johns Hopkins University Press, 1893. Reprint, Freeport, N.Y.: Books for Libraries Press, 1971.

Ingraham, Joseph Holt. *The Southwest.* New York: Harper Brothers, 1835.

James, Doris Clayton. *Antebellum Natchez.* Baton Rouge: Louisiana State University Press, 1968.

*Jet* 29 (August 1968): 45 (photo only).

Johnson, Michael P., and James L. Roark. *Black Slavemasters: A Free Family of Color in the Old South.* New York: Norton, 1984.

Jones, Edward A. *A Candle in the Dark: A History of Morehouse College.* Valley Forge, Pa.: Judson Press, 1967.
King, Martin Luther, Jr. "Showdown for Non-violence." *Look* 32, no. 8 (16 April 1968): 23–25.
Knox, Thomas W. *Camp-fire and Cotton-field: Southern Adventure in Time of War.* New York: Blelock and Co., 1865.
Koger, Larry. *Black Slaveowners: Free Black Slave Masters in South Carolina, 1790–1860.* Jefferson, N.C.: McFarland, 1985.
Logan, Rayford W. *Howard University: The First Hundred Years, 1867–1967.* New York: New York University Press, 1968.
Logan, Rayford W., and Michael R. Winston, eds. *Dictionary of American Negro Biography.* New York: W. W. Norton and Co., 1982.
Low, W. A., and Virgil A. Cift, eds. *Encyclopedia of Black America.* New York: McGraw Hill, 1981.
Macksey, Richard, and Frank E. Moorer, eds. *Richard Wright: A Collection of Critical Essays.* Englewood Cliffs, N.J.: Prentice-Hall, 1984.
Mandlebaum, Seymour J. *The Social Setting of Intolerance: The Know-Nothings, the Red Scare, and McCarthyism.* Chicago: Scott, Foresman and Co., 1964.
"Margurite Belafonte Tells—The Tragedy of Divorce," *Ebony,* August 1958, 25ff.
"The Mayor and the Keys to the City: A Parable." *Journal of the National Medical Association* 52, no. 1 (January 1960): 55–56.
Mays, Benjamin E. *The Morehouse Alumnus,* July 1965.
———. *Born to Rebel.* Athens: University of Georgia Press, 1987.
Mazique, Edward C. "A Physician Reflects on Alumni Day." *Providentially Speaking,* August/September 1984, 11.
———. "Doctors and Politics." *Journal of the National Medical Association* 52, no. 2 (March 1960): 136, 151.
———. "Health Care in Denmark." *Journal of the National Medical Association* 77, no. 1 (January 1985): 53–56.
———. "Integration Enters Medicine." *Journal of the National Medical Association* 51, no. 5 (September 1959): 381–87.
———. "Medical Dimensions in the Nuclear Age." Address of the Retiring President, Read at the Sixty-Fifth Annual Convention of the National Medical Association, Pittsburgh, Pa., August 8–11, 1960. Reprinted in *Journal of the National Medical Association* 52, no. 5 (September 1960): 352–60.
———. "Medicine in the Age of Stress and Star Wars." *Journal of the National Medical Association* 78, no. 3 (1986): 237–38.
———. "The Ojike Nigerian Hospital Project." *Journal of the National Medical Association* 56, no. 1 (January 1964): 112–14.
———. "Public Health and Medical Care in Russia." *Journal of the National Medical Association* 53, no. 4 (July 1961): 352–55.
———. "Statement by Edward C. Mazique, M.D., President, American Association for Social Psychiatry, before the Ways and Means Committee, U.S. House of Representatives, August 4, 1961." *Journal of the National Medical Association* 53, no. 6 (September 1961): 651–53.
———. "Statement by Representative of the National Medical Association before the Interstate and Foreign Commerce Committee, U.S. House of Representatives, January 30, 1962." Mazique papers.
———. "Trends and Transformations in Health Care." *Journal of the National Medical Association* 77, no. 5 (1985): 365–68.

McCormick, C. N., ed. *Natchez, Mississippi: On Top, Not "Under the Hill."* Natchez, Miss.: Daily Democrat Steam Print, 1897.
McNeil, Genna Rae. *Groundwork: Charles Hamilton Houston and the Struggle for Civil Rights.* Philadelphia: University of Pennsylvania Press, 1983.
"MDs Seek Insight into Illnesses of Poverty." *U.S. Medicine,* 15 June 1968, 38.
"Medical Care for Resurrection City." *Health Services World* 3, no. 7 (July–August 1968): 14–15.
"Medicine—Eliminating the Color Bar." *Time,* 28 June 1968, 61.
"Medics in Moscow." *Jet,* 29 September 1960, 26.
*The Memento: Old and New Natchez 1700–1897.* Vol. 1. Reprint, Natchez, Miss.: Myrtle Bank Publishers, 1984.
Mezerik, A. G., ed. *U-2 and Open Skies.* New York: International Review Service, 1960.
Morais, Herbert M. *The History of the Afro-American in Medicine.* Cornwells Heights, Pa.: The Publisher's Agency, 1976.
Mosley, Mrs. Charles C., Sr. *The Negro in Mississippi History.* Jackson, Miss.: Mrs. Charles C. Mosley, 1969.
Murray, Charles A. *Travels in North America During the Years 1834, 1835 & 1836.* 2 vols. London: R. Bentley, 1839.
*National Capital Planning Commission: Civil Disturbances in Washington, D.C.: April 4–8, 1968, A Preliminary Damage Report.* Washington, D.C., May 1968.
*The National Freedman, A Monthly Journal of The National Freedman's Relief Association,* New York.
"Negro Doctors Visit the Soviet Union." *New World Review,* September 1960, 27.
"NMA Past President Praises National Health Insurance." *Journal of the National Medical Association* 51, no. 2 (March 1959): 148–49.
"NMA Activities: Testimony at Congressional Hearings." *Journal of the National Medical Association* 51, no. 5 (September 1959): 408–9.
"NMA President's Testimony on Aid for the Aging. Statement of Dr. Edward C. Mazique." *Journal of the National Medical Association* 52, no. 4 (June 1960): 311–14.
Nordoff, Charles. *The Cotton States in the Spring and Summer of 1875.* New York: Appleton, 1876.
Olmstead, Frederick Law. *A Journey in the Back Country.* London: Sampson Low, Son and Co., 1860.
———. *The Cotton Kingdom: A Traveler's Observations on Cotton and Slavery in the American Slave States.* New York: Alfred A. Knopf, 1953.
Ploski, Harry A., and James Williams, eds. *The Negro Almanac: A Reference Work on the African American.* Detroit: GAR Research, 1959, 1971, 1989 editions.
"Poland Asks NMAA Aid On Pre-Natal Clinics." *Jet,* 22 September 1960, 16.
Price, Steven D., ed. *Civil Rights, Volume 2.* New York: Facts on File, 1973.
Reid, Whitelaw. *After the War: A Southern Tour.* Cincinnati: Moore, Wilstack and Baldwin, 1866.
Reitzes, Carl Dietrich, ed. *Negroes in Medicine.* Cambridge, Mass.: Harvard University Press, 1958.
*Report of City Council Public Hearings on the Rebuilding and Recovery of Washington, D.C. from the Civil Disturbances of April, 1968.* Washington, D.C.: City Council, 10 May 1968.
*Report of the National Advisory Commission on Civil Disorders.* New York: Bantam Books, 1968.

Ruetten, Richard T., and Donald R. McCoy. *Quest and Response: Minority Rights and the Truman Administration.* Lawrence: University Press of Kansas, 1973.

"Russian Operation." *Jet,* 22 September 1960, 16.

Schlesinger, Arthur M., Jr., ed. *History of U.S. Political Parties.* Vol. 4, *1945–1972, The Politics of Change.* New York: Chelsea House Publishers, 1973.

"Scudder Blood Controversy." *Journal of the National Medical Association* 52, no. 1 (January 1960): 56–58.

Scudder, John. "Practical Concepts in Modern Medicine." Sixth Annual Charles R. Drew Memorial Lecture at the Forty-Eighth Annual Meeting of the John A. Andrew Clinical Society, Tuskegee Institute, Alabama, April 23–29, 1960. Reprinted in *Journal of the National Medical Association* 52, no. 4 (July 1960): 266–77.

Scudder, John, and William D. Wigle. "Safer Transfusions through Appreciation of Variants in Blood Group Antigens in Negro and White Blood Donors." *Journal of the National Medical Association* 52, no. 2 (March 1960): 75–80.

*The Seventh Census of the United States, 1850.* Washington, D.C.: U.S. Printing Office, 1853.

Sewell, George Alexander. *Mississippi Black History Makers.* Jackson: University of Mississippi Press, 1977.

"Six Nominated to Board of Medicine." *Medical Society of the District of Columbia News* 19, no. 7 (July 1986): 1.

Sorenson, Theodore C. *Kennedy.* New York: Harper and Row, 1965.

"Statement of Seven Members of Columbia University Seminar on Genetics and the Evolution of Man." *Journal of the National Medical Association* 52, no. 4 (July 1960): 296.

Still, Larry. "What President's Medicare Means to Negroes." *Jet,* 14 June 1962, 16–19.

Swift, Leroy R. "Medical Mission to Moscow." *Journal of the National Medical Association* 53, no. 4 (July 1961): 346–51.

Sydnor, Charles Sackett. *Slavery in Mississippi.* New York: D. Appleton-Century Co., 1933.

Taylor, William Banks. *King Cotton and Old Glory.* Hattiesburg, Miss.: Fox Printing Co., 1977.

*Testimony Given in Hearings Before the Subcommittee on Obscene Literature of the Committee on Post Office and Civil Service of the House of Representatives,* 19 May 1959, Washington, D.C. Reprinted in "NMA Activities: Testimony at Congressional Hearings." *Journal of the National Medical Association* 51, no. 5 (September 1959): 408–9.

Torrence, Ridgely. *The Story of John Hope.* New York: Macmillan Co., 1948.

U.S. Congress, House Committee on the District of Columbia. *Civil Disturbances in Washington.* Washington, D.C.: U.S. Government Printing Office, 1968.

Washington, James Melvin, ed. *A Testament of Hope: The Essential Writings of Martin Luther King, Jr.* San Francisco: Harper and Row, 1991.

Wayne, Michael. *The Reshaping of Plantation Society: The Natchez District, 1860–1880.* Baton Rouge: Louisiana State University Press, 1983.

Wharton, Vernon Lane. *The Negro in Mississippi: 1865–1890.* Chapel Hill: University of North Carolina Press, 1947.

Whittier, C. Austin. "President's Address." *Journal of the National Medical Association* 41, no. 5 (September 1949): 229–30.

Wise, David, and Thomas B. Ross. *The U-2 Affair.* New York: Random House, 1962.

Wright, Richard. *Blackboy: A Record of Childhood and Youth.* New York: Harper and Brothers, 1945.

Yates, Elizabeth. *Howard Thurman: A Portrait of a Practical Dreamer.* New York: John Day Company, 1964.

Yeatman, James E. *A Report on the Condition of the Freedmen of the Mississippi.* St. Louis: Western Sanitary Commission Rooms, 1864.

Young, Murray. "West to East—East to West." *New World Review,* October 1960, 5–8.

## UNPUBLISHED AND MISCELLANEOUS SOURCES

"Going Home." *Sunday Morning with Charles Kuralt,* CBS television, 1990.

Hawkins, Ricardo. Document prepared by Mr. Hawkins for the author about his experiences with Dr. Mazique, 20 February 1985.

Mazique, Edward C. Papers. Includes newspaper clippings, photographs, press releases, memos, notes, programs, reports, letters, cards, travelogues, and speeches relating to all aspects of Dr. Mazique's life.

*Mazique, Jewell R. v. Edward C. Mazique.* Appeals records on microfiche at Superior Court of the District of Columbia, Washington, D.C.

Mazique, Maude. Personal diary for 1964–1965.

Miller, Mary Warren. "Black History of Natchez, Mississippi." 25 February 1983. Slide presentation for the Historic Natchez Foundation.

Moore, Edith Wyatt Collection. Judge George W. Armstrong Library, Natchez, Mississippi.

James Railey's Last Will and Testament. Probate box 126 (Will Book 3), 1861, Natchez Courthouse.

"Step into the Past with Natchez." Program for *The Confederate Pageant,* City Center Auditorium, 6 April 1990.

Will Book D, Natchez Courthouse.

## NEWSPAPERS AND NEWSLETTERS

*American Medical Association News*
*Atlanta Journal and Constitution*
*Baltimore Sun*
*Bulletin of the Medico-Chirugical Society of the District of Columbia*
*Bulletin of the National Medical Association*
*Capital Spotlight* (Washington, D.C.)
*Catholic Standard*
*Chicago Defender*
*Chicago Sun—Times*
*Cleveland Plain Dealer*
*Courier,* International
*Courier,* Washington Edition
*Crisis*
*Daily Worker*
*Dallas Morning News*
*Detroit Free Press*
*Detroit News*
*Detroit Times*
*Howard University Bulletin*
*Los Angeles Herald-Dispatch*
*Medical News: A Newspaper for Physicians*

*Medical Society of the District of Columbia News*
*Medical Tribune*
*Medical World News*
*Michigan Chronicle*
*Milwaukee Journal*
*Milwaukee Sentinel*
*Natchez Courier*
*Natchez Democrat*
*Natchez Free Trader*
*Natchez Southern Galaxy*
*National Medical Association, Inc. Bulletin*
*New York Times*
*Physician's Forum News*
*Pittsburgh Courier*
*Pittsburgh Post-Gazette and Sun-Telegraph*
*Pittsburgh Press*
*Scope Weekly*
*Tri-Weekly Democrat (Natchez)*
*Washington Afro-American*
*Washington Daily News*
*Washington Evening Star*
*Washington Gaily News*
*Washington Post*
*Washington Post and Times Herald*
*Washington Post and Times Star*
*Washington Star*
*Washington Times Herald*

# INDEX

Abernathy, Ralph, 258, 259, 262, 263–64, 267, 275, 292; on violence in Resurrection City, 265

Adams Co., Miss., 2, 3; ownership of land by blacks, 9

Adams, Numa P. G., 102, 103, 108

Agnew, Spiro T., 254

Aldrich, James T., 172, 190–92, 209, 211

Allegheny County Medical Society, 192

American Association for Social Psychiatry, 208

American Hospital Association, 165

*American Magazine*, **295**

American Medical Association (AMA), 142, 165, 177, 210, 292; black doctors not permitted to join, 124; and Kerr-Mills Bill, 205; opposition to Forand Bill, 174–76, 192; opposition to Medicare, 176, 182, 207, 211, 213; statement from Council on Medical Service, 292; use of scare tactic, 214

American Medical Association Political Action Committee (AMAPAC), 207

American Medical Political Action Committee (AMPAC), 176, 207

Anchorage plantation, 2, 16

Anderson, Brenda Boyd, **327**

Archer, Leonid "Josh", 69, 83–84

Archer, Samuel, 64, 68, 71

Arlington Cemetery, 104

Arlington County Medical Society, 142

Askenase, Philip, 272, 273

Atlanta University, 65, 81

Augusta, Alexander T., 138

Avedisian, Archie, 307–13

Baker, Joe, 26

Balewa, Abubakar Tafawa, 217, 218, 219

Baltimore, Md.: race riots in, 254

Barnes (murdered student), 66

Barry, Marion, 302

Bay Area Committee, 208

Beckett, Charles, 82, 91

Belafonte, Harry, 227, 229, 230

Belafonte, Margurite. *See* Mazique, Margurite

Bevel, James, 260

Birmingham, Al.: attacks on demonstrators in, 239

Black United Front (BUF), 288

Blackburn, Ben, 56–57

Bloedorn, Walter, 155

Bluegart, Julian, 275–76

Bowen, Anthony, 166

Boyd, Alice, 17

Boyd, James, 15, **16**, 33–34

Boyd, James, Jr., **16**, **327**

Boyd, Mary Mazique, 15, **16**

Boyd, Samuel S., 33

Boyd, Seward, **16**

Boyd, Wilbur, **16**, 45

Boys and Girls Clubs of America, 307–8

Brady (school superintendent), 81

Brawley, Benjamin G., 68

Brazael, Brailsford R., 76

Brown, Edmund, 232

Build Black Incorporated, 288

Bull Throwers Award, 297
Bunche, Ralph, 101, 106, 246
Bunting, James, 168
Burch, Mildred, 74
Burney, Leroy E., 181, 189–90
Burton, Alice, **16**
Bush, Barbara, 321
Bush, George H. W., 311
Byrd, Frances Margurite, 227
Byrd, Robert, 278
Byrnes, John F., 214

Califano, Joe, 276
Carter, Alma, 226
Carter, Raymond, 70
Carver, George Washington, 71
Catholic Church: and education of ECM's children, 163–64; racism within, 161–62
Caulfield, Philip, 161, 162–63
Chambers, Whittaker, 134
Cheek, James, 302
Chiang Kai-shek, 133
China Grove plantation, 1–2, 7, 8, 12, 16, 114, 327
CIBA Pharmaceutical Products, Inc., 174
Citizens Advisory Council, 146, 152–53
Civil Rights Act of 1875, 97
Civil Rights Act of 1964, 165, 242
Civil Rights Bill, 255
Civilian Conservation Corps, 99
Clement, Kenneth W., 213
Cobb, Montague, 103, 139–40, 141, 153, 154, 165, 177, 184, 209, 214, 218
Cohen, Wilbur, 205, 262
Committee on African Affairs, 216
Congress of Racial Equality (CORE), 238
Consolidated Parents Group, 163
Cornely, Paul, 101, 102, 103, 106, 107, 177
Costanbader, Frank D., 142–43
cotton farming, 19–20, 21
Crawford, Jewell. *See* Mazique, Jewell Crawford
Crockett, Ethelene, 198
Crockett, George, 72, 74, 76
Cushenberry, Kent, 313–15, 317
Czechoslovakia, 198

Dansby (professor), 73
Davidson, Eugene, 154
Davis, Benjamin O., 152
Davis, Murray B., 188
Davis, P. Wilkins, 154
Dawson, Clara Newkirk, 223
D.C. Department of Public Health, 270–71
D.C. General Hospital, 270
De Priest, Oscar, 98
Delaney Amendment, 181
District Medical Society, 96, 140, 141, 153, 268, 274; dinner given by, 293; integration of, 146
District of Columbia. *See* Washington, D.C.
District of Columbia Political Action Committee, 294
Divine, Father, 113–14
Donaldson, John S., 189, 190
Donohue, Joseph, 133, 151
Dooley, Thomas, 217
Drew, Charles, 101, 103, 111, 184, 186
DuBois, W. E. B., 81; on philosophy of education for blacks, 62
Dunbar, Paul Laurence, 117

Eagleston, Halston, 106
Eastland, James O., 163, 240, 265
Edward C. Mazique Parent Child Center, 326

Eisenhower, Dwight D., 133, 134, 177, 205
Eleanor, Sister, 160
El Khodary, Ashraf, 297
Ellington, Duke, 230
Elmore, Joyce, 276
emancipation papers, 5
Epps, Charles, 325
Equal Services Acts, 148–49
Evers, Medgar, 238
Evers, Medgar, Mrs., 260
Ewing, Oscar R., 140

Farmer, James L., 101
Fauntroy, Walter E., 240–42, 243, 246, 249, 252, 254, 264, 288, 290, 323, 328; mediates dispute over park permit for Resurrection City, 258; and plan to improve conditions for inner-city dwellers, 285-86
Federation of Citizens Associations, 143
Ferriday, La., 32–33, 41
Fleming, Arthur S., 181, 190, 205
Fleming, Robert I., 218
Fleming, Robert V., 146, 151
Forand, Aime, 175–76
Forand Bill, 173, 174, 177, 181–82, 191–92
Ford, P. W., 219
Foreign and International Health Program, 215
Forsyth, Ga., 83–86
Foster, Woo, 79
Franklin, John Hope, 185
Frazier, E. Franklin, 101, 106
Frazier, Tip, 47–48
Freedmen's Hospital, 109–116, 139, 155, 263, 268, 270
Freeman (DMS president), 141

Gaffney, Leo, 158
Gallinger Hospital, 140, 153
Garne, Johnny, 128
Gasset, Skipper, 63–64
George Washington University Hospital, 155, 156
Georgetown University Hospital, 154
Giles, Lewis, Jr., 196, 197
Gloster, Hugh, 67, 302, 304
Glover, Iris, 85
Grant, Murray, 270, 274, 276
Gray, Jimmy, 121
Green, Clarence, 111
Green, Constance McLaughlin, 246
Gregory, Dick, 127, 295, 321
Grigsby, Margaret, 198

Hadley (doctor), 153
Hadley Hospital, 153–54
Hall, Woolsey W., 146, 150
Hanks, Alex, 41
Hardin, Clifford, 281
Hastie, William, 100, 101
Hawkins, Ricardo, 127
Health Services Coordinating Committee (HSCC), 268, 269, 270, 271
Heath, Frederick, 271
Henry, Mary, 56
Hiss, Alger, 134
Holman, Mary, 272, 273
Homeopathic Hospital, 156
Hope, John, 61–66, 68, 81, 124
Hopkins, Harry, 99
House Un-American Activities Committee (HUAC), 134, 151
Houston, Charles Hamilton, 100, 102, 122–28, 130, 133, 135–38
Houston, Henrietta, 136
Houston, Ulysses, 125, 137, 138, 141
Howard University, 90, 98, 101–2, 132, 303

Howard University Medical School, 105, 281, 322
Howard, William Schley, 67
Hubbard (Forsyth president), 89
Hubert, Dennis, 67
Hughes, Charles Evan, 64
Hughes, Langston, 117
Humberto, Jack, 45
Humphrey, Hubert, 183, 295
*Hurd v. Hodge*, 123, 127

Ickes, Harold, 99–100, 110
Imhotep Conference, 165, 177, 211

Jackson, Alvin, 263
Jackson, Jesse, 279
Jason, Robert, 103
Jim Crowism, 66, 97, 135, 163
John R. Thompson Restaurant Company, 148
Johnson, J. T., 266
Johnson, Joseph L., 103, 106, 108–9
Johnson, Lyndon B., 102, 165, 207, 213, 239, 242, 244, 252, 280, 287, 295
Johnson, Mordecai, 98, 101–2
Johnson Publishing, 200, 201
Johnson, William, 3, 4, 5; murder of, 6
Joint Committee on National Recovery, 100
Jones, Frank, 154
Jones, Lucias, 78
Just, Ernest, 102

Kane, James, 158, 159
Karpman, Benjamin, 106–7
Kaufmann, Joseph A., 147, 152
Kelly, Shipwreck, 84
Kennedy, Ethel, 260
Kennedy, John F., 183, **206**, 206, 208, 213, 239–40, 240, 286
Kennedy, Robert F., 254, 260
Kennedy-Anderson Bill, 206
Kerner Commission, 244–45
Kerr, Lorin E., 208
Kerr-Mills Bill, 205, 206
Khrushchev, Nikita S., 196
Kilgore, Thomas, Jr., 217
Kilmarnock plantation, 42
King-Anderson Bill, 209, 211
King, Coretta Scott, 260, 261–62
King, Martin Luther, Jr., 217, 237, 238, 242, 244, 254, 257–58, 290; rationale for Poor People's Campaign, 247–48
Kirchner (doctor), 156
Klaus, Irene, **298**
Ku Klux Klan, 98, 243
Kuralt, Charles, 326

Larson, Leonard, 209, 210
Latimer, John W., 271
Lawson, Belford, 169
Lawson, Belford, Jr., 285
Lawson, Marjorie McKensie, 285–86, 290, 291
Lincoln Memorial: 1922 dedication of, 98
Longdon, Chauncey, 166

Mandela, Nelson, 328
Manhattan Central Medical Society, 187
March on Washington, 238, 240, 242–43
Marks, Miss., 280–81
Marshall, Herbert, 177, 209
Marshall, Thurgood, 172, 245
Mason, Vaughn, 209
Mays, Benjamin E., 31, 65, 76, 217, 280
Mazique, Addie Birdie, 49
Mazique, Addie Wilkerson, **20**, 21, 28, 114, **115**, 115, **129**; with ECM,

**227**; with ECM and Maude, **225**

Mazique, Alex (Grandpa Alex), 7, 12, 13, **14**, 14, 16, 17, 18, 42

Mazique, Alex, III, **20**, **21**, 21, 22, 35, 49, 51, 56, 114

Mazique, Alex, Jr., 16, 17, **20**, 21, **23**, 34, 44, **129**; death of, 86; and logging, 39

Mazique, August, 7, 8, 12, 13

Mazique, Douglas, **20**, **21**, 21, 35, 49, **55**, 91, 114, 306, 307; with family, **129**; as salutatorian (Natchez College), 55

Mazique, Edna, **20**, 21, 49, 52–53

Mazique, Edward Craig: with Abraham Ribicoff, **212**; addressing Arkansas Medical Association, **179**; admitted to staff of Georgetown University Hospital, 154; appointed to Citizens Advisory Council, 146; awards presented to, 297, 317; and blood transfusion controversy, 184–88; as bookstore manager, 108; and Boys Club, 308–13; called before the HUAC, 135; and Catholicism, 163; as child with family, **20**; chosen president of National Medical Association, 171; on cover of *American Magazine*, **295**; death of, 317; death of sisters and desire to become a doctor, 54; on debating team, 76; divorce from Jewell, 221–25; with dog, **42**; eating pigeons with Grandpa Alex, 18; with family, **21**, **129**, **307**, **327**; and founding of bank, 246; with G. M. Sampson, **92**; graduation from Howard University, 109; graduation from Natchez College, **55**; and health care for the elderly, 182–83, 189, 198–99, 204, 214; "Integration Enters Medicine" speech, 173; involvement with Resurrection City, 267; with Jewell, **104**; job at cleaners, 46–48; with John Kennedy, **206**; with Margurite and Irene Klaus, **298**; marriage to Jewell Crawford, 103; marriage to Margurite, 233–35; with Maude, **303**; with Maude and Florence Ridlon, **329**; as Morehouse undergraduate, **75**; with mother and sister Maude, **225**, **227**; with mother and wife, **115**; named to Morehouse Board of Trustees, 303–304; odd jobs held at Morehouse, 70–71; in office, **118**; office spared riot damage, 251, 253; with officers of senior class at Morehouse, **77**; picketing of YMCA, 168; plowing experience, 37; portrait of, **318**; and principalship of Athens, Ga. school, 90; receives honorary doctorate from Morehouse, 302, 305; receives Outstanding Achievement Award from NMA, 282; on recruitment of blacks for HSCC, 273; relationship with father, 38–41; starts *Mississippi World* newspaper, 79; suffers from malaria and phlebitis at Morehouse, 70; suffers from phlebitis as intern at Freedmen's Hospital, 111; summers at Oakland with Grandpa Alex, 17; support of flouridation, 147, 150; trip to Eastern Europe, 195–204; as valedictorian (Natchez College), 55; walks out on government briefing, 197; and wedding party, **234**

Mazique, Edward "Skip", 126, 163

Mazique, Eloise, **129**

Mazique family, 2–17, **20**, **227**; reunion of 1990, 326-28

Mazique, Hubbard, 13

Mazique, Ike, 13

Mazique, James, 15, 16, 42, 52

Mazique, Jeff, 126

Mazique, Jewell Crawford, 89, 91, 103, **115**, 129–31, 163, 164, **179**, 183–84, 226, 287; divorce from ECM, 221–25; with ECM, **104**; removal of fibroids, 126

Mazique, Jim, 13, 16
Mazique, Juanita, **129**
Mazique, Laura Craig, **14**, 17
Mazique, Margurite, 223, 229, 231–33, 251, 276, 293, **298**, 299, 304–5, 317; and wedding party, **234**
Mazique, Mary, 34
Mazique, Maude, 17, **20**, 21, 22, 33, 44, 49, 51–52, 114–15, **129**, 223, 224, 226, **307**, 326, **327**; with ECM, **303**; with ECM and Florence Ridlon, **329**; with ECM and mother, **225**
Mazique, Robert, 15, 16, 42
Mazique, Rudolph, 13
Mazique, Sadie, **20**, 21, 49, 52–53
Mazique, Sarah, 7, 8, 12, 13, 17
Mazique, Shirley, **129**
Mazique, Theodore, 49, 114, 115, **129**
Mazique, Walter "Jack", **20**, 49
Mazique, William, 15
Mbadiwe, K. Ozuomba, 217, 218, 219
McCarthy, Eugene, 160
McCarthy, Joseph, 134, 152
McMurtry, Affie Mazique, 14
McMurtry, Lycurgus, 14
McNamara, Pat, 205, 208
McNamara, Robert, 239
Meany, George, 157
Medicaid, 214
Medical Aged Assistance, 205
Medical Committee for Human Rights, 272, 292
Medical Society of the District of Columbia, 138–39, 143
Medicare, 182, 195, 203, 205, 207–15, 292, 296; AMA opposition to, 176, 182, 207, 211, 213; ECM gives political support to those backing, 206
Medico-Chirurgical Society, 96, 98, 125, 138, 139, 140, 141, 143, 146, 153, 154, 163, 165, 268; endorsement of national health insurance, 176
Meharry Hospital, 109
Meharry Medical College, 91
Meredith, James, 238, 244, 324
Miller, Kelly, 102
Milloy, Courtland, 324–25, 326
Mills, Wilbur, 176, 213, 214
Minor, John, 141
Miriani, Louis C., 172
Mishell, Robert, 208
*Mississippi World*, 79
*Missouri ex rel. Gaines v. Canada*, 122
Model Inner City Community Organization (MICCO), 286, 288, 290, 292
Mody, Vinod R., 279
Montrose plantation, 16
Morehouse College, 59–93, 302
Morehouse Medical School, 306
Morse, Wayne, 183
Moten, Robert R., 56, 98
Moultrie, H. Carl, 328
Murray, Peter Marshall, 126, 209, 210
Myers, Randolph, 167, 168

Nader, Ralph, 273
Nagle, Patrick, 149
Natchez College, 54–56
Natchez, Miss., 1–4; Confederate Pageant in, 327
National Association for the Advancement of Colored People (NAACP), 97, 122, 154, 165, 177, 230, 238, 287; and Freedom Fund, 229
National Medical Association (NMA), 140, 165, 174, 177, 182, 211, 213, 274, 282, 295; failure to support Ojike Memorial Medical Center, 218; international program of, 195; and

medical missions, 216; support for federal financing of medical care for elderly, 214
National Medical Political Action Committee (NMPAC), 189, 294
National Medical Society of the District of Columbia, 138
National Urban League, 165
nationalized medicine, 196, 198, 202, 204
New Negro Alliance, 100
Niagara Movement, 62, 97
Norton, Catherine, 299, 302

Oakland plantation, 2, 7, 12, 13, 18, 42, 327
Occidental Restaurant, 147–48
Offutt, Dorsey, 142
Ojike, Mazi Mbonu, 217
Ojike Memorial Medical Center, 217, 218, 223, 230
Olney Inn, 118
Osborn, Jerome, 103
Owen, S. H. C., 15, 16, 55
Owen, Sarah Mazique, 15
Oxley, Lawrence, 211

Parks, Rosa, 237
Passavanti, Sam, 48
Payne, Ethel L., 272
Pelham, Delores, **307**, 326
Perkins, Emmie, 116
Perry, John Sinclair, 141
Pike, James, 217
plantations, 1–2, 8, 16. *See also named plantations*
Poindexter, Hildrus A., 100, 105–106
Poor People's Campaign, 247–50, 255, 257, 259, 277, 280, 283, 292; concessions won by, 262; and D.C. Department of Public Health, 271; failure of, 266–67
Powell, Adam Clayton, 183, 229, 249
Powers, Gary, 196
Progressive Party, 133
Providence Hospital, 158, 160, 163, 297–302
Purvis, Charles B., 138

race riots: in Baltimore, Md., 254; in Washington in 1919, 98; in Washington in 1963, 249–55
Railey, Charles, 8
Railey, James, 4, 8; last will and testament of, 7, **8**
Railey, Logan, 8
Railey, Matilda, 9
Rakestraw, Colley, 87–88
Rakestraw, Lafayette, 87
Randolph, A. Philip, 238, 240
Rathe, Barbara, 183
Rayburn, Sam, 207
Read, Florence, 81, 82
Reeves, Gary, 328
Resurrection City, 257–83; disorganization and violence in, 261, 263–64; exposure to tear gas, 277; and health van controversy, 269–70; and immunizations, 274; meeting medical needs of, 268; and National Park Service, 258
Rhyne, Joseph, 272
Ribicoff, Abraham, 213; with ECM, **212**
Ridlon, Florence, **329**
Robertson, Eugene, 108
Robeson, Paul, 133, 134
Robinson, Jackie, 135, 230
Rodgers, Jimmy, 87
Rogers, William P., 183
Roosevelt, Eleanor, 99, 217
Roosevelt, Franklin D., 124, 175
Ross, Norman, 252
Rowan, Carl, 246
Roy, Celestine Mazique, 13

Roy, Haywood, 13
Ruhland, George C., 139–40
Rustin, Bayard, 240, 248, 260

Sampson, G. M., 85, **92**, 92, 166
Scales, Gag, 39
Scherle, William J., 250
Scott, Bud, 45
Scudder, John, 184–88
segregation, 97; in Atlanta, 66; in churches, 101; in contemporary America, 323–24; in hospitals, 153; in restaurants, 101, 148–49
Selma-Montgomery March, 243
Shadd (minister), 112, 113
Shaw Health Center, 289
Shields, Wilmer, 9
Shilo Baptist Church, 309
Sibley Memorial Hospital, 156–57, 168
Sidwell Friends School, 163
Simmons, Roscoe Conklin, 31
Sims, Berta Mazique, 15
Sims, C. S., 15
Smith, R. Stillmon, 172–73
Smith, Robert D., 4
Solidarity Day, 259, 260, 261, 267, 270
Sorensen, Theodore, 239
Southeastern University, 167, 168
Southern Christian Leadership Conference (SCLC), 238, 247, 250, 257, 258
Sparkman Bill, 178
Spellman, Mitchell Wright, 160–61, 165, 293
Spelman College, 60, 65, 69
Stamps, Herman, 119
Stanley (slave), 18
Statom (plantation overseer), 21, 28–29
Still, Larry, 196–97, 199–204, 211
Stokes, Alvin, 134
Street, Elwood, 99
Student Non-Violent Coordinating Committee (SNCC), 238
Sullivan, Louis, 306
Sumner, Charles, 138
Suzette, Catherine Boyd, 34
Swan, Lionel, 293
Swift, Leroy R., 197, 199
Symington, Stuart, 183

Talmadge, Eugene, 89
Taylor, Norman, 315–16
Terrell, Mary Church, 117
Terry, Luther, 214
Thomas, Riley, 112
Thurman, Howard W., 73–74, 101, 106
Tillman, Nathaniel P., 76
Trippe, Juan, 218, 219
Truman, Harry, 133, 175; Civil Rights Message, 132
Truman Health Insurance Bill, 177
Tucker, A. W., 138
Tucker, Sterling, 245, 260, 261, 314
Turner, J. C., 147, 149–50, 152

United National Bank of Washington, 246
United Nations, 133, 196, 197
Urban League, 238
urban renewal, 287–88
USSR, 196, 197, 199

Van Croft, Ruby, 313
Vance, Cyrus, 254
Voting Rights Act of 1965, 242, 243

Wallace, George, 242, 243
Wallace, Henry A., 124, 133, 135
Walton, Charlotte, 126

 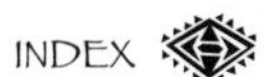


Ward, Francis, 323
Washburn, Laura Mazique, 15
Washington, Booker T., 63, 97, 117; on philosophy of education for blacks, 61–62
Washington, D.C., 95–119, 237–55; and discrimination in housing, 122; and home rule, 145–46; race riots in, 98, 249–55; segregation and black culture, 132
Washington Hypnotic Medical Society, 113
Washington, John, 117
Washington, Walter, 246, 254, 264, 267, 275
Watts riots, 244
Weaver, Robert C., 100, 245
Webb, Harvey, Jr., 272
Webber, Charles, 157, 168
Welsh, Mother, 117
Welsh, William, 116
Wexler, Charles, 21, 233
White Apple Village plantation, 7, 13, 17, 42
White Citizens Council, 165
Whittico, James, Jr., 282
Whittier, C. Austin, 176
Wilds, Richard, 28–29
Wildsville, La., 21, 25–28, 30, 41; flooding in, 43–44
Wilkerson, Bud, 32
Wilkerson, Caroline, 28
Wilkerson, Douglas, 28
Wilkins, Roy, 211, 248
Williams, E. Y., 112–13, 223–24
Williams, G. Mennen, 180, 190, 239
Williams, Hosea, 277
Wilson, Woodrow, 97
Wiprud, Theodore, 141, 142, 143
Wisner, La., 34, 39
Wolfe, Sidney, 272, 273
Woodlands plantation, 16
Woodville, Miss., 7
Woodward School for Boys, 167, 168

Young, Andrew, 260, 266
Young, M. Wharton, 106
Young Men's Christian Association for Colored Men and Boys, 166
Young Men's Christian Association (YMCA), 165